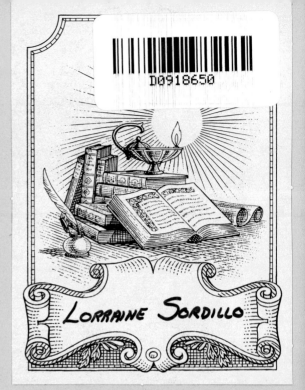

BIOLOGY OF LACTATION

A SERIES OF BOOKS IN ANIMAL SCIENCE

Editor: G. W. Salisbury

BIOLOGY OF LACTATION

G. H. Schmidt

CORNELL UNIVERSITY

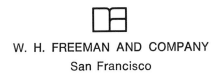

W. H. FREEMAN AND COMPANY
San Francisco

Printed in the United States of America

Library of Congress Catalog Card Number: 78-150409
International Standard Book Number: 0-7167-0821-3

1   2   3   4   5   6   7   8   9

CONTENTS

PREFACE

This book is intended to serve as a textbook for students of the physiology and biochemistry of lactation and as a general reference book for research workers in this field. It is an attempt to bring together the pertinent and the most recent literature on lactation. Because the primary intent was to write a textbook, dogmatic statements were made whenever the results in the literature appeared to warrant them. In most cases, these statements are substantiated by references. If a clear-cut interpretation of the literature could not be made by the author, the significant literature was reviewed and a tentative conclusion was reached. As additional information is gathered, these conclusions may have to be changed. These cases in which no hard and fast conclusions were reached emphasize the lack of a complete understanding of the mammary gland and of its functions and the difficulty of interpreting conflicting results in the literature.

An exhaustive citation of references is not included. Whenever possible, review articles or research articles with brief reviews have been cited. Most of the references are listed at the end of each paragraph. It is hoped that the references will direct the reader to the important literature on lactation.

The book is intended for use by advanced undergraduates and graduate students who have had some previous training in biochemistry and physiology. It has been impossible to review all of the basic principles in these subjects before relating them to the function of the mammary gland.

An effort was made to cover all areas of study relating to the mammary gland, including development, secretion, milk removal, and common abnormalities of the udder and its secretion. For this reason, information on many species was used. In some cases, most of the information came from studies of laboratory animals, especially in the biochemical area, where most of the work has been done on rat and mouse mammary tissue. In other areas, the knowledge comes almost exclusively from studies of the cow. This is true in such areas as milk removal, milk secretion rate, and udder abnormalities. Information on the human mammary gland has received limited attention in this book for several reasons. The amount of controlled research work on human lactation is small; and much of the present work is concerned with the cessation of secretion after parturition instead of increasing it, since, in many western countries, breast feeding has ceased to be a major method of nourishing the young.

I wish to thank the many people who have made the book possible, especially Professors R. P. Natzke and J. E. Kinsella for their comments and constructive criticisms of parts of the book. Special thanks are due to my secretary, Mrs. Virginia Ross, for the large job of typing the drafts and final copy, and to Mrs. Jane Tutton for doing three of the drawings.

December 1970

G. H. Schmidt
CORNELL UNIVERSITY

BIOLOGY OF LACTATION

1

THE MAMMARY GLAND
AND ITS SECRETION

Nature has provided some of the species in the animal kingdom with mammary glands for the nourishment of their offspring after birth. Animals having hair and mammary glands belong to the class Mammalia. The word *mammal* comes from the latin word *mamma*, which means breast, or milk gland. In most mammals, the young develop in a placenta and are born in a rather helpless state. After birth, the young are nourished by milk, the physiological fluid of the mammary gland. Milk has a rather high calorific value and a balance of nutrients so that it satisfies the nutritional needs of the young during their early critical period of development and provides for their adequate growth until they are able to consume solid foods. Milk has been described as nature's most perfect food.

Man has domesticated some of the mammals and over the years has selected and bred them to produce volumes of milk far in excess of that needed to nourish the young. This excess is the basis of the dairy industry, which is one of the most important agricultural enterprises in North America, Europe, Australia, and New Zealand. The dairy cow is the predominant animal used for this purpose, but the goat, sheep, and water buffalo are also kept and bred for their milk-producing ability.

TABLE 1-1
Composition of milk from different species.

Species	Fat %	Protein %	Lactose %	Ash %	Total solids %	Reference
Antelope	1.3	6.9	4.0	1.30	25.2	7
Ass (donkey)	1.2	1.7	6.9	0.45	10.2	7
Bear, polar	31.0	10.2	0.5	1.2	42.9	2
Bison	1.7	4.8	5.7	0.96	13.2	7
Buffalo, Philippine	10.4	5.9	4.3	0.8	21.5	4
Camel	4.9	3.7	5.1	0.7	14.4	7
Cat	10.9	11.1	3.4	—	—	7
Cow						
Ayrshire	4.1	3.6	4.7	0.7	13.1	1
Brown Swiss	4.0	3.6	5.0	0.7	13.3	1
Guernsey	5.0	3.8	4.9	0.7	14.4	1
Holstein	3.5	3.1	4.9	0.7	12.2	1
Jersey	5.5	3.9	4.9	0.7	15.0	1
Zebu	4.9	3.9	5.1	0.8	14.7	9
Deer	19.7	10.4	2.6	1.4	34.1	8
Dog	8.3	9.5	3.7	1.20	20.7	7
Dolphin	14.1	10.4	5.9	—	—	7
Elephant	15.1	4.9	3.4	0.76	26.9	7
Goat	3.5	3.1	4.6	0.79	12.0	7
Guinea Pig	3.9	8.1	3.0	0.82	15.8	7
Horse	1.6	2.7	6.1	0.51	11.0	7
Human	4.5	1.1	6.8	0.20	12.6	7
Kangaroo	2.1	6.2	trace	1.20	9.5	7
Mink	8.0	7.0	6.9	0.7	22.6	6
Monkey	3.9	2.1	5.9	2.60	14.5	7
Opossum	6.1	9.2	3.2	1.60	24.5	5
Pig	8.2	5.8	4.8	0.63	19.9	7
Rabbit	12.2	10.4	1.8	2.0	26.4	3
Rat	14.8	11.3	2.9	1.5	31.7	7
Reindeer	22.5	10.3	2.5	1.40	36.7	7
Seal, grey	53.2	11.2	2.6	0.70	67.7	7
Sheep	5.3	5.5	4.6	0.90	16.3	7
Whale	34.8	13.6	1.8	1.60	51.2	7

1-1   COMPOSITION OF MILK

Milk contains three characteristic components: lactose, casein, and milk fat. The quantities of these and other components of milk vary among species, although the composition is affected by many genetic and environmental factors. Table 1-1 shows the composition of milk of some animals. The percentages given are average figures and can be used only to make a general comparison of composition among species. The greatest variation in composition occurs in the milk fat percentage; this results in comparable changes in the percentage of total solids. Both percentages are high for mammals that live in water; the milk of some has a fat content above 40%, giving it the consistency of thick cream.

1-2   IMPORTANCE OF MAMMARY GLAND STUDIES

Study of the mammary gland anatomy, histology, physiology, and biochemistry is important for many reasons. For example, greater knowledge in these areas would allow dairymen to alter the environment and conditions under which the mammals are kept, especially the nutrition and milking procedures, thereby inducing them to produce larger volumes of milk and, in some cases, effecting a change in the composition of the milk to better meet the needs of the human population. An understanding of the function of the mammary gland is also of definite help in the control of some of the diseases and conditions that adversely affect the gland, diseases such as mastitis, edema, and cancer.

The mammary gland tissue also lends itself very well to the study of basic physiological functions of cells and organ systems. Mammary gland tissue is different from most tissues in that most of its growth occurs after the animal approaches maturity. The mammary gland is usually classified as an accessory gland to the reproductive system. Under normal conditions, it develops only after the reproductive system becomes operative. In the placental animals, most of the major development occurs after the start of pregnancy. It is therefore possible to study the growth of an organ system in the animal after fetal development. Thus, the experimental conditions to evaluate the growth of the mammary gland can be applied directly to the animal being studied. In contrast to most of the fetal growth of tissue, which appears to be the result of inductor growth of the tissue itself, the growth of the mammary gland is under the control of hormones. It is not known whether the levels of hormones in the blood during pregnancy control the extent of mammary gland growth or whether the hormones serve only as an inducer or "key" to allow the genetic material in the deoxyribonucleic acid within the cell concerned with cell division for gland growth to express itself. If the amount of growth were dependent upon the levels and combination of hormones in the blood, it might be possible to increase the amount of mammary growth in domestic animals by hormone administration with a possible concomitant increase in level of milk production. It is now possible to culture mammary gland tissue *in vitro* and change the hormonal environment to induce the tissue to secrete milk.

The initiation of the milk secretion process is definitely under the influence of hormones. The mammary gland, therefore, provides a tissue system in which the action of a hormone on the tissue can be isolated and the exact role of a hormone in inducing the synthesis process may be studied. This system has also been used as an assay for prolactin.

The continued secretion of milk is controlled by several factors. The amount of milk produced and the composition of milk can be altered by changes in the hormonal and nutritional status of the animal. The hormones, somatotrophin and thyroxine, increase the level of milk production of the dairy cow. For the secretion of milk to continue, the secretory products must be periodically removed. The evacuation of milk from the mammary gland of most mammals requires the stimulation of the nervous system through suckling or milking procedures. The nervous stimulus induces the release of the hormone, oxytocin, which causes the myoepithelial cells surrounding the milk-producing alveoli to contract, thus forcing the milk from the alveoli into the ducts. If the milk is not evacuated, the secretion process decreases and eventually stops with the complete involution of the secretory tissue. Thus, the secretion process of developed mammary gland tissue requires the interplay of hormonal, nutritional, and neurohormonal processes in addition to the evacuation of the milk by the suckling of the young or the milking of the mammal by man.

Another unique aspect of the mammary gland is that a drop in the level of milk production occurs after the peak level of secretion. This happens regardless of the nutritional regimes of the animals or the intensity of the suckling stimulus. It thus appears to be a normal involution process, which leads to the complete cessation of the secretion process. Under normal conditions the secretion process resumes only after another pregnancy, during which the secretory tissue has developed in the udder. Thus, the mammary gland is a tissue that develops during pregnancy, undergoes an active secretory status, and then almost completely degenerates after the young are mature enough to exist on solid foods. This may happen many times during the lifetime of the female. The mammary gland therefore provides a tissue for the study of the factors that are responsible for the developmental and involutional processes.

Since the status of the mammary gland changes markedly during the developmental, secretory, and involutional processes, the cell physiologist can study the changes in the cell components as they relate to the different physiological stages. Current emphasis has been related to the study of the changes in nucleic acid content and the enzyme levels in the cells. From these studies, it may be possible to relate specific changes in the cell components to changes in the secretion process.

Mammary gland tissue has also been used to study biochemical pathways, because some of the secretory products, particularly casein and lactose, are primarily limited to the mammary gland.

Because the mammary gland is a skin gland, its major vascular connections to the body are limited to a few arteries and veins. This has made it possible to measure the blood flow through the organ as well as changes in the composition of blood as it enters and leaves the mammary gland. Such measurements have aided scientists in establishing definite precursor-product relationships for blood and milk and a quantitative relationship between the two.

A greater understanding of the function of the mammary gland is thus important to explain more fully the nature of the universe; and to allow man to manipulate the animal population to produce greater quantities of "Nature's most perfect food" and to treat and prevent some of the maladies affecting the human population, especially cancer.

REFERENCES

1. Armstrong, T. V. 1959. *J. Dairy Sci.* 42:1.
2. Baker, B. E., C. R. Harrington, and A. L. Symes. 1963. *Canad. J. Zool.* 41:1035.
3. Bergman, A. J., and C. W. Turner. 1937. *J. Biol. Chem.* 120:21.
4. Dittmer, D. S., ed. 1961. *Blood and other Body Fluids.* Federation of American Societies for Experimental Biology, Washington, D.C.
5. Gross, R., and A. Bolliger. 1959. *J. Dis. Child.* 98:768.
6. Jorgensen, G. 1960. *Nutr. Abstr. Rev.* 30:1218.
7. Smith, V. R. 1959. *Physiology of Lactation*, 5th ed. Ames, Iowa: Iowa State University Press.
8. Spector, W. S., ed. 1956. *Handbook of Biological Data.* National Research Council, Washington, D.C.
9. Verdiev, Z., and D. Veli-Zade. 1960. *Nutr. Abstr. Rev.* 30:1216.

MAMMARY GLAND ANATOMY

Before considering the function of the mammary gland, it is necessary to understand its anatomy and histology and its relationship to the rest of the body. The mammary glands of mammals are found in various sizes, shapes, and locations; however, the function of all mammary glands is the secretion of milk for the nourishment of the offspring.

Mammals include a variety of species, ranging from the monotremes, which are the most primitive phylogenetically, to man, who has the most complex nervous system. The Mammalian class includes 3,500 existing species and 1,000 living genera. This class is divided into two subclasses, the Prototheria, the egg-laying mammals, and the Theria, mammals that bear live young. There are 18 living orders in these two subclasses. Monotremeta is the only order under the Prototheria subclass. The monotremes, which have the most primitive mammary glands, are egg-laying mammals that have no placenta for the development of the young. One species, the duck-billed platypus, is a fur-covered animal that lays its eggs in a moist underground tunnel and hatches them in a manner comparable to that of a bird. The young platypus lives entirely on the milk secreted by its mother. The platypus's mammary glands are located on each side of the midline of the abdominal wall. There are about 100 to 150 separate glands, each composed of a simple-branched and convoluted tube. The walls of the tube have a membrana propria with an internal layer of secretory cells and an external contractal layer. The milk secreted by each gland moves to the surface of the abdomen and oozes onto a stiff mammary hair, from which the secretion is licked off by the young. In contrast to the higher forms of mammary gland, there is no nipple.

Another species of the Monotremeta order is the porcupine anteater. It develops a pouch on the surface of the abdomen and the egg is transferred to the pouch immediately after ovulation. The egg is hatched and the young live on the milk secreted by the dam. The anteater's mammary gland differs from that of the platypus in that the milk oozes into a small depression within the pouch instead of being secreted onto a hair.

The subclass Theria has two infraclasses, the Metatheria, which are pouched animals, and the Eutheria, the placental animals. A single order, Marsupialia, is classified under the Metatheria. These animals have somewhat more complex mammary glands than the monotremes. The marsupials are pouch-bearing animals that give birth to live young; however, the young are developed in a primitive type of placenta and are born in a very immature state. This order includes the kangaroo and the opossum. At birth the young are transferred to the pouch, the marsupium, and the young remain semipermanently attached to a mammary gland nipple until they are well grown. The mammary glands of the marsupials are more highly developed than those of the monotremes in that the ducts of the simple glands come together into a teat or nipple through which the milk is secreted. The nipples are usually located in a depression in the pouch. The marsupials may have as many as 20 nipples in the gland pouch.

Most of the existing orders of mammals belong to the infraclass Eutheria. These animals have highly developed placentas and give birth to live young. The mammary glands of these mammals are highly developed and all have teats. The sizes and shapes vary in the different species, but in most cases, the mammary gland is composed of a teat, a duct system, and lobes and lobules of secretory tissue drained by the duct system. Some animals have a series of mammary glands on each side of the midline of the abdominal wall. Others have a grouping of two or four glands that form an udder, which is usually located in the inguinal region. For details on the anatomy of some of the species, see the reviews by Raynaud (14), Smith (17), and Turner (20, 21). The anatomy of the mammary glands of some of the common domestic animals and the laboratory animals commonly used for milk secretion studies will be reviewed in this book.

2-1   COW

In the western world, most of the dairy industry is based on the dairy cow. Consequently, much attention has been directed to detailed studies on the anatomy and function of the mammary gland of this species. For this reason, considerably more information is available on this species than on most others.

External Appearance

The anatomy of the cow's udder has been reviewed by Turner (21). Four mammary glands join together to form the udder. The udder is a skin gland and is covered with hair, except for the teats. The udder has been described as being square in appearance or as having a more or less rounded saccular appearance.

The udder is separated into two halves by a longitudinal groove, the intermammary groove. In some udders the fore and rear quarters are also separated by a groove; however, this characteristic is not desired. The rear quarters make up the largest portion of the udder and secrete approximately 60% of the milk. In addition to the four teats that drain the mammary glands, some cows have extra teats, the supernumerary teats. These are usually located posterior to the two rear teats, but in some cases they are located between the fore and rear teats. The extra teats are usually removed when the calf is less than one year of age, because of their unsightly appearance and the possibility of infection with mastitis organisms.

The weight of the udder varies with the age of the cow, the stage of lactation, the amount of milk in the udder, and inherited differences among cows. In one study (10), it was found that the average empty weight of the udders of 78 Holstein cows was 49.4 lb with a range from 14.4 lb to 165.7 lb. The capacity of these udders was determined by measuring the amount of fluid that could be injected at 10 lb of pressure into the empty amputated udder. The average capacity was found to be 67.9 lb. The capacity of each udder exceeded the amount of milk obtained from the udder at any milking. The weight and capacity of the udders increased with age for animals up to 6 years of age, with the greatest increases occurring between the first and second lactations. There were no significant increases in either udder weight or capacity after cows reached 6 years of age. The weight decreased with advancing lactation for all lactations, the most pronounced decrease occurring during the first two months of lactation. The capacity did not change during the first two months, after which it decreased 6 lb per month.

The teat varies in shape from cylindrical to conical. The rear teats are usually shorter than the fore teats. Since the advent of machine milking, cows with shorter teats have been selectively bred, because they have been shown to have a more rapid milk-flow rate than those with longer teats (15).

One of the most important concerns to the dairyman is to have cows with udders that are large enough to produce large volumes of milk and, at the same time, not to have them excessively large or with poor udder attachments, conditions that create management problems. The dairy cow score card created by the Purebred Dairy Cattle Association describes the desirable shape of the udder as being long, wide, and of moderate depth. The udder should extend well forward, be strongly attached, and have a reasonably level floor. The rear attachment should be high and wide and the quarters should be evenly balanced and symmetrical. An outstanding cow with a desirably shaped udder is shown in Figure 2-1.

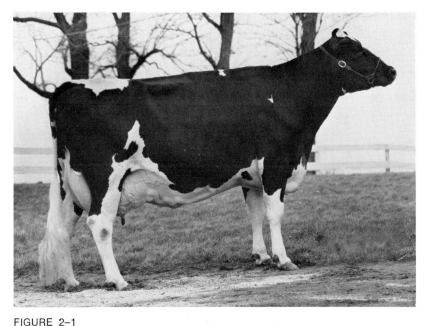

FIGURE 2–1
Collins-Crest Ivanhoe Triune J, a cow that combines excellent type and production. She was classified excellent (2E-96) and produced 31,028 lb of milk and 1020 lb of milk fat in 365 days as a 5-year old.
(Courtesy of Donald S. Collins family, Perry, N. Y.)

Interior Structure

The right and left halves of the udder are separated internally by the medial suspensory ligament, which is made up of two sheets of dense connective tissue (see Figure 2-2). Although no specific membrane separates the fore and rear quarters of each udder half, the duct systems are independent of each other. A longitudinal section of udder cut through the fore and rear teats is shown in Figure 2-3.

The udder is composed of small areas of flesh-colored secretory tissue surrounded by connective tissue capsules. The secretory tissue is made up of alveoli. A number of alveoli are joined together by a common duct and are surrounded by connective tissue to form a lobule. Many lobules are again surrounded by connective tissue to form lobes (see Figure 2-4). The white strands of connective tissue throughout the mammary gland serve to support the secretory tissue within the udder. The small visible whitish tissue separating the fore and rear quarters is the connective tissue capsule between the lobes of the two quarters. An udder commonly referred to as a "hard" udder is one with a large amount of connective tissue in comparison to secretory tissue. This may be an inherited characteristic or brought about by mastitis, a disease in which the secretory tissue is replaced by connective tissue.

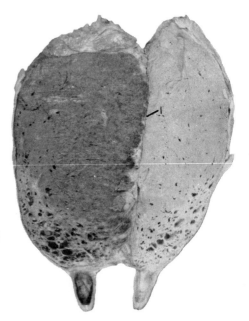

FIGURE 2–2
Cross section of the bovine mammary gland through the rear quarters, which are separated by the medial suspensory ligament (I) The quarters had been injected with two different color dyes.

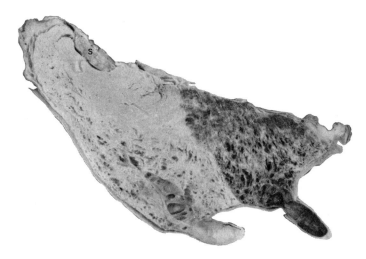

FIGURE 2-3
Longitudinal section of the bovine udder through the fore
and rear quarters. Two different colored dyes were injected into
the two quarters. s, Supramammary lymph node.

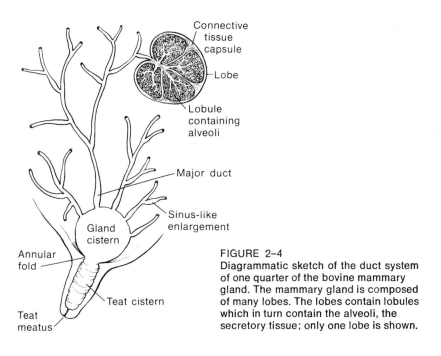

Connective
tissue
capsule

Lobe

Lobule
containing
alveoli

Major duct

Sinus-like
enlargement

Gland
cistern

Annular
fold

Teat cistern

Teat
meatus

FIGURE 2-4
Diagrammatic sketch of the duct system
of one quarter of the bovine mammary
gland. The mammary gland is composed
of many lobes. The lobes contain lobules
which in turn contain the alveoli, the
secretory tissue; only one lobe is shown.

Duct System   The lobes empty into ducts that in turn drain into larger ducts (see Figure 2-4). These join the major ducts that enter the gland cistern above the teat. The duct system and the gland cistern carry the milk from the secretory tissue to the teats, where it can be obtained by machine or hand milking or by the calf. The ducts and gland cisterns also serve as collecting vessels for part of the milk between milkings. This allows the udder to secrete larger volumes of milk than that which could be stored in the secretory tissue only. At the point where a duct sends off a branch, the branch usually has a narrow opening and then forms a sinus-like enlargement before it narrows again. In some cases the ducts divide into two branches of the same size. This constriction at the point of branching prevents the milk from flowing by gravity to the teat and gland cisterns.

The larger ducts in the lower portion of the fore quarters are concentrated on the lateral surfaces, whereas the distribution of ducts is more uniform in the upper part of the fore quarters and in the rear quarters. The larger ducts have a tendency to be short and wide and the smaller ducts are more rounded. Usually 10 to 12 ducts lead into each gland cistern, but as many as 20, and in rare cases even higher numbers, have been found.

Gland Cistern   The size and shape of the gland cistern (lactiferous sinus) for each quarter vary considerably. In some cases, the cistern is circular; in others, it appears to be nothing more than pockets of various sizes formed from the terminations of the major ducts. The capacity of the gland cisterns varies from 100 to 400 g of milk. No relationship exists between the size of the cistern and the amount of milk secreted by the quarters.

Teat   The teat cisterns (sinus papillaris) are cavities within the teat and are located just below the gland cisterns. The gland and teat cisterns are continuous; however, in most cows a definite circular construction, the annular fold, is located between the two cavities (see Figure 2-4). It is composed of dense connective tissue and is 2–6 mm in width. In exceptional cases, a horizontal septum forms at the annular fold and prevents milk flow, resulting in a blind quarter. The teat cistern is lined with numerous longitudinal and circular folds in the mucosa (Figure 2-5). These tend to overlap each other to form pockets in the side of the teat and may serve as storage places for bacteria.

The end of the teat of the cow has one opening, the streak canal (also called teat meatus or ductus papillaris), which has a usual length of 8–12 mm, but may range from 5–13 mm. The circumference of the streak canal varies from 4–11 mm. The streak canal shortens in length when

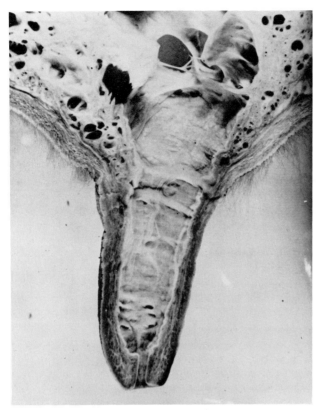

FIGURE 2–5
Section of the teat of a bovine mammary gland showing
numerous circular folds in the teat cistern. (Courtesy of Babson
Bros. Company, Oak Brook, Illinois.)

pressure is applied to the teat during milking and at the same time the cistern of the teat tends to balloon out, because of the pressure within the udder. The streak canal appears to lengthen and dilate with each additional lactation, with the greatest increase occurring from the first to second lactations (4, 5, 11, 12).

The streak canal is composed of 5 to 7 convex epithelial projections that form a star-shaped slit. The projections are held closed by involuntary, circular sphincter muscles. The streak canal retains the milk in the udder against the pressure developed by the accumulation of milk. In addition, it keeps dirt and bacteria out of the udder between milkings. It has also been shown that the size of the streak canal and the tautness of the sphincter muscle surrounding the meatus play an important role in determining the rate of milk flow. This appears to be an inherited condition (1, 13).

Located just above the streak canal are a series of 4 to 8 folds radiating in all directions. This is known as Fürstenburg's rosette, named after the man who first described it. The larger folds are accompanied by smaller accessory folds. Pressure from the accumulation of milk within the teat and glands causes the folds to smooth out, which aids in the retention of milk.

Suspensory Apparatus

Swett et al. (18) studied the suspensory apparatus of the udder of a Holstein cow and separated the tissues into seven parts. Tissue 1 was described as the skin, which serves in a minor capacity to suspend and stabilize the udder. The fine areolar subcutaneous tissue or superficial fascia that attaches the skin to the underlying tissue was described as tissue 2. Tissue 3 is the cordlike (coarse areolar) tissue that forms a loose bond between the dorsal surface of the front quarters and the abdominal wall (see Figure 2-6). A weakening of this tissue causes the udder to break away from the abdominal wall.

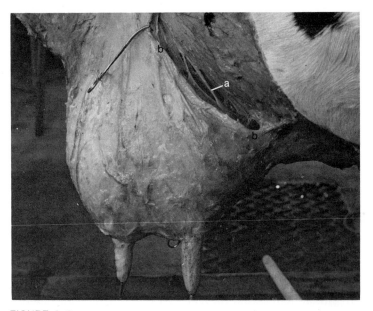

FIGURE 2–6
Suspensory apparatus of the udder. Cordlike tissue (a) (Tissue 3) that holds the udder in contact with the abdominal wall. Deep layer of lateral suspensory ligament (b). (From Swett, et al. 1942. *J. Agr. Res.* 65:19.)

Tissue 4 is the pair of superficial layers of the lateral suspensory ligaments, partially composed of elastic tissue. These ligaments arise from the subpelvic tendon and extend downward and forward over the udder and reflect off the inner face of the thigh. These layers are fairly close to the median line at the rear of the udder and then flare out towards the anterior portions of the udder. This is one of the primary supporting ligaments of the udder. The pair of deep, somewhat thicker layers of the lateral suspensory ligaments (Figure 2-7) are defined as tissue 5 and they also have their origin on the subpelvic tendon. These deeper lateral sheets extend down over the udder and virtually envelop it. They attach to the convex lateral surfaces of the udder by numerous lamellae, which pass into the gland and become continuous with the interstitial framework of the udder. This too forms an important part of the suspensory apparatus of the udder. Tissue 6 is the subpelvic tendon (Figure 2-8), which in itself is not a part of the suspensory apparatus of the udder, but it gives rise to the superficial and deep layers of the lateral suspensory ligaments. The subpelvic tendon is not a continuous sheet of tissue but is attached at a number of separated points along the ventral side of the pelvis.

Two adjacent sheets of heavy yellow elastic tissue make up the median

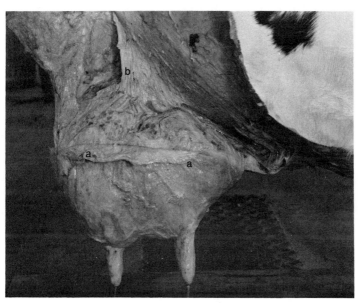

FIGURE 2-7
Suspensory apparatus of the udder. Deep layer of the lateral suspensory ligament (a). A portion of the median elastic suspensory ligament (b). (From Swett et al. 1942. *J. Agr. Res.* 65:19.)

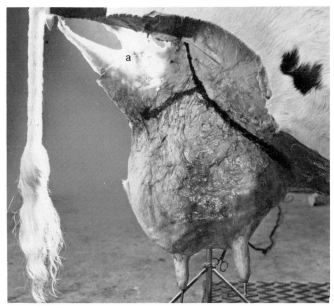

FIGURE 2–8
Subpelvic tendon (a), which gives rise to the two sheets of the
lateral suspensory ligaments. (From Swett et al. 1942.
J. Agr. Res. 65:19.)

suspensory ligament, tissue 7. They arise from the abdominal wall and
attach to the medial flat surfaces of the two halves of the udder to form a
septum between them. The medial suspensory tissue possesses great ten-
sile strength. It is located over the center of gravity of the udder to give
a nearly perfectly balanced suspension of the udder after the other tissues have been removed (see Figure 2-9). The medial suspensory ligaments again play an important role in the suspension of the udder. A
weakening of tissue 3 and the lengthening of the medial and lateral suspensory ligaments cause the udder to drop and, in severe cases, to become
pendulous.

Blood Circulation

Arterial System   Most of the blood is supplied to the udder by the two
external pudendal (external pudic) arteries, one for each half of the
udder (Figure 2-10). The arteries enter the mammary gland from the
abdominal cavity through the inguinal canal. As they enter the mammary gland, the arteries form a sigmoid flexure, which probably allows
for the lowering of the udder when it becomes filled with milk. The external pudendal arteries are branches of the external iliac arteries, which

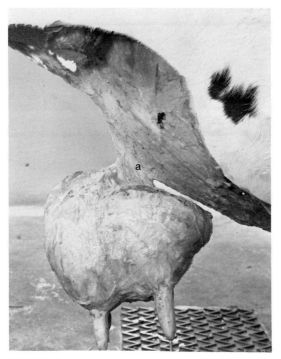

FIGURE 2–9
Medial suspensory ligament (a) of the udder gives a
nearly perfect balanced suspension of the udder.
(From Swett et al. 1942. *J. Agr. Res.* 65:19.)

arise from the aorta. The internal iliac arteries, which supply blood to the genitalia and the pudendal region, are also branches of the aorta. The perineal arteries arise from the internal iliacs and supply blood to a very small portion of the posterior dorsal part of the rear quarters.

The mammary arteries are continuations of the external pudendal arteries after they enter the mammary gland. The mammary artery for each half gives off a small branch to the supramammary lymph node and the upper part of the rear quarters. The mammary artery then branches into two large arteries, the anterior, or cranial, mammary artery and the posterior, or caudal mammary artery. A small branch, the subcutaneous abdominal artery, arises from the mammary artery before it divides into the anterior and posterior arteries. This travels anteriorly and supplies blood to the ventral abdominal wall just anterior to the udder and to the basal part of the udder. It is questionable whether this artery supplies blood directly to any of the secretory tissue. In some animals, the subcutaneous abdominal artery is a branch of the cranial mammary artery.

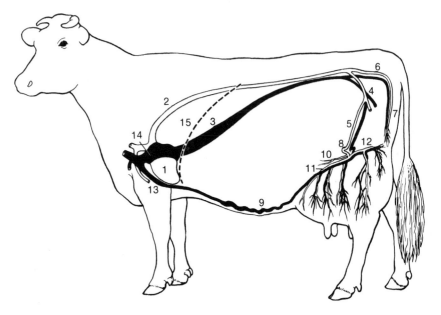

FIGURE 2–10
Blood circulation to and from the udder. 1—Heart, 2—Abdominal aorta,
3—Posterior vena cava, 4—External iliac artery and vein, 5—External pudendal
artery and vein, 6—Internal iliac artery and vein, 7—Perineal artery and vein,
8—Sigmoid flexure of the external pudendal artery and vein, 9—Subcutaneous
abdominal vein, 10—Subcutaneous abdominal artery, 11—Cranial mammary
artery, 12—Caudal mammary artery, 13—Internal thoracic artery and vein,
14—Anterior vena cava, and 15—Diaphragm.

Branches of the cranial and caudal mammary arteries spread ventrally
and laterally and divide and subdivide many times so that eventually
small arterioles surround each alveolus. They also supply blood to the
connective tissue and the teats. There appears to be no anastomosing
between the arteries of the two halves of the udder.

Venous System   The blood from each half of the udder leaves by two
veins, the external pudendal and the subcutaneous abdominal, or milk
vein. The external pudendal vein forms a sigmoid flexure just below the
inguinal canal, divides into the cranial and caudal branches, and then
divides and subdivides and its branches follow the paths of corresponding
arteries and arterioles. The blood leaving the udder through the external
pudendal vein flows through the external iliac vein and the posterior vena
cava to the heart. The subcutaneous abdominal vein is a continuation of
the cranial branch of the mammary vein and leaves the udder at the

anterior border of the udder. It travels along the ventral surface of the abdominal cavity just below the skin. The subcutaneous abdominal veins move anteriorly and penetrate the abdominal wall on each side of the xiphoid cartilage. The places where veins enter the abdominal cavity are referred to as the milk wells. After entering the abdominal cavity, the veins pass forward to join the internal thoracic veins, which then travel to the anterior vena cava.

A small perineal vein is located towards the posterior dorsal area of each half of the udder and drains the area of the udder to which the perineal artery supplies blood—this area is, again, a very small portion of each half of the udder.

A venous circle at the base of the udder is formed by branches of the right and left cranial and caudal mammary veins. Branches of the caudal mammary veins anastomose at the posterior base of the udder and branches of the subcutaneous abdominal veins anastomose a few inches anterior to the base of the udder. It is questionable whether free movement of blood occurs between the two halves of the udder because of the direction of the valves in the veins (Figure 2-11).

The blood can leave the udder by either the subcutaneous abdominal vein or the external pudendal vein in the lactating ruminant. The exact route is probably dependent upon the position of the animal, for it appears that the blood leaves the udder via the subcutaneous abdominal vein in the standing animal. When either of the major veins is compressed, the blood flows in the other vein. Linzell (8) made a detailed anatomical and blood flow study of the veins of sheep, goats, and cows of various ages. He found that the cranial portion of the subcutaneous abdominal vein of the cow had 6 to 14 valves pointing towards the heart and the caudal portion had 1 to 5 valves pointing towards the udder. In the young animal

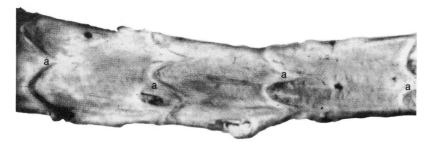

FIGURE 2–11
One of the veins of the udder that has been opened up to show the valves (a),
which allow the blood to flow in one direction.
(From *Linzell*, 1960. *J. Physiol.* 153:481.)

the blood is carried towards the udder in the caudal portion of the vein. Pregnancy and lactation cause the veins to increase in size and the valves cease to function, thus allowing the blood to flow in either direction.

Lymphatic System

The lymphatic system of the udder is composed of lymph vessels and nodes. The vessels carry tissue fluid, or lymph, from the tissue spaces to the lymph nodes and return the fluid to the venous circulation. A valve-like structure, located at the end of the thoracic duct, prevents the blood from being regurgitated into the lymphatic system. This valve and additional valves in the lymph vessels cause the lymph to flow only in the direction of the venous blood system. The lymph nodes filter the fluid by removing foreign material and pass it to larger lymph vessels, which transfer it to the venous blood via the thoracic duct just anterior to the heart. The lymph nodes also add leucocytes to the lymph. The udder usually has one large lymph node for each half. It is the supramammary lymph node and it lies just posterior to the inguinal canal. In some cases, as many as seven smaller lymph nodes have been counted for each half of the udder. After passing through the supramammary lymph node, the lymph leaves the udder by one or two lymph vessels and these pass through the inguinal canal to join other lymph vessels.

The lymph enters the node through the afferent vessels on the node's convex border, passes through a network of sinuses in the node, and emerges from the hilus into the efferent vessel. The lymph vessels are difficult to identify, because they have a small amount of connective tissue in their walls and because the lymph in them has a very clear color.

Lymph is moved by a pressure differential caused by breathing, the pressure in the blood capillaries, and the contraction of the muscles. When an excessive amount of lymph accumulates between the skin and the secretory tissue of the udder, udder edema develops. This is most serious in first-calf heifers and in older cows with pendulous udders at the time of calving.

The subcutaneous lymph ducts under the skin of the udder are very prevalent and in the mature cow become quite large. Some attain a diameter of 5–7 mm. These vessels run in a dorsal caudal direction to the supramammary lymph nodes (Figure 2-12). The lymph from the glandular tissue is carried by a variable number of deep and superficial lymph vessels and their size varies from 2–6 mm in diameter. The teats have an abundant supply of lymph vessels. These are separate for each teat and are slightly larger than the subcutaneous lymph vessels. The lymph vessels from the teats join either the deep or the subcutaneous vessels, or both.

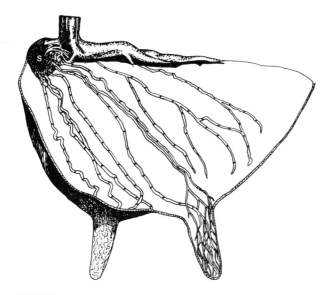

FIGURE 2–12
Diagrammatic sketch of the subcutaneous lymph vessels
traveling in a dorsal-caudal direction to the supramammary
lymph node(s). The vessels have valves in them that
allow the lymph to move only in one direction—toward
the lymph node.

Nervous System

The udder is supplied with two types of nerves, the afferent, or sensory, fibers and the efferent sympathetic fibers. Afferent nerve fibers originate from the dorsal root of the spinal cord and the efferent, or motor, fibers arise from the ventral root. After leaving the vertebral column, they join to form spinal nerves. These are paired and in cattle the nervous system consists of 37 pairs of spinal nerves and 12 cranial nerves.

Only a few of the spinal nerves are involved in innervating the udder. The first lumbar nerves send fibers to the anterior surface of the udder and the adjacent abdominal wall (Figure 2-13). It is questionable whether these fibers enter the udder. The second lumbar nerves descend from the vertebral column to the flank and innervate the anterior parts of the udder. These fibers may enter the glandular tissue of the fore quarters. Branches of the second, third, and fourth lumbar nerves join to form the inguinal nerves and enter the udder through the inguinal canal. These fibers do not unite as a single nerve for each udder half, but are usually joined together as a group. The inguinal nerves divide into anterior and posterior nerve fibers at the inguinal ring. Branches of these nerves are found throughout

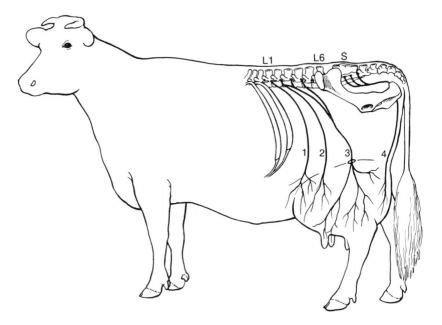

FIGURE 2–13
Nervous system of the udder. 1—First lumbar nerve, 2—Second lumbar nerve,
3—Inguinal nerve, 4—Perineal nerve, L1—First lumbar vertebra,
L6—Sixth lumbar vertebra, and S—Sacrum.

the glandular tissue, the milk collecting system, the teats, and the skin of
the udder. A small branch of each posterior inguinal nerve innervates the
supramammary lymph gland area.

The perineal nerves arise from the second, third, and fourth sacral
nerves and enter the udder at its posterior caudal portion along with the
perineal arteries and veins. The perineal nerves supply nerve fibers to
the posterior part of the udder. The sacral nerves are considered to be
part of the parasympathetic nervous system, and some workers have
thought that these nerves bring parasympathetic nerve fibers to the udder.
These fibers have not been found in the udder, however, and it is generally
concluded that they are not present within the mammary gland of the cow.

The motor or efferent nervous supply to the udder is confined to the
inguinal nerves. Cutting the inguinal nerves or removing the sympathetic
trunk in the lumbar area removes all efferent nervous stimuli to the
udder, as is shown by vasodilation of the vessels in the udder. Russian
workers have indicated that secretory nerve fibers are present in the
glandular tissue of the udder; these findings have not been verified, however (3). The primary functions of the sympathetic nerve fibers to the
udder are control of the blood supply to the udder and innervation of

smooth muscles surrounding the milk-collecting ducts and the sphincter muscles within the teat. Stimulation of the sympathetic nervous system causes a vasoconstriction of the blood vessels and this has an inhibiting effect on milk secretion instead of a stimulatory one.

2-2 GOAT AND SHEEP

The udders of the goat and sheep are quite similar, therefore they will be discussed together. The anatomy of the mammary glands of these species has been reviewed by Turner (21). The udders of these animals consist of two mammary glands, each drained by a teat. The teats of the goat vary tremendously in size, with some being small and difficult to milk and others being extremely large. The teats of the sheep are uniformly smaller than those of the goat. The goat's teats have a tendency to be wide at the base and protrude like funnels from the udder without any marked point of connection. Hair is present on the teats of both species, but it is very fine in texture. Supernumerary teats are quite common in both species.

Both animals have one streak canal per teat. The boundary between the streak canal and the teat cistern can be easily distinguished by the naked eye. In the goat the pavement epithelium of the streak canal has a white color and the epithelium of the teat cistern has a yellowish color. The epithelium of the teat cistern of the sheep is yellowish; however, the streak canal has a darkly pigmented epithelial lining. At the point between the streak canal and the teat cistern in the goat, a rosette similar to that of the cow is found.

The gland cistern of the sheep is irregular in shape and relatively small in size. The cisterns of the teat and the gland of the goat are large in comparison to the amount of gland tissue. The gland cisterns of both species act as collecting vessels for the large milk ducts that lead into them. The ducts carry the milk from the alveoli and small ducts in the secretory tissue.

The arterial circulation of the udders of the goat and sheep is similar to that of the cow. The external pudendal artery supplying blood to the udder becomes the mammary artery after it passes through the inguinal canal. After passing into the udder tissue for a short distance, the mammary artery inclines cranially.

The external pudendal arteries and veins differ from those of the cow in that they do not branch into cranial and caudal mammary arteries and veins as they enter the udder. The external pudendal arteries and veins of the goat and sheep enter the udder close to the posterior basal border rather than about two-thirds of the distance from the anterior border as in the cow. As the mammary artery passes cranially, it gives off a deep medial branch. It continues anteriorly and sends off deep lateral and cranial branches and finally terminates in the anterior basal border of the udder.

The blood is removed by two veins. One of these, the external pudendal vein, leaves the udder and runs parallel to the external pudendal artery. As it enters the udder at the posterior basal border, it turns sharply anteriorly and sends branches into the udder parallel to those of the arteries. The mammary vein travels cranially and leaves the udder at its anterior basal border as the subcutaneous abdominal vein, which passes forward and enters the thoracic cavity just behind the sternum. The perineal arteries and veins in the goat are much less well developed than in the cow.

The lymphatic vessels from each mammary gland of the sheep and goat pass to the superficial inguinal lymphatic glands (supramammary lymph gland) on each side of the udder. From here a single lymphatic trunk passes through the inguinal canal into the abdomen and runs parallel and caudal to the external pudendal blood vessels (9).

The udders of the goat and sheep are supplied with inguinal nerves (external spermatic), which divide into two branches. The superficial branch innervates the abdominal wall muscles, whereas the deep branch passes through the inguinal canal and follows the external pudendal artery and vein to the udder. In the udder, it sends off two branches that innervate the arterial walls, the milk ducts, and the teats.

Perineal nerves run with the perineal vessels from the side of the vulva. They divide into a number of branches and supply nerve fibers to the skin and back of the udder. Branches of these nerves enter the glandular tissue (7, 21).

2-3 HORSE

The anatomy of the udder of the mare has been reviewed by Turner (21). It consists of two mammary glands that are located in the inguinal region. The teat of each gland is canalized by two streak canals, which are 5–10 mm in length. The streak canals lead into separate teat cisterns, which join independent gland cisterns that have systems of ducts leading into them. The streak canals have heavy lengthwise folds, which securely close the openings. The many-layer epithelial lining of the streak canal has a blackish pigmentation. The transition between the lining of the streak canal and the two-layer lining of the gland cistern is gradual. A rosette is found above the streak canal, and just above this is a funnel-shaped teat cistern. The gland cisterns form at approximately right angles to the teat cisterns with the cranial gland cistern turning forward and the caudal gland cistern turning posteriorly. The cistern membrane has many folds.

The teats of the lactating mares are rather flat and broad with blunted tips and are not spherical in shape. The skin covering the teats and udder is pigmented and covered with thin fine hairs. Sebaceous and sweat glands are also present in the udder and teats.

The vascular system of the mare is similar to that of the cow, sheep, and goat except that perineal arteries and veins have not been described. The external pudendal artery passes through the inguinal canal to become the mamamary artery at the base of the udder. It gives off a branch to the supramammary lymph node. As the mammary artery moves cranially in the mammary gland, it gives off lateral and ventral branches, which supply blood to the secretory tissue, the connective tissue, and the teat.

The blood is drained from the udder by an external pudendal vein and the subcutaneous abdominal vein. The external pudendal vein follows the same course as the external pudendal artery. The subcutaneous abdominal vein arises from the anterior branch of the external pudendal vein, which passes through the anterior base of the udder. The subcutaneous abdominal vein then travels underneath the skin of the abdominal wall and unites with the internal thoracic vein.

The lymphatic system is similar to that of the cow. A supramammary (superficial inguinal) lymph node for each half of the udder is located between the udder and the ventral abdominal wall. Lymphatic vessels carry lymph from the skin, the mammary gland, and the teats to these nodes, which in turn filter the lymph and return it to the general blood circulation. The nerves to the udder are derived from the inguinal nerve.

2-4 GUINEA PIG

The mammary apparatus of the guinea pig consists of two mammary glands and teats located in the inguinal region. The nipples are canalized by a single duct, which consists of a constricted entrance composed of pavement epithelium, the streak canal, and an ampullary dilation, which corresponds to the cistern of the teat in the larger animals. The ducts turn caudally at the base of the nipple and then divide into two secondary ducts. The two secondary ducts give rise to the tertiary and smaller ducts, which in turn give rise to the lobulo-alveolar system of the mammary glands (23).

The blood is supplied almost entirely by the external pudendal arteries, some branches of which extend beyond the glands anteriorly (Figure 2-14).

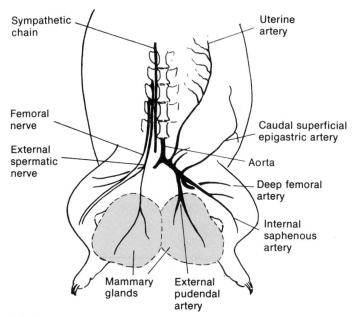

FIGURE 2–14
Blood and nerve supply to the guinea-pig mammary gland.
(From Tindal and Yokoyama, 1962. *Endocrinology* 71:196.)

The superficial vessels of the thoraco-abdominal wall are of little importance in supplying blood to the mammary gland, although anastomosis between these vessels and the branches of the external prudendal vessels does occur. The veins parallel the arteries except for an additional vein (unaccompanied by an artery) that drains the posterior part of the glands and joins the perineal branch of the external pudendal vein (6, 19, 23).

The external spermatic nerve sends two large branches to the gland. One accompanies the external pudendal vessels and the second leaves the abdominal cavity laterally above the inguinal ligament and enters the gland a short distance in front of the other vessels and nerves (6).

2-5 RABBIT

The rabbit has two rows of glands and teats, which extend from the thoracic to the abdominal region (Figure 2-15). The anterior pair of teats are usually found on the loose skin of the neck. The second pair of teats are located over the thoracic cavity and the third pair at the point of the last rib. The rabbit usually has 3 to 5 pairs of glands. The fourth pair, when only 4 pairs are present, is located in the inguinal region.

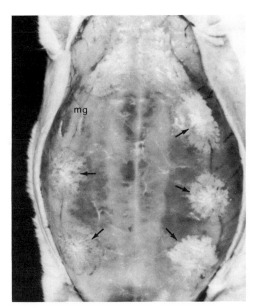

FIGURE 2-15
Mammary glands of the rabbit (↑). The anterior
pair of glands are not exposed. In this rabbit
the mammary gland just anterior to the inguinal
mammary gland on the animal's left
side is missing (MG).

When 5 pairs are present, the fifth pair is located anterior to the inguinal pair. Most of the teats have 5 or 6 ducts with a range of from 5 to 13. Each teat is connected to and drains a lobe of mammary gland tissue. The lobes are arranged in a radial manner from the teat, as shown in Figure 2-16 (20).

Blood is supplied to the mammary glands by several vessels. The caudal superficial epigastric vessels leave the femoral vessels in the thigh and anastomose with the external pudendals within the inguinal mammary glands. The caudal superficial epigastrics anastomose with the lateral thoracics and these vessels supply blood to all the mammary glands. Superficial extensions of the deep circumflex iliac and subscapular arteries also join the lateral thoracic arteries. Cutaneous branches of the phrenico-abdominal vessels supply the abdominal and inguinal glands. Branches of the internal thoracics, the cranial epigastric, and cranial superficial epigastric arteries also supply blood to the thoracic and cranial abdominal mammary glands. The cranial thoracic gland also receives blood from the axillary arteries, which emerge just behind the clavicle, and from the subclavian arteries in front of the clavicle. These

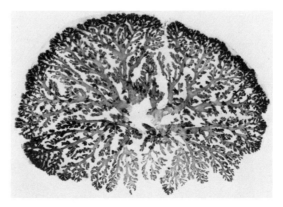

FIGURE 2–16
Mammary duct and lobulo-alveolar arrangement in
the rabbit. Each lobe is drained by a duct, which
extends to the exterior of the teat. (From Norgren
1967. *Acta Univ. Lund,* II, No. 11.)

vessels usually do not supply blood to the mammary glands in other
species. The venous system parallels the arterial system.

The mammary glands of the rabbit are innervated by fibers from
several nerves: the subcutaneous nerve from the fourth cervical nerve,
lateral cutaneous nerves from the third lumbar nerve to the third thoracic
nerve, the external spermatic nerve, and ventral cutaneous branches of
intercostal nerves (6).

2-6 RAT AND MOUSE

The rat usually has 6 pairs of mammary glands. Three of these pairs
are thoracic glands, 1 pair is abdominal, and 2 pairs are inguinal glands.
The mammary apparatus of the mouse is comparable to that of the rat
except that, normally, only 5 pairs of mammary glands are found. The
3 pairs of thoracic glands and 2 pairs of inguinal glands are comparable
to those in the rat; however, the abdominal glands are absent. In the
lactating rat, the separate glands are indistinguishable. The mammary
glands appear as a sheet of tissue extending from the neck to the anus,
interrupted only in the region of the lower ribs. The separate glands
can be delineated by injecting dye into each duct. The absence of the
abdominal pair in the mouse causes a considerable space on the abdominal wall that is free of mammary gland tissue. These glands form two
V-shaped areas. The 3 pairs of thoracic glands form a V with the point
of the V directed anteriorly. The 2 inguinal pairs and the abdominal pair
in the rat form a V with the point of the V directed caudally (2, 22, 24).

The teats are canalized by a single duct. A constricted entrance is found at the tip of the teat and this is called the streak canal. In addition, the single duct has an ampullary dilation corresponding to the cistern of the teat in the larger animals. At the base of the teat, the single duct turns laterally (except those of the inguinal glands) and then divides into 2 or 3 secondary branches. These give rise to the numerous tertiary ducts, which drain the lobes composed of alveoli (20, 22, 24).

The thoracic glands receive branches of the internal thoracic, cranial, and epigastric arteries and veins. The anterior gland also receives superficial cervical vessels and the posterior thoracic gland receives branches from the lateral thoracic vessels. The latter vessels anastomose with the caudal superficial epigastric vessels. Lateral cutaneous branches of the intercostals join the thoracic vessels. The abdominal and inguinal glands receive their blood supply from the superficial epigastric artery, the superficial and deep external pudendal arteries, and occasionally from the iliac branch of the ilio-lumbar (deep circumflex iliac) artery and lateral cutaneous branches of the phrenico-abdominal arteries (Figure 2-17).

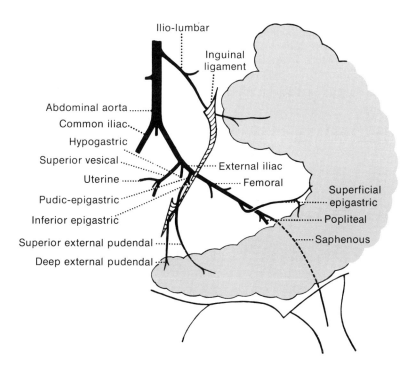

FIGURE 2–17
Arterial blood supply to the abdominal and inguinal mammary glands (gray areas) of the rat. (From Bisset et al. 1967. *Brit. J. Pharmacol. Chemother.* 31:537.)

Free anastomoses between branches appear within the gland mass. The larger veins usually parallel the arteries; however, the smaller arteries and veins are less apt to do so. The nerves to the mammary gland resemble those of the rabbit, except that the rat and mouse do not have a branch from the fourth cervical nerve (2, 6, 22).

2-7 SWINE

The sow has two parallel rows of mammary glands and teats that extend over the entire abdominal wall from the pectoral to the inguinal regions (Figure 2-18). The first pair of glands lie immediately behind the connection of the ribs with the sternum. Each gland is separate and appears as a half spherical-shaped elevation on the body. The number of teats and glands vary between 8 and 18 with 12 teats being most common. Over 95% of the animals possess between 10 and 14 teats. The teats are free of hair and sebaceous glands (21).

Each teat is transversed by two streak canals and two small teat cisterns. The streak canals are 3–4 mm long and are tightly closed by longitudinal folds which come from the teat cistern.

The teat cistern is an elliptical dilation or sinus of the duct instead of a larger cistern as is present in the ruminants. The walls of the cistern contain many longitudinal folds. The cisterns extend into the glands to

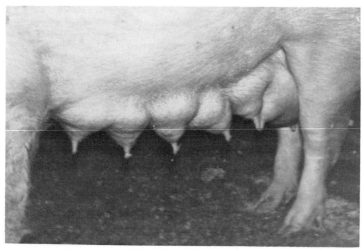

FIGURE 2–18
Mammary glands of the sow.

become the gland cisterns. These cisterns in turn give rise to the ducts that drain the milk from the alveoli located within the lobules and lobes. There are two separate duct systems within each mammary gland (21).

The anterior mammary glands are supplied with blood from the external thoracic arteries (anterior mammary arteries). The posterior mammary glands receive blood from the external pudendal arteries similar to those in cattle. The external pudendal arteries become the posterior abdominal arteries and continue anteriorly to supply the abdominal and inguinal mammary glands. They then anastomose with the external thoracic arteries. The blood leaves the mammary glands by veins that parallel the major arteries. These are the external thoracic veins and the posterior mammary veins (21).

Three groups of lymph nodes filter lymph from the mammary glands. They are the superficial inguinal lymph nodes (supramammary) located between the posterior mammary glands and the abdominal wall, the mediastinal cranial lymph nodes situated ventral to the anterior vena cava at the entrance to the thoracic cavity, and the ventral superficial lymph nodes located cranio-dorsal to the shoulder joints. These lymph nodes receive lymph from the skin, the teats, and the glandular tissue (21).

2-8 DOG AND CAT

The lactating mammary glands in the dog and cat form two parallel rows located on each side of the midline from the axilla to the inguinal region. The mammary glands of a lactating bitch are shown in Figure 2-19. The cat normally has 4 pairs of glands and the dog most commonly has 5, but ranges between 4 and 6 pairs. The usual pairs of glands in the dog are 1 inguinal, 2 abdominal, and 2 thoracic. The cat has only 1 pair of abdominal glands. The teat of the dog contains 8 to 22 ducts and the cat has 4 to 8 ducts. The streak canals of the ducts are lined by a squamous epithelium and open in a roughly circular pattern on the end of the teat. Above each streak canal is a teat sinus, which continues into a lobule of the gland (6, 16, 20).

The basic vasculature and direction of blood flow is about the same in lactating and nonlactating glands of the dog and cat. The arterial supply of the thoracic glands is (1) perforating branches of the internal thoracic arteries, (2) cutaneous branches of the intercostal arteries from the seventh thoracic artery caudally and (3) the lateral thoracic arteries (16).

The cranial abdominal glands are supplied by the cranial superficial epigastric arteries and the cutaneous branches of the caudal intercostal arteries. The caudal abdominal and inguinal glands are supplied by the

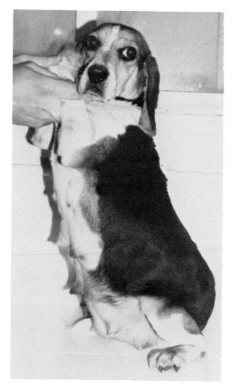

FIGURE 2–19
Mammary glands of a lactating bitch.

caudal superficial epigastric arteries, which are branches of the external pudendal arteries. The two epigastric arteries anastomose at the umbilicus. The caudal abdominal glands also receive cutaneous branches of the phrenico-abdominal arteries and the inguinal glands receive cutaneous branches of the deep circumflex iliac arteries. The blood is drained by veins that run parallel to the arterial supply. A valve is usually present in the external pudendal vein just outside of the inguinal canal, but it is the only valve encountered in the mammary veins (6, 16).

Lymph vessels from the teats, skin, and glandular tissue associated with the thoracic and cranial abdominal mammary glands travel to the axillary lymph node on each side of the body. The caudal abdominal and inguinal glands drain to the superficial lymph nodes on each side. Sometimes there is a connection between the lymphatics of the cranial and caudal abdominal mammary glands in the dog (16).

Lateral cutaneous branches of the ventral divisions of the third thoracic to third lumbar spinal nerves enter the glands laterally. The inguinal gland also receives innervation from the external spermatic nerve and this nerve supplies most of its vasomotor innervation. Ventral cutaneous branches of the intercostal nerves, which accompany vessels from the internal thoracic artery and vein, also supply the thoracic glands (6).

2-9 SUMMARY

The internal functional structure of the mammary glands of most domestic and laboratory animals is similar. The milk is secreted by alveoli, which are grouped in small clusters (lobules). They are surrounded by connective tissue capsules and drained by small ducts. Groups of lobules form larger clusters, a lobe, and these in turn are again surrounded by connective tissue capsules. The entire mammary gland is composed of lobules and lobes. The ducts draining the lobules and lobes become larger towards the teat as more and more secretory tissue is drained by them. The duct system can be compared to a tree, which has a trunk with large branches and an ever decreasing size of small branches as they move towards the periphery of the tree. Differences among animals appear in the duct systems and cisterns in each gland, the number of openings in each teat, and the number and location of the glands.

The cow, sheep, goat, horse, and guinea pig have a grouping of mammary glands that are located in the inguinal region. The udder of the cow has four glands, whereas the other species only have two glands. The teats of the guinea pig, goat, sheep, and cow are canalized by a single duct, the streak canal, or teat meatus, whereas the horse has two canals leading to the duct system. Above the streak canal are located teat cisterns or ampullary dilations, which lead to the cisterns or larger ducts of the mammary gland.

The rat, mouse, rabbit, dog, cat, and sow have a series of mammary glands located on each side of the midline and extending from the thoracic region to the inguinal region. The teats of the rat and mouse have a single streak canal, the sow has two per teat, and the rest of these animals have four or more in the end of each teat. The teat canals of animals with many openings in each teat drain a large lobe, whereas a single streak canal leads to a cistern, which acts as a collecting vessel for all the lobes in the gland.

The major blood supply to the mammary glands located in the inguinal region comes from the external pudendal arteries or some of their branches. Blood coming to the mammary glands located on the abdominal and thoracic regions of the animal is supplied by blood vessels that supply blood to the body walls in these regions. The veins, except the subcutaneous abdominal veins, follow the same pathways as the arteries. The subcutaneous abdominal veins are found in most animals whose mammary glands are grouped in the inguinal region. They leave the anterior border of the udder, travel along the ventral surface of the abdominal cavity just below the skin, and penetrate the abdominal wall on each side of the xiphoid cartilage. After penetrating the abdominal wall, the veins pass forward and join the internal thoracic veins.

The mammary glands are supplied with afferent sensory fibers as well as sympathetic efferent fibers. Parasympathetic fibers are not present in the mammary gland. An elaborate lymphatic system is also present for the drainage of the lymph from all mammary glands. Most species have superficial inguinal (supramammary) lymph nodes that play an important role in filtering lymph from the mammary glands.

REFERENCES

1. Baxter, E. S., P. M. Clarke, F. H. Dodd, and A. S. Foot. 1950. *J. Dairy Res.* 17:117.
2. Bisset, G. W., B. J. Clark, J. Haldar, M. C. Harris, G. P. Lewis, and M. Rocha e Silva, Jr. 1967. *Brit. J. Pharmacol. Chemother.* 31:537.
3. Cross, B. A. 1961. In S. K. Kon and A. T. Cowie, eds., *Milk: The Mammary Gland and Its Secretion,* Vol. I. New York: Academic Press. Ch. 6.
4. Espe, D., and C. Y. Cannon. 1942. *J. Dairy Sci.* 25:155.
5. Johnston, T. 1938. *J. Comp. Path. Therap.* 51:69.
6. Linzell, J. L. 1953. *Brit. Vet. J.* 109:427.
7. Linzell, J. L. 1959. *Quart. J. Exptl. Physiol.* 44:160.
8. Linzell, J. L. 1960. *J. Physiol.* 153:481.
9. Linzell, J. L. 1960. *J. Physiol.* 153:510.
10. Matthews, C. A., W. W. Swett, and M. H. Fohrman. 1949. *USDA Tech. Bull.* 989.
11. McDonald, J. S. 1968. *Amer. J. Vet. Res.* 29:1207.
12. McDonald, J. S. 1968. *Amer. J. Vet. Res.* 29:1315.
13. Naito, M., Y. Shoda, H. Kobayashi, Y. Fukushima, and S. Nomura. 1965. *Jap. J. Zootech. Sci.* 36:496.
14. Raynaud, A. 1961. In S. K. Kon and A. T. Cowie, eds., *Milk: The Mammary Gland and Its Secretion,* Vol. I. New York: Academic Press. Ch. 1.
15. Schmidt, G. H., R. S. Guthrie, and R. W. Guest. 1963. *J. Dairy Sci.* 46:1064.
16. Silver, I. A. 1966. *J. Small Animal Pract.* 7:689.
17. Smith, V. R. 1959. *Physiology of Lactation,* 5th ed. Ames, Iowa: Iowa State College Press.
18. Swett, W. W., P. C. Underwood, C. A. Matthews, and R. R. Graves. 1942. *J. Agr. Res.* 65:19

19. Tindal, J. S., and A. Yokoyama. 1962. *Endocrinology* 71:196.
20. Turner, C. W. 1939. *The Comparative Anatomy of the Mammary Glands.* Columbia, Mo.: Univ. Coop. Store.
21. Turner, C. W. 1952. *The Mammary Gland.* Columbia, Mo.: Lucas Brothers.
22. Turner, C. W., and E. T. Gomez. 1933. *Mo. Agr. Expt. Sta. Res. Bull.* 182.
23. Turner, C. W., and E. T. Gomez. 1933. *Mo. Agr. Expt. Sta. Res. Bull.* 194.
24. Turner, C. W., and A. B. Schultze. 1931. *Mo. Agr. Expt. Sta. Res. Bull.* 157.

MAMMARY GLAND HISTOLOGY AND CYTOLOGY

Even though the mammary glands of species differ in number, location, size, and shape, the histology and cytology of the secretory tissue appear similar. The secretory tissue forms the milk, and the rest of the mammary gland structure provides precursors to the secretory tissue, removes the milk from the tissue and transports the milk to the exterior of the gland. Thus, there are differences in the anatomy of the gland in terms of the movement of milk from the lobes and lobules of the secretory tissue to the exterior of the gland. In some animals, the milk from the lobes moves directly to the exterior of the teat through the many canals in the teat, whereas in others, the milk from the lobes empties into a collecting vessel, such as the gland cistern, and moves to the exterior of the teat through a single opening.

With the advent of the electron microscope, it has been possible to identify the sites of synthesis of some of the milk components within the cell and to study the expulsion of milk particles from the secretory tissue, the epithelial cells in the alveoli. Electron microscopy and histochemistry have given us considerable information on the synthesis of proteins and fat droplets in the cell. A fuller understanding of the histology and cytology of the cell will allow us to identify the sites of formation of most milk components synthesized in the cell and the processes involved in the movement of nonsynthesized milk components from the blood into the alveolar lumina. The histology and cytology of the mammary gland have been reviewed by Mayer and Klein (17) and Turner (28).

3-1 MAMMARY GLAND HISTOLOGY

The Alveolus

The basic component of the secretory tissue is the alveolus. A diagrammatic sketch of an alveolus is shown in Figure 3-1. Each alveolus is roughly spherical and is composed of a single layer of epithelial cells that surround a cavity, or lumen. The epithelial cells rest on a basement membrane (membrana propria), which is rather ill-defined in histological sections, but can be clearly seen by electron microscopy. Milk from the

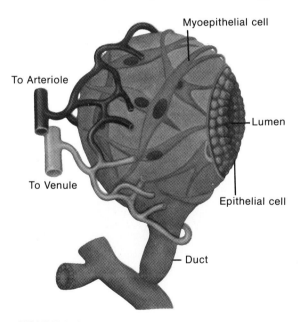

FIGURE 3–1
Diagrammatic sketch of an alveolus and its blood supply. (From Morrow and Schmidt. 1964. CIBA Veterinary Monograph Series/one. CIBA Pharmaceutical Company, Summit, New Jersey.)

epithelial cells is secreted into the alveolar lumen and is drained away by a small duct, an intercalary duct. These ducts join to form several intralobular ducts, which carry milk to the exterior of the lobule, which is a cluster of alveoli.

Myoepithelial cells are located between the basement membrane and the epithelial cells. When activated by oxytocin, these specialized cells cause milk ejection from the lumina of the alveoli. Myoepithelial cells are devoid of lipid granules and are alkaline phosphatase positive. These have been studied and identified with silver nitrate impregnation techniques by Richardson (21) (Figure 3-2).

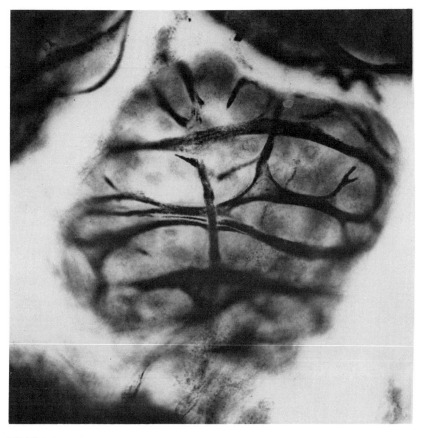

FIGURE 3–2
Myoepithelial cells surrounding an alveolus. (From Richardson. 1949. *Proc. Royal Society (London), Ser. B,* 136:30.)

Each alveolus is surrounded by capillaries that supply blood, containing milk precursors, to the epithelial cells for the synthesis of milk. Venuoles drain the excess blood from each alveolus and return the blood to the general venous circulation. The alveolus is rarely surrounded by connective tissue. The only membranes separating the alveoli within the lobule are the arterioles, venuoles, and the membrana propria.

The epithelial cells within the alveolus are usually columnar in shape when little or no secretion is present in the lumen. As the lumen fills with milk, the alveolus stretches, causing the epithelial cells to become flattened. A cross section of alveoli containing flattened epithelial cells caused by the accumulation of milk in the lumina of the alveoli is shown in Figure 3-3.

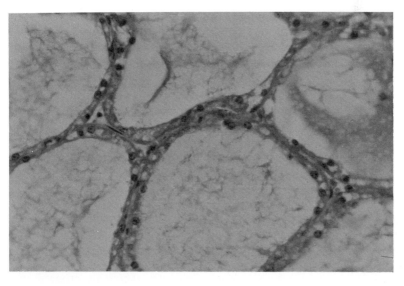

FIGURE 3–3
Cross section of goat mammary gland tissue showing alveoli filled with milk.

Lobules and Lobes

Groups of alveoli are located in functional units, called lobules, which are drained by a common duct and encapsulated by connective tissue. One lobule in the lactating cow is composed of 150 to 220 alveoli and has

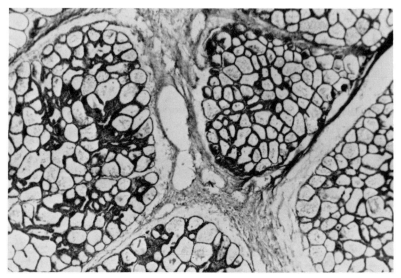

FIGURE 3–4
Goat mammary gland alveoli arranged in lobules and surrounded
by connective tissue capsules.

a volume of 0.7–0.8 mm^3 (29). The arrangement of alveoli within lobules is shown in Figures 2-4 and 3-4. Lobules of mouse mammary gland tissue that are filled with milk are shown in Figure 3-5.

A series of lobules join together and are drained by a larger duct. The lobules form a lobe and are surrounded by a larger connective tissue capsule. In the cow the connective tissue appears to be a pearly white and the secretory tissue is a flesh or orange-yellow color. These small differences can be seen by the naked eye in a cut section of mammary gland.

In animals, such as the rat, mouse, and rabbit, that have flat sheets of mammary tissue, the lobules of the mammary glands are primarily two-dimensional. They lack the three-dimensional orientation found in the goat, sheep, and bovine mammary glands.

There are no true lymphatics in the connective tissue surrounding the small lobules. The interlobular connective tissue septa have occasional bundles of smooth muscles scattered irregularly in them as well as some isolated smooth muscle cells. These muscles rarely come in contact with the outer layer of alveoli in the lobule. The concentration of the smooth muscles and their irregular distribution indicate that they do not play a major role in milk ejection (21).

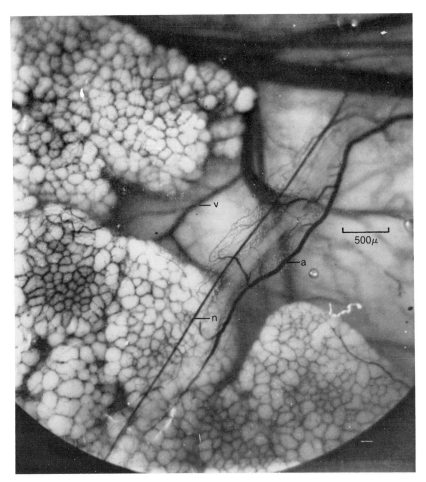

FIGURE 3–5
Lobules of mouse mammary gland tissue filled with milk with an artery (a),
vein (v) and a nerve (n). (Courtesy of J. L. Linzell, Institute of Animal
Physiology, Babraham, Cambridge, England.)

Ducts

The presence of the lobes and lobules and their ducts leads to the
identification of intralobular ducts (within a lobule), interlobular ducts
(between lobules), intralobar ducts (within lobes), and interlobar ducts
(between lobes).

The lining of the ducts depends upon their location within the mammary gland. The smaller ducts, the intercalary and intralobular ducts,

consist of a basal membrane with a layer of columnar epithelial cells that give the lumen of the duct a distinct and rounded appearance. The outer surface of the basal membrane is surrounded by myoepithelial cells oriented with the long axis of the ducts. The interlobular ducts have the same structure and general appearance as the intralobular ducts although their lumina are not as rounded because of the presence of longitudinal folds. It is generally believed that the ducts with a single layer of epithelial cells are capable of secretion.

The larger ducts differ from the smaller ducts in that they have two or more layers of cells in their lining. A cuboidal layer of cells rests on the basement membrane and these are covered by an inner layer of columnar cells. The ducts with a two-layer lining are incapable of milk secretion.

The entire duct and cistern epithelium of the bovine is covered with myoepithelial cells, which appear to be slightly denser and are much more difficult to identify than those on the alveoli. A gradual increase in the mixed muscle fiber layers, as well as a decrease in the amount of connective tissue, occurs as the ducts become larger. Elastic fibers surround the milk ducts and smaller ductules. The amount of elastic tissue surrounding the ducts is greatest in the larger ducts and decreases in amount with a decrease in size of ducts, becoming just a few fibrils around the intercalary ducts. Collagen fibers are also found with the elastic tissue (18).

Teat and Gland Cisterns

The teat and gland cisterns, like the larger ducts, are also lined with a two-layer epithelium. The deep layer is composed of cuboidal cells and the upper layer is composed of cylindrical cells. These cells rest upon a loose connective tissue layer. Mixed muscular fibers are predominant in this area and a few longitudinal muscular fibers are present. Figure 3-6 shows the two-layer lining of the teat cistern in the goat.

Small accessory glands are found in the wall of the teat cistern and in the gland cistern in the cow. These are small and have the general appearance of a lobule of secretory tissue (Figure 3-7). The accessory gland is made up of small alveoli-like structures with a lumen and a single layer of cuboidal epithelial cells. These cells are imbedded in the tunica propria. The larger accessory glands have a duct lined by a two-layer epithelium leading into either the teat or the gland cisterns. No exact function has been determined for these glands, but it is probable that they secrete milk. In the mare, the small accessory glands do not appear in the teat cistern and are only slightly developed in the gland cisterns. Accessory glands are often found in the cistern wall and beneath the pavement epithelium in the sow.

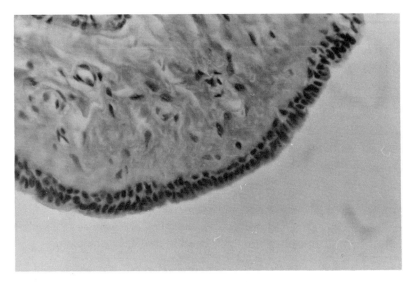

FIGURE 3–6
Two-layer epithelial lining of the teat cistern of the goat.

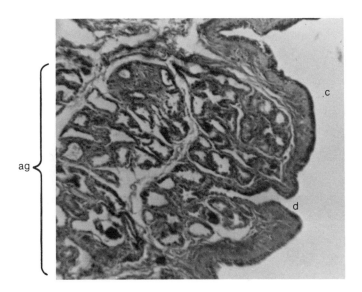

FIGURE 3–7
Accessory gland (ag) in the wall of the teat cistern (c)
of the goat. A duct (d) is apparently leading to
the accessory gland.

The cistern of the teat is lined by the two-layer epithelium that rests upon a membrana propria of wavy connective tissue. This is very distinct from the deeper tunica propria because of a lack of cells in the membrana propria. The Fürstenburg's rosette in the cow is also covered with the same epithelium as that of the teat cistern.

The cisterns of the goat and sheep are similar to that of cattle except the lining membrane of the sheep has one peculiarity. At the point of constriction between the gland and teat cisterns, the epithelium is transformed into a multilayer pavement epithelium. A gradual transition then occurs to the two-layer lining epithelium of the teat and gland cisterns.

The sinuses (teat cisterns) of the cat and dog have a two-layer, columnar epithelium. The sinuses of the bitch show circular smooth muscle sphincters, but these are absent in the cat (23).

Teats—Epithelial Lining, Muscles, and Structure

The epidermis of the skin is composed of at least three distinct parts (Figure 3-8). The germinal layer from which all the other layers develop is the stratum germinativum or Malpighian layer. Located above the

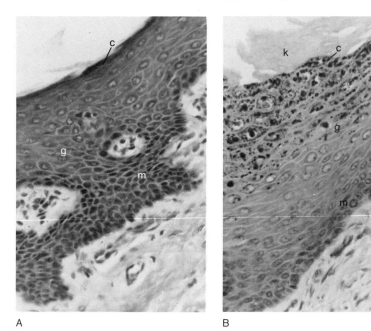

A   B

FIGURE 3–8
Epithelial lining of the teat. A. Epidermis of the skin. B. Epithelial lining of the teat meatus, showing k, Keratin; m, Malpighian layer (stratum germinativum); g, Stratum granulosum; c, Stratum corneum.

germinal layer is the stratum granulosum, which is composed of several layers of somewhat flattened but still nucleated cells. These cells contain irregularly shaped granules in the cytoplasm. As the size and number of granules within the cells increases, the nucleus becomes pale and disintegrates; thus, the stratum lucidum is formed. It is a pale strip of tissue made up of several layers of closely packed flattened, nonnucleated cells. It may or may not be present in the epidermis of the udder. The outer layer is the stratum corneum and consists of layers of flat, elongated, cornified cells.

The epithelium that lines the teat meatus is similar to the epidermis of the skin of the teat except the stratum corneum of the teat meatus is much thicker (Figure 3-8). Within the mammary gland there is a transition from the multilayer epithelium lining the teat meatus to the single-layer epithelium lining the lumina of the alveoli. The material lining the teat canal is keratin. It is part of the stratum corneum of the lining of the teat meatus that is sloughed off into the lumen of the teat meatus. Keratin plays an important role in preventing the entrance of mastitis-causing bacteria. The layers beneath the keratin in the teat meatus are the same as those of the epidermis.

The teat wall of the cow consists of an abundance of elastic connective tissue interspersed with muscle fibers in which longitudinal fibers predominate. Some circular and oblique muscle fibers are also found in this area. The middle portion of the teat wall, the corpus cavernosum, is a vessel zone and has a large number of longitudinal blood vessels and lymph vessels (Figure 3-9). The veins are very numerous in this area and, because of their thick walls, are hard to distinguish from arteries. The main characteristic difference between arteries and veins in this area is that arteries have rounded lumina and veins have oblong or flat ones. Another distinguishing characteristic is that the arteries have no valves whereas the veins have numerous valves.

The muscle components of the bovine teat end consist of two types. Inner longitudinal muscles are found under the epithelium of the papillary eminences. These muscles are abundant and are found in small bundles. Superimposed upon these is a circular layer of muscle fibers that form the sphincter muscle to keep the teat meatus closed (Figure 3-10). This sphincter is kept under constant tension from nerve impulses from the sympathetic nervous system.

The streak canals of the sheep and goat are lined by a multilayer pavement epithelium, which rests upon a membrana propria. Below the membrana propria are the papillary eminences, which are rather slender. A dense connective tissue layer follows the papillae. Logitudinal muscle bundles also surround the streak canal which are in turn surrounded by circular muscle layers. The transition from the multilayer epithelium of

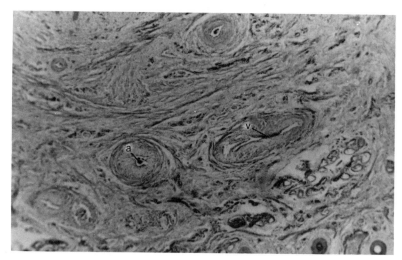

FIGURE 3–9
Corpus cavenosum area of the goat teat with arteries (a) and veins (v).

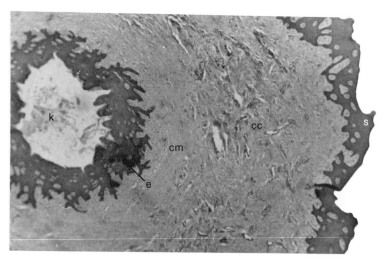

FIGURE 3–10
Cross-section of the teat of the goat showing k, keratin in teat meatus; e, epithelial lining of the meatus; cm, circular muscle fibers surrounding meatus; cc, corpus cavenosum; s, epidermis of the skin.

the streak canal to the two-layer epithelium of the teat cistern is as abrupt in the sheep and goat as it is in the cow. The teats of sheep differ from those of cattle and goats by a slight development of the smooth muscles and a large amount of elastic connective tissue.

The streak canals of the mare are lined with a multilayer pavement epithelium. These cells rest on the tunica propria, which forms high thin papillae. The stratum granulosum is absent in the streak canal. The connective tissue surrounding each streak canal contains many elastic fibers. Heavy lengthwise folds securely close the streak canal. The longitudinal muscle layer surrounding each streak canal is much more prominent than in cattle and the circular muscle fibers are not as distinct. A rosette is present between the streak canal and the teat cistern.

The two streak canals of each teat of the sow are 3–4 mm long and are lined by a multilayer pavement epithelium with stratum granulosum and a highly cornified layer. The streak canals are held tightly closed by longitudinal folds coming from the teat cistern. Strong circular fibers enclose each streak canal and form a sphincter; however, it includes only a few muscle fiber bundles and the elastic fibers in the circular fibers are primarily responsible for closing the streak canals. The longitudinal muscle fibers found in cattle are absent in the tip of the teat in swine. The transition from the pavement epithelium of the streak canal to the two-layer epithelial lining of the teat cistern is much more gradual than that found in cattle.

The streak canal of each duct in the cat is lined by a multilayer pavement epithelium similar to the other animals. The streak canals lack papillae in the tunica propria. Around each streak canal is a closely woven circular network consisting entirely of elastic tissue. The cat's teat does not have a true muscular sphincter nor does it have the longitudinal muscle fibers below the streak canal epithelium (27).

The streak canals of the dog are similar to those of the cat in that both have the multilayer epithelial lining and a network of elastic fibers but no smooth muscle fibers, around the streak canals, and both lack the papillary bodies and the longitudinal muscle fibers below the epithelium in the streak canals. Considerable muscular tissue is found in the outer zone of the teats between the canals and the skin (27).

The nipples of the rat, mice, and guinea pigs are canalized by a single duct, which is covered by a multilayer epithelium similar to that found in other animals. The constricted entrance to the teat meatus serves as a sphincter to prevent milk escape between nursings (27).

3-2   MAMMARY GLAND CYTOLOGY

Observations of the epithelial cells of the mammary gland with the use of the electron microscope indicate that the components of these cells are comparable to those found in most cells. For details on the structure of the "typical" cell, see the textbooks on cellular physiology by Campbell

(3), Davson (5) and Giese (10). A diagram of a cell is shown in Figure 3-11.

Early histologists describe the cell as having two major parts, the nucleus and the cytoplasm. It was generally concluded that the nucleus contained the genetic material, was involved in cell division, and deter-

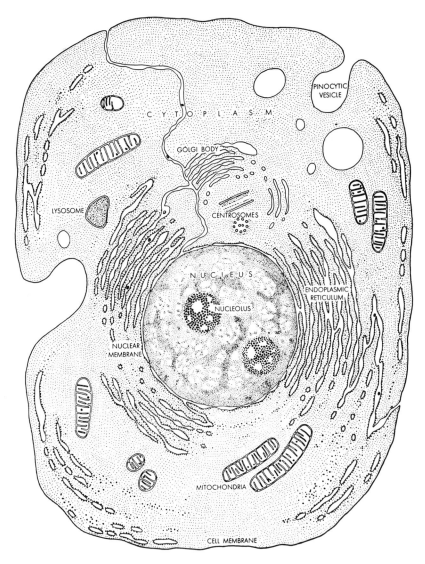

FIGURE 3–11
Diagrammatic sketch of a typical cell (From "The Living Cell" by Jean Brachet. Copyright © 1961 by *Scientific American*, Inc. All rights reserved.)

mined the activity of the cytoplasm. The cytoplasm carried out the metabolic function of the particular cell. This general relationship is still valid; however, studies from electron microscopy and new biochemical and cytochemical procedures have produced more detailed information on the structure and function of the cell. The cytoplasm is the microenvironment for the nucleus and there is a continued communication between the cytoplasm and nucleus. In multicellular organisms the cells are differentiated to carry out specific functions, such as secretion, absorption, maintaining structure, and conveying impulses. An electron microscopic photograph of an epithelial cell is shown in Figure 3-12.

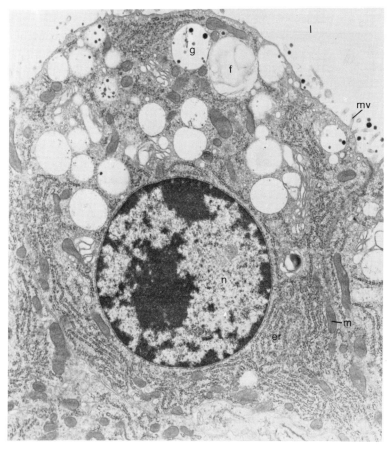

FIGURE 3–12
An electron micrograph of an epithelial cell of the lactating cow.
l, Lumen; g, Golgi with protein droplets; f, Fat droplet; mv, Microvillus;
n, Nucleus; m, Mitochondria; er, Endoplasmic Reticulum. (Courtesy
of L. F. Hood, Pennsylvania State University and Cornell University.)

Structure of the Epithelial Cell

Plasma Membrane   The entire cell is surrounded by a plasma membrane, which is between 75 and 100 Å in width. The classical concept of this membrane is that it is made up of a double layer of lipid molecules oriented parallel to each other with a layer of protein adsorbed on both surfaces of the membrane (6). The bilayer of lipids has nonpolar carbon chains at the center of the membrane with the polar ends pointing outwards. The plasma membrane also has a number of pores, lined with protein molecules, leading to the interior of the cell.

Within recent years, another concept of the cell membrane has been proposed (11). Most of the experimental evidence for this concept is based on studies of the membranes of mitochondria; however, it is believed to be the model for membranes in general. In this concept, the membrane is visualized as a continuum, one particle thick, made up of fused repeating particles. The particles are lipoprotein macromolecules, all identical or nearly identical in form and size, but chemically and functionally different. In many membranes, especially those of mitochondria, the repeating unit is composed of a basepiece linked to a projectory headpiece. The basepieces make up the continuum and the headpieces project into the interior of the cell or the organelle. Lipid is required to compel the repeating units to form a two-dimensional alignment. In the absence of lipid, the repeating units stack up in a three-dimensional form and cannot perform the functions of a membrane.

The endoplasmic reticulum and the Golgi apparatus of the cytoplasm are continuous with the pores of the plasma membrane. The cell membrane itself forms an almost impermeable barrier between the aqueous portion of the cytoplasm and the aqueous solution surrounding the cell. However, the barrier is modified by pores, carriers, and pumps requiring energy for operation that move individual ions or molecules. The luminal cell membranes of mammary gland epithelial cells have a large number of microvilli, the function of which is not known. The basal portion of the cell rests on a basement membrane that is about 600 Å thick (1, 13).

Nucleus   The nucleus is a roughly spherical body in the cell with a diameter of 5–7 μ. Most cells have one nucleus. This is especially true of the mammary gland epithelial cells. The nucleus is surrounded by a double membrane with the outer membrane being continuous with the endoplasmic reticulum. The nucleus is connected with the cytoplasm by a system of pores in the two-layer membrane. It has been estimated that the nuclear membrane has pores ranging in diameter from 400–800 Å and that these pores cover approximately 10% of its surface area. These pores are large enough to permit the passage of protein molecules (26).

The nucleus contains the genetic material, which is made up of chromatin material. This is primarily deoxyribonucleic acid (DNA) that is complexed with a basic protein, a histone. The combination of these two form nucleohistones. The DNA molecule, which has a molecular weight in the millions, contains a combination of four bases, the pentose sugar deoxyribose, and phosphate groups. The four bases are composed of two purines, adenine and guanine, and two pyrimidines, cytosine and thymine. Each base is attached to the 1-carbon position of deoxyribose. The pentose sugars are joined in a strand by a phosphodiester bond between the 3- and 5-carbon atoms of the adjacent pentose sugars. The genetic information is coded by the sequence of bases on the polynucleotide. DNA is composed of two strands that curl around each other to form a double helix. The strands are joined together by hydrogen bonding between the pairs of bases. Adenine is always bonded to thymine and guanine is always bonded to cytosine. Prior to mitosis the chromatin material congregates into the chromosomes, the number of chromosomes being specific for each species.

The DNA is responsible for the activity of the cytoplasm and accomplishes this by the synthesis of ribonucleic acid (RNA). RNA is comparable to DNA, except the pyrimidine uracil replaces the thymine of DNA, and the pentose sugar ribose replaces deoxyribose. Three types of RNA are present in the cell. Messenger RNA (mRNA) carries the coded information from the DNA to the ribosomes on the endoplasmic reticulum and there serves as a template for the synthesis of proteins and enzymes from amino acids. This synthesis is controlled by the particular sequence in the mRNA. A triplet of bases on mRNA serves as the code for the placement of amino acid, i.e., a triplet of adenine-adenine-adenine is the code for lysine, and the code adenine-uracil-guanine is specific for methionine. The sequence of bases in mRNA is determined by a portion of the DNA strand in which the bases of the mRNA being synthesized line up opposite the bases of DNA, similar to the arrangement in the double stranded DNA, except that uracil lines up opposite adenine.

The second RNA is the ribosomal RNA (rRNA), which becomes part of the ribosomes lining the endoplasmic reticulum. The third type, transfer or soluble RNA (tRNA), recognizes specific amino acids in the cytoplasm, activates them, and carries them to the specific sites on the mRNA. The recognition of the amino acid and the site on the mRNA is determined by a specific triplet of bases on each tRNA. There is at least one specific tRNA for each amino acid. The triplet of bases on the tRNA pairs with the triplet on the mRNA, and in this way the mRNA determines the sequence of amino acids in a protein.

It is generally believed that the amount of DNA per cell is constant for a species; however, recent evidence on rabbit mammary gland tissue questions this basic assumption (24). DNA can be demonstrated in the nucleus by the Fuelgen stain and other basic stains. The nucleoli do not have a membrane separating them from the nucleus but are intermeshed with the chromosomal DNA. The nucleoli appear to be primary sites for protein and ribosomal RNA synthesis.

The nucleus contains 5–10% of the RNA in the cell. The nucleus is capable of performing all of the metabolic reactions of the cytoplasm but at a much lower level of activity. The principal function of the nucleus is to serve as the site for the regulation and transmission of heredity characteristics.

Electron microscopic studies of mammary gland epithelial nuclei are limited. From the studies conducted, it appears that the nucleus has more than one nucleolus and that these nucleoli are rich in RNA material. Cytologists have argued about the involvement of nuclei in the secretion process, but it is generally agreed that the RNA molecules are synthesized in the nucleus and transported to the cytoplasm and the endoplasmic reticulum, where they carry out their metabolic functions.

Endoplasmic Reticulum and Ribosomes   The endoplasmic reticulum (ER) is a series of membrane-bounded tubules, vesicles, and cisternae that extend from the nuclear membrane outward to the plasma membrane. The ER is dispersed in parallel rays in the basal portion of the cell as well as the sides of the nucleus. Most of the tubules are rough surfaced and have dense particles attached on the outer surface of the membrane. The dense particles are ribosomes and take up basophilic dyes, because of their high RNA content. Ribosomes that are not attached to the endoplasmic reticulum are found throughout the cytoplasm. The ribosomes are the major sites of protein formation within the cell. The protein molecules to be exported from the cell are transferred to the interior of the membrane and apparently travel to the Golgi apparatus before being released from the cell (16).

Prior to the advent of electron microscopy, it was thought that the cytoplasm was a homogeneous mass of material. It now appears that the entire cytoplasm consists of a series of membranes and much of the secretion process and functional work of the cell is done by the passage of micromolecules through membranes. This is particularly true of the large amount of ER, which divides the cytoplasm into compartments. The ER allows the cell to maintain efficient contact with its environment. It has been estimated that 40% of the liver cell is composed of membranes (3).

The ribosomes not attached to the ER are probably sites where proteins are synthesized for use in the cell. Vacuoles as part of the ER or of the Golgi apparatus or located throughout the cell may be reservoirs for essential secretory materials or for waste products of the cells. All ribosomes that have been isolated from animal cells have a sedimentation constant of 75–85 Svedberg units. Animal ribosomes consist of approximately equal amounts of RNA and protein. The ribosome is composed of two subunits and has an approximate size of 230 Å. The epithelial cells during lactation have an abundant endoplasmic reticulum.

Golgi Apparatus The Golgi apparatus is a series of smooth membrane-lined tubules and cavities that are continuations of the lipoprotein membranes of the endoplasmic reticulum. The Golgi apparatus appears to play no direct part in protein synthesis, but is involved in exporting protein synthesized by the ribosomes. It is the first area in the cell in which electron microphotographs can identify protein particles. It has been suggested that the Golgi may function as a condensation membrane to concentrate smaller proteins into larger drops or granules, which can be observed with the electron microscope. It may also function by removing water from the maturing secretions (1, 13, 15, 31).

Zymogen granules of the pancreatic cells take on an identifiable form in the Golgi apparatus of the pancreas by a progressive concentration of secretory products, which then move to centrally located condensing vacuoles. From there, they move away from the Golgi zone and accumulate in the apical region of the cell and wait to be released after the intake of food. The membrane of the Golgi vacuole becomes the limiting membrane of the zymogen granule. The membrane surrounding the zymogen granule fuses with the plasma membrane and then discharges its granule into the lumen without rupture of the cell membrane. The Golgi apparatus plays a role in the export of steriods and protein in the rat liver, since lipoprotein molecules apparently are exported through the Golgi apparatus (4, 22, 25).

The Golgi apparatus of the mammary gland epithelial cell is located in the apex of the cell and on both sides of the nucleus. It consists of parallel arrays of flattened sacs, large vacuoles, and numerous microvesicles. The vacuoles of the Golgi apparatus contain protein droplets measuring 40–300 Å in diameter. These vacuoles open at the cell apex (13, 16, 20, 30, 31).

The Golgi apparatus is also related to the transport of products to the ribosomes. Injections of ^{3}H-labeled leucine were given to lactating mice and the mammary glands were removed for electron microscope and autoradiographic studies. Seventy percent of the radioactivity was found in the Golgi apparatus for the first 30 minutes, but by 50 minutes, 28% of the radioactivity was present in the protein appearing in the vacuoles. The radioactivity within the Golgi apparatus had dropped to 50% (9).

The Golgi apparatus of the lactating cow mammary gland occupies one-half to two-thirds of the cytoplasm and the material is primarily distributed around the nucleus. This tissue contains a string of progessively enlarging vacuoles, apparently starting in the nuclear region and extending outward to the luminal border. The vacuoles have thin single-membrane walls and contain a loose network of very fine fibrils or a few dense droplets, or both (8).

Mitochondria Located throughout the cytoplasm are the mitochondria, sausage-shaped objects measuring about 15,000 Å in length and 5,000 Å in diameter. Mitochondria have a two-layer wrapping with the inner membrane projecting into the interior by a number of sacs or protrusions called cristae. The cristae are transverse to the long axis of the mitochondrion. The surface of both the outer and inner membranes and cristae are sprinkled with small particles that carry out the chemical activities of mitochondria. The inner membranes contain the enzymes involved in the citric acid cycle (see Chapter 11).

Mitochondria are considered the power houses of the cell in that they supply over 90% of the energy requirements. The mitochondria, regardless of the cell species or type, have the same basic structure and apparent function. Their size and the shape vary with the isolation procedure and whether the cells are viewed *in situ*. It has been calculated that mitochondria make up 18% of the total volume and 22% of the total cytoplasmic volume of the rat liver cell (3).

The mitochondria supply energy to the cell by the oxidation of subtrates and the conversion of released energy into the form of bond energy of adenosine triphosphate (ATP). This involves three steps: (1) carrying out oxidation reactions that supply electrons; (2) transferring the electrons along a chain of intermediates that synthesize ATP; and (3) catalyzing synthetic reactions that are powered by ATP. These processes appear to be located on both the inner and the outer membranes of the cells. Mitochondria can actively accumulate certain ions from the surrounding cytoplasm in a process that appears to be related to the respiratory chain phosphorylation. Mitochondria also oxidize and actively synthesize fatty acids.

It has been questioned whether the mitochondria are self-reproducing or whether they arise from other organelles. Recent evidence indicates that mitochondria contain DNA that can be used as a template to synthesize messenger RNA for protein formation. It also appears that mitochondria arise from *de novo* synthesis within the cell.

The mitochondria of the lactating mammary gland cells have the same appearances as those of other cells. A large number of these have been reported and would be expected during secretion, because of the large amount of energy required for the secretory processes. The mitochondria are located throughout the epithelial cell; however, Feldman (8) reported that they appeared to be most conspicuous at the basement membrane surface in the lactating cow mammary gland.

Lysosomes   Another particle scattered throughout the cell is the lysosome. They are slightly smaller than mitochondria and contain most of the active degradative or hydrolytic enzymes of the cell. The lysosomes have a dense matrix with vacuoles or droplets in them and a very dense peripheral rim. The lysosomal membrane usually remains intact, but is extremely sensitive to rupture under a variety of physiological conditions. Its rupture causes the release of the enzymes, which can cause a breakdown of the cell. DeDuve (7) divided the cellular lysosomes into four categories: storage granules, digestive vacuoles, autophagic vacuoles, and residual bodies. Lysosomes also engage in intracellular digestive processes in which material is taken into the cell, broken down after the release of the hydrolytic enzymes, and the breakdown products excreted. Lysosomes also function as scavengers for removing unneeded or foreign material from the cell. The particular function of the lysosomes in a cell may vary with the type of cell. They may have an entirely different function in a cell concerned primarily with absorption in contrast to one concerned with secretion.

Lysosomes have also been demonstrated in the mammary gland epithelial cells of rats and mice. These particles have distinct enzymatic composition and are intermediate in size between microsomes and mitochondria. The lysosomes have a low level of enzymatic activity when they are isolated undamaged from the cell. However, rupture of the lysosomes causes a considerable increase in enzymatic actvity (12, 19).

Lipid Secretion

Fat droplets are easily recognized in histological sections with the use of special dyes, such as Sudan IV. They are also visible in the electron microscope slides, because of their homogeneity and their high electron density. Fat droplets are considerably larger in size than protein droplets and range in diameter from 500 $m\mu$ to 8 μ with an average of 3–4 μ in diameter. The larger fat droplets are usually seen in the apex of the cell; however, they show no constant topographical relationship to any cell organelle (20, 31).

The site of origin of fat droplets within the epithelial cell is not known. They apparently are not associated with the Golgi zone as are the lipoproteins of the rat liver cells. Stein and Stein (25) injected ^{3}H-labeled fatty acids into lactating mice, removed the mammary glands and studied the tissue with electron microscopy and radioautography. The labeled fatty acids were esterified almost immediately after they entered the cell. The esterification appeared to occur in the rough endoplasmic reticulum and the esterified acids then moved to the lipid droplets in the cell. Lipid droplets were never seen in the Golgi apparatus.

Other Secretion Processes

Recently, Brew (2) has postulated that lactose is synthesized in the cisternae of the Golgi apparatus. The final step of lactose synthesis requires the enzyme, lactose synthetase. Lactose synthetase is made up of two proteins, the A and B proteins. The B protein is one of the milk proteins, α-lactalbumin. The α-lactalbumin is transported through the channels of the ER to the Golgi where the A protein is situated. The combination of the two proteins creates the necessary enzymatic conditions for lactose synthesis. Little information is available on the place or areas of transfer of water, minerals, vitamins, and the nonsecreted protein droplets through the epithelial cells.

Myoepithelial Cells

The myoepithelial cells have been described in electron photographs (13). They have a clear appearance with a filamentous cytoplasm and a highly indented oval nucleus. The myoepithelial cell has no secretory function and is involved primarily in contraction of the alveolus during milk ejection.

Release of Secretory Products

Early cytologists identified three types of secretion within the mammary gland (28). The holocrine type occurs when the entire epithelial cell disintegrates to become part of the secretion. This is not an important form of milk secretion, because the epithelial cells do not divide rapidly enough to produce a large volume of milk. The presence of cytoplasmic fragments and nuclei in the milk can best be explained by a daily disintegration of some epithelial cells during the course of lactation. The apocrine type of secretion involves the migration of the secretory products to the apex of the epithelial cell, where rupture of the cell membrane takes place to release the secretory products. In this, part of the cytoplasm is exposed and a small part of it is released with the secretory droplets. The merocrine secretion involves the movement of the secretion products through the epithelial cell membrane without injury to the membrane itself. At least part, if not most, of the secretion of milk particles occurs by this method.

The only two components of milk for which observations on the extrusion of products into the lumen of the alveolus have been made are protein and fat droplets. The milk protein molecules move to the Golgi apparatus and are concentrated in terminal dilations of the flattened Golgi sacs. These dilations subsequently detach to form closed vacuoles containing protein particles. The closed vacuoles migrate towards the cell apex with a further concentration of the products within the vacuoles. The vacuoles open at the cell surface, releasing the droplets into the lumen, where they are readily visible (16, 30, 31). Brew (2) proposed a similar movement of lactose to the lumen of the alveolus.

Large fat droplets appear in the apex of the epithelial cells and are released through the plasma membrane. The lipid particles leave the cytoplasm and are surrounded by a double-cytoplasmic membrane that is 170–290 Å thick. The plasma membrane constricts below the fat droplet as it moves from the apex of the cell (Figures 3-13, 3-14). The plasma membrane joins together below the fat droplet before it is released from

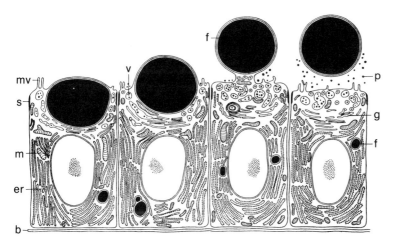

FIGURE 3–13
The process of excreting the fat droplet without exposure of the cytoplasm to the lumen of the cell. mv, Microvillus; s, Terminal Bar;
m, Mitochondria; er, Endoplasmic reticulum; b, Basement membrane;
f, Fat droplet; v, Vacuole; p, Protein granule; and g, Golgi apparatus.
(From Bargmann and Knoop. 1959. Z. Zeilforsch. 49:34.)

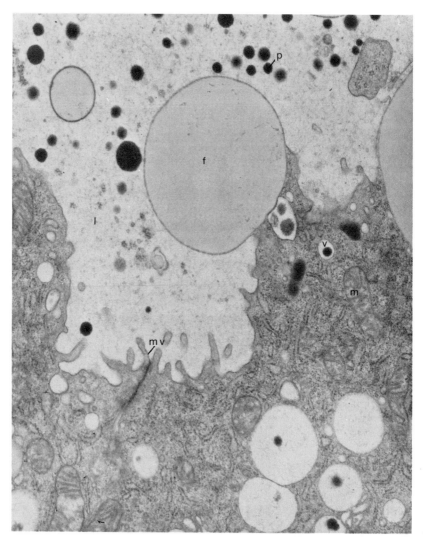

FIGURE 3–14
Electron microphotograph of an epithelial cell excreting a fat droplet. I, Lumen of
alveolus; f, Fat droplet; mv, Microvillus; p, Protein granule; v, Vacuole;
m, Mitochondria. (Courtesy of S. R. Wellings, University of California, Davis.)

the cell, consequently the cytoplasm is not exposed. In this way the fat
particles are released without the fragmentation of large masses of apical
cytoplasm. A small amount of cytoplasm with some vacuoles containing
protein granules is entrapped with the fat droplet during the constriction
of the plasma membrane. This is extruded with the fat droplet. Most of

the fat particles in the lumen of the alveoli have a plasma membrane surrounding them (1, 13, 16, 20, 31).

Changes in Epithelial Cells Occurring During Mammary Gland Development

Several studies describe the cytological changes in the epithelial cells that occur during the various physiological stages of the mammary gland. The changes appear similar in the cow, rat, and mouse. Virgin mouse tissue has ducts with one or two layers of cuboidal cells. The cell membranes are distinct and microvilli are present at the luminal surfaces. The cytoplasm contains small particles that appear to be ribonucleoprotein particles. There is very little endoplasmic reticulum and the few small mitochondria are either oval or rod-shaped. A relatively small amount of Golgi apparatus is located in the apical region. The nuclei have peripheral condensations of chromatin and large nucleoli. The ductal lumina are nearly empty or contain a very small amount of amorphous granular material. Lipid inclusions in the virgin rat mammary tissue are limited; the endoplasmic reticulum is not yet folded nor well developed and the Golgi zone contains no protein granules (1, 31).

The mammary duct epithelium of the early pregnant mouse tissue has similar characteristics to that of virgin tissue. The cytoplasm is filled with small ribonucleoprotein particles and the mitochondria appear larger and show more distinct internal cristae. The Golgi is still inconspicuous (31).

Mouse mammary gland tissue taken on the 14th day of pregnancy shows numerous alveoli with small lumina. The alveoli contain a single layer of cells, with secretory droplets similar to casein appearing in the apex of some of the cells. Some of the cells contain lipid droplets. The endoplasmic reticulum is more abundant than in the early stage of pregnancy and consists of scattered flattened sacs whose outer surfaces are covered with ribosomes. Numerous ribonucleoprotein particles are scattered throughout the cytoplasm. The mitochondria are numerous in all parts of the cell and exhibit the characteristic two-layer membrane with internal cristae. The Golgi apparatus is still relatively small. Similar observations on tissue obtained from bovine mammary gland tissue during the dry period have been made. Both protein and lipid droplets are present. Ribonucleoprotein particles are located throughout the cytoplasm and a relatively small number of mitochondria with their characteristic lining are present. Microvilli are present in the lumen (8, 31).

The mammary gland cells during late pregnancy and early lactation are characterized by having highly developed cells similar to those found during later lactation. The epithelial cells are very numerous with fat and protein droplets appearing in the apex of the cells. The endoplasmic reticulum is well developed and the number of mitochondria is large. The Golgi apparatus is considerably larger than that of midpregnancy and is located in the apex of the cell and on both sides of the nucleus. The size of the mitochondria of the lactating bovine tissue is double that of mitochondria in the dry tissue. A detailed study of the mitochondria of mammary gland tissue of guinea pigs at the end of pregnancy and during lactation showed a constancy in the amount of mitochondrial substance per unit area of cytoplasm. With the advent of secretion, the cells increase in volume and, coincidentally to this, the mitochondria elongate and some increase in diameter. The average number of mitochondria per cell showed a twofold increase at the start of secretion. The increase in number of mitochondria per cell is the principal change occurring at the onset of lactation (1, 3, 14, 31).

3-3 SUMMARY

The basic secretory tissue of the mammary gland is made up of alveoli. These are located in clusters, lobules, and are drained by a common duct and encapsulated with connective tissue. An alveolus is made up of a single layer of epithelial cells, which absorb precursors from the blood, secrete the milk components, and release them into the lumen of the alveolus. From the lumen the milk is transferred by a small duct to the larger ducts. The epithelial cells are located on a basement membrane. Enmeshed between the basement membrane and the epithelial cells are myoepithelial cells, which are involved in the contraction of the alveoli during the milk-ejection process. Arterioles and venuoles surround each alveolus and supply blood to the epithelial cells and remove the blood that is not used for milk synthesis.

The smaller ducts within the lobules are lined with a single layer of epithelial cells and are capable of secretion. The larger ducts and the gland and teat cisterns are lined with a basal layer of cuboidal cells and upper layer of columnar cells. Some animals, especially the cow, have accessory glands located in the walls of the teat and next to the gland cisterns. They have the histological structure of a lobule, but their exact function is not known. The teat meatus is lined with a type of tissue transitional between the epidermis of the skin and the two-layer epithelial lining of the teat cistern. Keratin is located within the teat canal and it is part of the stratum corneum, the upper layer of the epidermis. The teat meatus is held closed either by circular muscle fibers that are under constant tension from nerve impulses or by strong elastic fibers.

The epithelial cells are similar to most cells found in the body in that they have the same organelles and structural components of the other cells. The epithelial cell is surrounded by a plasma membrane that is between 75 and 100 Å in width. There are two concepts of the structural configuration of the cell membrane; however, the prevalent one is that it is made up of a double layer of lipid molecules with a layer of protein adsorbed on both surfaces of the membrane. The plasma membrane has a number of pores, carriers, and energy-driven pumps by which the cytoplasm within the cell communicates with the environment on the outside of the cell. Each epithelial cell has one nucleus that has a diameter of 5–7 μ. The nucleus contains deoxyribonucleic acid (DNA), which is made up of four bases, a pentose sugar, and phosphate groups. DNA is arranged in two strands that are curled around each other to form a double helix. DNA is responsible for the activity of the cytoplasm and does this by directing the synthesis of a second nucleic acid, ribonucleic acid (RNA). RNA is synthesized within the nucleus and directs protein synthesis within the cytoplasm. DNA is also responsible for cell division and for transmitting the same genetic material to each of the dividing cells.

RNA travels to and is involved in protein synthesis in the endoplasmic reticulum, which is a series of membrane-bounded tubules located throughout the basal portion of the cell and on the sides of the nucleus. The proteins are synthesized on the ribosomes lining the endoplasmic reticulum. The synthesized protein moves to the lumen of the endoplasmic reticulum and is then transferred to the Golgi apparatus, from which it is released into the lumen of the alveolus. Mitochondria are large organelles whose primary function is to provide energy for the energy-requiring processes within the cell. Mitochondria supply energy by the oxidation of substrates absorbed by the cell and conversion of the released energy into the form of bond energy of ATP. The bond energy of ATP is used for the chemical reactions requiring energy. Lysosomes are found throughout the cell, but their exact function is not known. They contain enzymes that can cause breakdown of the cell. They also contain enzymes that are probably involved in acting as scavengers or removing unneeded or foreign material from the cells.

Electron micrographs have shown the release of lipid and protein droplets from the cells. Protein droplets are encased in smooth, lined vesicles. These vesicles or closed vacuoles migrate toward the cell apex and the vacuoles open to the cell surface, releasing the droplets into the lumen without rupture of the plasma membrane. Lipid particles come together to form larger droplets as they migrate from the base to the apex of the cell. During release of the fat droplet into the lumen of the alveolus, the plasma membrane constricts below the fat droplet and joins together before the droplet is released into the lumen. In this way, the cytoplasm is not exposed to the lumen.

REFERENCES

1. Bargmann, W., and Knopp, A. 1959. *Z. Zellforsch,* 49:344.
2. Brew, K. 1969. *Nature* 223:671.
3. Campbell, P. N. 1966. *The Structure and Function of Animal Cell Components.* Oxford: Pergamon Press.
4. Caro, L. G., and G. E. Palade. 1964. *J. Cell Biol.* 20:473.
5. Davson, H. 1964. *A Textbook of General Physiology,* 3rd ed. Boston: Little Brown.
6. Davson, H., and J. G. Danielli. 1952. *The Permeability of Natural Membranes.* London: Cambridge Univ. Press.
7. de Duve, C. 1963. *Lysosomes.* CIBA Foundation Symposium. London: J. and A. Churchill.
8. Feldman, J. D. 1961. *Lab. Invest.* 10:238.
9. Fiske, S., V. Courtecuisse, and F. Haguenau. 1966. *Compt. Rend.* 262D: 126.
10. Giese, A. C. 1968. *Cell Physiology,* 3rd ed. Philadelphia: W. B. Saunders Co.
11. Green, D. E., and A. Tzagoloff. 1966. *J. Lipid Res.* 7:587.
12. Greenbaum, A. L., T. F. Slater, and D. Y. Wang. 1960. *Nature* 188:318.
13. Hollman, K. H. 1959. *J. Ultrastructure Res.* 2:423.
14. Howe, A., K. C. Richardson, and M. S. C. Birbeck. 1956. *Exptl. Cell Res.* 10:194.
15. Kirkman, H., and A. E. Severinghaus. 1938. *Anat. Rec.* 71:79.
16. Kurosumi, K., Y. Kobayashi, and N. Baba. 1968. *Exptl. Cell Res.* 50:177.
17. Mayer, G., and M. Klein. 1961. In S. K. Kon and A. T. Cowie, eds., *Milk: The Mammary Gland and Its Secretion,* Vol. I. New York: Academic Press. Ch. 2.
18. McFarlane, D., J. C. Rennie, and P. S. Blackburn, 1949. Cited by C. W. Turner. 1952. *The Mammary Gland.* Columbia, Mo.: Lucas Brothers. P. 135.
19. Miyawaki, H. 1965. *J. Nat. Cancer Inst.* 34:601.
20. Patton, S., and F. M. Fowkes. 1967. *J. Theoret. Biol.* 15:274.
21. Richardson, K. C. 1949. *Proc. Royal Soc. (London) Ser. B,* 136:30.
22. Siekevitz, P., and G. E. Palade. 1960. *J. Biophys. Biochem. Cytol.* 7:619.
23. Silver, I. A. 1966. *J. Small Animal Pract.* 7:689.
24. Sod-Moriah, U. A., and G. H. Schmidt. 1968. *Exptl. Cell Res.* 49:584.
25. Stein, O., and Y. Stein. 1967. *J. Cell Biol.* 34:251.

26. Stern, H., and D. L. Nanney. 1965. *The Biology of Cells*. New York: John Wiley.
27. Turner, C. W. 1939. *The Comparative Anatomy of the Mammary Glands*. Columbia, Mo.: Univ. Coop. Store.
28. Turner, C. W. 1952. *The Mammary Gland*. Columbia, Mo.: Lucas Brothers.
29. Weber, A. F., R. L. Kitchell, and J. H. Sautter. 1955. *Amer. J. Vet. Res.* 16:255.
30. Wellings, S. R., and K. B. De Ome. 1961. *J. Biophys. Biochem. Cytol.* 9:479.
31. Wellings, S. R., K. B. De Ome, and D. R. Pitelka. 1960. *J. Nat. Cancer Inst.* 25:393.

4

MAMMARY GLAND DEVELOPMENT

Mammary gland growth in the female takes place during five distinct phases of the development: prenatal, prepubertal, postpubertal, pregnancy, and early lactation. During fetal development, hormonal influences are not necessary for the development of the gland. In most species the male mammary gland has structures similar to those of the female gland; however, the male gland does not have as much growth as the female gland. The extent of nonhormonal development of the mammary gland in the fetus is a very small portion of the growth found in the lactating gland, but the basic structures of the gland are formed during fetal development. These are then more fully developed under hormonal influences after puberty.

Prepubertal development is generally confined to the growth of the parts of the mammary gland that are not clearly defined at birth, such as the sphincter around the teat meatus and smooth muscle fibers. This growth is probably not under hormonal control, but the growth occurring after puberty is thought to be due almost entirely to hormonal influences. The bulk of the growth takes place during pregnancy and then regresses after the peak of lactation. This cycle repeats itself with each pregnancy and lactation period.

The normal development of the mammary gland during fetal growth, before and after puberty, and during pregnancy will be described. In addition, the extensive literature in the field of the hormonal control of mammary gland growth will be reviewed.

4-1 FETAL DEVELOPMENT OF THE MAMMARY GLAND

The development of the mammary anlage in the placentalia appears to be comparable in all species. The first mammary growth in the fetus occurs as a raised area of ectoderm on both sides of the midline in either the inguinal region or on the entire abdominal surface. When this area of ectoderm narrows, it is referred to as the mammary band. The band narrows further to form the mammary line. This is usually supported by a ridge of underlying dermis. The mammary buds develop along the mammary line and correspond to the number of mammary glands and accessory glands characteristic of each species. The buds are formed by the congregation of the mammary line cells into a definite collection of ectodermal cells to form an epithelial nodule. The mammary buds then sink into the mesenchyme to form the secretory and duct systems of the mammary gland. The mammary bud is first lenticular, then hemispherical, and then spherical in shape (67).

Cow

Turner (92) has outlined the fetal and postnatal development of the mammary gland in the cow. The following is a summary of his report. The embryonic development of the mammary gland begins at a very early fetal age. The first signs of mammary gland development occur during the first month of embryonic life and consist of a single layer of cuboidal cells that forms from the ectoderm and differentiates from the underlying mesenchyme tissue. The superficial layer of flattened cells forms the mammary band in the inguinal region. The formation of the mammary lines begins about the 4th to 5th weeks of fetal age when the embryo is 1.4–1.7 cm in length. These are composed of several layers of cells that have developed from the Malpighian or germinal layer, the lower layer of the ectoderm. The mammary lines are transient in nature for they soon give rise to the mammary buds. Two intermediate stages in development between the mammary line and the mammary bud are the mammary crest and the mammary hillock (Figure 4-1). Two mammary buds form on each mammary line and these give rise to the fore and rear quarters of each half of the udder. The mammary buds are formed by the time that

Mesenchyme   Basement membrane

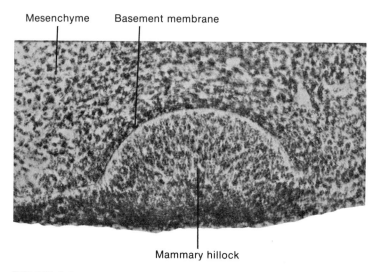

Mammary hillock

FIGURE 4-1
The mammary hillock of a bovine fetus, which is 2.1 cm in length.
(From Turner. 1930. *Mo. Agr. Expt. Sta. Res. Bull.* 140.)

the embryo is 2.1 cm in length, early in the second month of the fetal life. The cells continue to proliferate and cause the mammary bud to become spherical in shape and sink into the mesenchyme. The mammary bud may sink entirely into the mesenchyme except for a small opening at the outer pole causing a depression or dimple, the mammary pit. Up to this stage the male and female embryos have comparable mammary gland development. Differences in growth rates between sexes occur with the advent of teat development.

The formation of the teat begins during the 2nd month of embryonic life, when the fetus is approximately 8–9 cm long. This begins by a very rapid development of the mesenchyme tissue beneath and surrounding the mammary bud that forces the mammary bud to be raised above the surface of the surrounding epithelium. At the same time, there is a slight opening in the distal end of the bud. Prior to this time the mammary bud is oval in shape, but the movement to the surface causes the shape of the bud to be changed. The development of the male mammary gland teat now becomes somewhat slower than that of the female.

The formation of the teat and gland cisterns begins during the 3rd month of fetal development. This is brought about by an invagination of the deeply staining Malpighian layer of cells. A solid core of these cells forms the primary sprout (Figure 4-2), which invaginates the mammary bud and follows the path of least resistance, pushing the mesenchyme cells

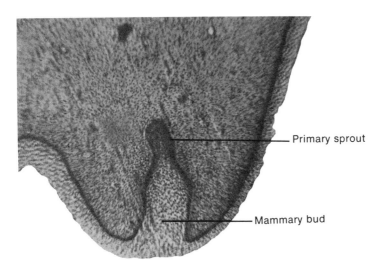

FIGURE 4–2
Development of the primary sprout in the bovine fetus. (From
Turner. 1930. *Mo. Agr. Expt. Sta. Res. Bull.* 140.)

aside. The primary sprout gives rise to the teat cistern, the gland cistern, and major ducts in the udder. The primary sprout is canalized when the embryo is about 19 cm in length, at fetal age of approximately 100 days. The canalization is brought about by a separation of the cells in the center of the primary sprout at the proximal end (the area closest to the center of the body) and proceeds towards the distal end. The teat lumen is formed by a separation of cells without disintegration. The development and canalization of the primary sprout occurs somewhat later in the male.

As the teat grows, the tip of the mammary bud is opened. The cells of the bud become cornified and take the appearance of the epidermal layer of the skin. The cistern of the gland is formed by a continual growth of the lumen, which is done by the cells pushing the mesenchyme cells in all directions. The gland cistern is well outlined by the time the fetus is 4 months of age. The number of layers of cells lining the cavity is reduced to 2 or 3. The formation of the teat cistern occurs with the progressive canalization of the primary sprout towards the distal end. The teat cistern can be seen when the fetus is approximately 30 cm in length, at fetal age of 16 weeks. At this stage it is more of a duct than an actual cistern; however, the progressive movement of the cells in a horizontal direction causes the cavity of the teat cistern to become larger and the number of layers of cells lining the cavity to be reduced to 2 or 3. The duct then narrows at its distal end to form the streak canal. The streak canal is the last part of the primary sprout to become canalized. The lining of the streak canal consists of the multilayer epithelium comparable to that seen in the skin covering the teat.

After the primary sprout has reached its greatest extension at about 16 cm in length (about 13 weeks of fetal age), several secondary sprouts are given off from the terminal end of the primary sprout (Figure 4-3). These grow upward, at various angles to the direction of the primary sprout, and into the underlying mesenchyme tissue and give rise to the duct system of the udder. The secondary sprouts are composed of a solid core of cells before they canalize, comparable to the primary sprout in its development. The secondary sprouts develop tertiary sprouts and these in turn send off sprouts until the final duct system of the udder is developed. There is, however, very little growth beyond the secondary sprout stage in the fetus. The secondary sprouts then become canalized and develop a two-layer epithelial lining. The canalization of the secondary sprouts begins at the cisterns and works through the periphery of the sprout development.

The mesenchyme tissue lying below the Malpighian layer is made up of loosely connected spindle-shaped cells. This develops into the dermis of the skin. When the fetus is 8–12 cm in length, the mesenchyme tissue begins to differentiate into fibrous tissue, which has a tendency to form threads or bundles that are located perpendicular to the base of the udder. Blood vessels form and run perpendicular to the base of the udder. At

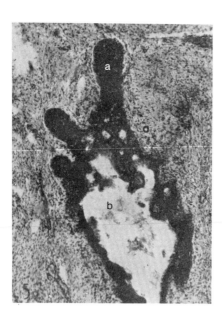

FIGURE 4–3
Development of several secondary sprouts (a) from the primary sprout, which has become canalized to form the gland cistern (b). (From Turner. 1931. *Mo. Agr. Expt. Sta. Res. Bull.* 160.)

about 12–13 cm fetal length, a series of connective tissue cells begin to form a series of whorls. These are composed of an aggregation of cells in the center with circularly disposed cells on the periphery (Figure 4-4). With further development of the gland, second and third rows of whorls appear and soon the entire mammary gland appears to be filled with an aggregation of whorls. These are essentially connective tissue cells, but gradually lipids are stored in the cytoplasm. It is assumed that these whorls are replaced by secretory tissue when the alveoli develop.

The further development of the teat takes place by the growth of all of the tissues involved. The teat meatus takes on its characteristic multilayer epithelium and the lining of the teat cistern changes to a two-layer epithelium. The sphincter muscle fibers around the streak canal are not well developed, but the vascular zones in the midsection of the teat are well developed by birth. The quarters of the bovine mammary gland form independently, but with further growth they join together and are covered by the skin. Part of the median suspensory ligament has been developed by the time the fetus is 60 cm long.

Most of the mammary gland development described previously is completed during the first 6 months of fetal growth. Very little further devel-

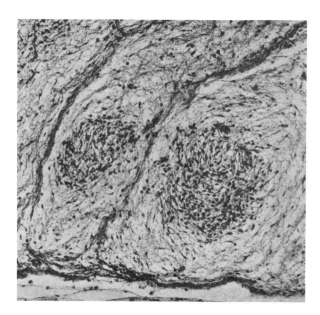

FIGURE 4-4
Development of connective tissue whorls in the mammary gland of an embryo, which is 16 cm in length.
(From Turner. 1931. *Mo. Agr. Expt. Sta. Res. Bull.* 160.)

opment takes place prior to birth. At birth the teat is well developed and
definite outlines of the teat and gland cisterns are seen. The secondary
sprouts are developed and some of the sprouts are canalized; however, a
solid core of cells still persists on the terminal ends. The growth of the
sprouts is limited to a small area around the gland cistern. The nonsecre-
tory tissues in the udder are quite well formed at birth. The basic vascular
system of the udder, as well as the lymphatic system, is comparable to
that in the mature udder. The skin and hair covering the udder are comparable to those of the adult. The adipose tissue and connective tissue
make up distinct fatty pads or cushions surrounded by connective tissue
septa. The four mammary glands are distinct entities and are not yet
formed into an udder.

Mouse

The mammary gland in the mouse embryo arises as a zone of raised
epidermal cells on each side of the trunk; this zone is apparent in the
11-day embryo. (This development has been summarized by Raynaud
(67).) A mammary line is formed from the raised epidermal cells. The
formation of the mammary line is brought about by the congregation of
neighboring ectodermal cells, which in turn separate into individual buds
along the line. The migration of cells takes place towards centers that
determine the location of the mammary glands. The migration is brought
about by inductor action of the underlying mesenchyme in contrast to
hormonal action which causes growth in the adult mammary gland. From
the 12th to the 14th day of fetal age, the mammary bud changes from a
flat convex shape to a more spherical form. Up to this time the male and
female fetuses develop at the same rate. At the 15th day, the female gland
is differentiated by the mammary bud sinking into the mesenchyme
tissue but remaining connected to the epidermis by a neck of ectodermal
cells. During this phase the mammary bud lengthens and assumes the
shape of a band of epithelial cells, referred to as the primary mammary
cord. Its base is still attached to the epidermis. At term, the distal end
begins to branch to form the lobulo-alveolar system of the mammary
gland.

Other Animals

The development of the mammary gland of the ewe and the goat are
comparable to that of the bovine except the goat fetus has hair anlagen
on the skin of the teat. The mammary development of the pig proceeds
along the same lines as that of the mouse, except the teat has two ducts.

4-2 MAMMARY GLAND GROWTH
FROM BIRTH TO PUBERTY

Most of the increase in mammary gland growth from birth to puberty is due to an increase in connective tissue and deposition of fat in the mammary gland; however, a certain amount of secretory tissue growth does take place. The growth of the mammary gland area in the rat parallels the increase in the metabolic weight from birth until the 22nd to the 23rd day of life and it is referred to as isometric growth. At this time there is a marked increase in the mammary gland growth rate that is about three times faster than that of the body surface. This growth is referred to as allometric growth. This precedes puberty by 13–19 days. Castration of the rats prevents the allometric phase of growth indicating that the ovaries play a significant role in mammary growth before puberty (10). Sinha and Tucker (75) confirmed these results with respect to mammary area but found that the mammary gland DNA content (an indicator of new cell growth) increased at a constant rate in rats between 10 and 100 days of age, a rate that was 1.96 times faster than the rate of increase in body surface area. Comparable findings on mammary gland area have also been found in mice in which the mammary glands grow isometrically from the 7th to 21st days of life, at which time a marked allometric growth takes place. The allometric growth in the mouse mammary gland is over 5 times as great as that of the body surface area. This again precedes puberty, which occurs at about 28 days in the strain of mouse tested. The change from isometric to allometric growth closely follows weaning and there is a possibility that the mouse secretes a substance in her milk that antagonizes the role of estrogen in mammary gland growth. A change from isometric to allometric mammary growth also occurs in the bovine at 3 months of age. This measure is based on the DNA content of the mammary gland (21, 26, 77).

The development of the mammary glands from birth to puberty continues at the same rate as that of body growth. In the calf, the ducts continue to grow and assume the shape of those found in the mature udder. The quarters continue to grow in size, partially due to the deposition of adipose tissue, until the front and rear quarters approach each other and finally become joined at the base. In addition to an increase in the udder weight of calves from birth to puberty, there is an increase in the udder capacity, determined by the amount of formalin solution that can be injected into an excised udder of calves of different weights (92).

Palpation of the glandular growth of the mammary gland from birth to 6 months of age has been used to predict the milk production of the mature animals. A low correlation has been found between the amount of glandular growth and the mature milk production. A high correlation would not be expected since the environment plays a major role in determining the milk production records of a cow. This form of selection probably has little importance in trying to predict the milk-producing potential of young calves (40, 83).

4-3 MAMMARY GLAND DEVELOPMENT DURING RECURRING ESTROUS CYCLES

Further development of the mammary gland takes place after puberty with each estrous cycle due to the hormones of the ovary, estrogen and progesterone, in conjunction with prolactin and somatotrophin (STH) from the anterior pituitary. This is accomplished by the growth of buds and branches from the sides and terminal ends of the secondary and tertiary sprouts. These branch and rebranch many times until the final buds develop into alveoli. It is questionable whether alveoli *per se* develop during estrous cycles and prior to pregnancy. The small ducts have the same characteristic one-layer lining of the alveoli and, consequently, cross sections of mammary gland tissue may reveal ducts that are mistaken for alveoli. In most species it is possible to detect growth of the duct system shortly prior to and during estrus by the detection of newly formed buds. Most of the growth attained during each estrous cycle appears to be lost by regression after the end of the estrous cycle. A certain amount of positive growth does take place during recurring estrous cycles since the amount developed is somewhat more than the amount that regresses. Sinha and Tucker (76) studied the mammary gland development of rats during the estrous cycles, using total mammary gland nucleic acid content as an index of cellular proliferation. They found that there was an increase in the deoxyribonucleic acid (DNA) content per 100 g of body weight during the first four estrous cycles and no further increases occurred after the fourth cycle. The mammary gland DNA content was 8% higher at estrus in comparison to proestrus and some regression of the DNA content occurred after estrus. Similar results have been obtained in the dairy heifer (77). It appears that most of the growth occurs during the estrogenic phase of the estrous cycle.

Histological changes in the bovine mammary gland are also observable at various stages of the estrous cycle. Just prior to and during estrus, the alveolar lumina are large and filled with secretion. The epithelial cells are cuboidal in shape. During diestrus, the cells are columnar in shape, the lumina are shrunken with no secretion in them, and the lobules are relatively small (31, 77). Laguchev (38) studied the mitotic activity of the mouse mammary gland during the estrous cycles and found the activity to reach a maximum on the day of estrus and fall thereafter to a low level at diestrus.

The epithelial cells of the ducts and alveoli of the mammary gland prior to pregnancy have the same characteristics as those found during pregnancy and lactation. The major ducts have the characteristic two-layer lining resting upon a membrana propria. The ducts are surrounded by connective tissue of varying thickness. Where alveoli are present, the connective tissue septa are present with thin septa separating the lobules and thicker septa separating the lobes. The majority of the tissue within the mammary gland, however, is made up of adipose tissue (92). The extent of the duct growth of a nonpregnant dairy heifer is shown in Figure 4-5.

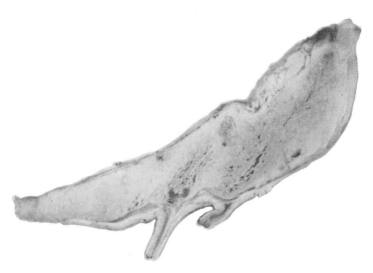

FIGURE 4–5
Section showing duct growth in the mammary gland of a nonpregnant heifer.

4-4 CHANGES OCCURRING
DURING PREGNANCY

The majority of the mammary growth occurs during pregnancy. The extent of the duct growth occurring in early pregnancy is primarily dependent upon the amount present at the onset of pregnancy. Hammond

(31) described the changes occurring in the bovine mammary gland during pregnancy. He states that there is little increase in duct length during pregnancy, the maximum being only 3.0 cm. The average initial length of the ducts was 9 cm. The ducts develop by growing along the connective tissue bands that divide the adipose tissue in the udder.

The size of the gland cistern is small during the first few months of pregnancy and a marked increase in its size occurs during the 5th and 6th months of pregnancy.

There is very little increase in the amount of secretory tissue in the udder during the first few months of pregnancy. During the 4th month, there is a slight increase in the proportion of secretory tissue and most of this is found in the vicinity of the large ducts entering the gland cistern. During development the tissues within the udder take on the characteristic appearance of those found during lactation. The large ducts have the characteristic two-layer lining with an underlying connective tissue. The smaller ductules and alveoli have the one-layer cuboidal-shaped epithelial cells. During the 5th month, the secretory tissue begins to become quite prominent. The secretory tissue is developed by a further branching of the ducts and formation of the end buds. The secretory tissue replaces the fatty tissue to form definite lobules. At this time the lobules are in evidence, but they are still very small. The connective tissue fibers separating the lobules and lobes are in evidence and have been organized into distinct layers. These contain numerous blood capillaries. During the 6th month of pregnancy the gland tissue has swollen to the

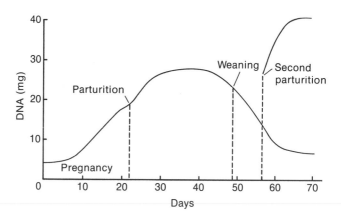

FIGURE 4–6
Changes in the DNA content of the six abdominal-inguinal mammary glands of rats during pregnancy, lactation, after weaning, and a second lactation. (Adapted from references 64, 87, 88, 89.)

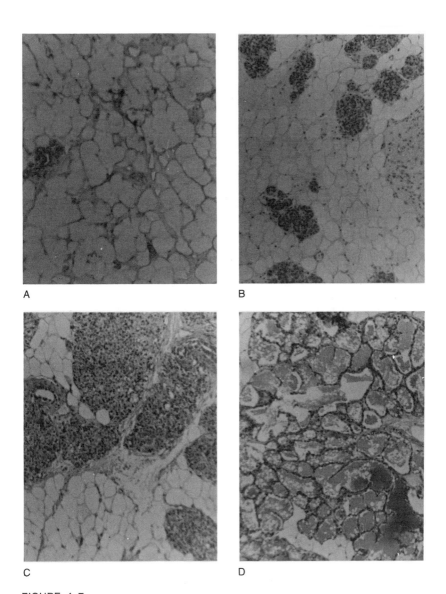

FIGURE 4–7
Histological changes in rat mammary tissue during various physiological
states. A. Tissue from a virgin rat showing cross-section of ducts and abundant
adipose tissue. B. Tissue from a 10-day pregnant rat showing some growth
of the lobulo-alveolar system. C. Tissue from an 18-day pregnant rat, showing
more extensive lobulo-alveolar growth. D. Tissue from a rat taken shortly
after parturition. The alveoli are developed and filled with milk.

extent that it has crowded out almost all of the adipose tissue, especially in the areas around the cisterns and the larger ducts.

Secretory tissue continues to grow throughout the remainder of pregnancy. Along with the development of the ducts and the secretory tissue, the vascular and lymphatic systems take on definite forms. During the 9th month of pregnancy, the alveoli begin to show secretory activity. The epithelial cells become distended, with the cytoplasm appearing granular. Fat droplets are noted in the cells and some may be found in the lumen of the alveoli. The marked increase in udder size during the terminal part of pregnancy is probably due to accumulation of secretory material within the mammary gland.

Kwong (37) found that most of the duct proliferation occurred during the first 3 months of pregnancy in the heifer. Growth during the 4th to 7th month consisted of the development of the secretory tissue. Secretion was noted during the later part of the 7th month of pregnancy. The alveoli became distended with secretion during the terminal 2 months of pregnancy.

Some authors state that mammary growth is complete by midpregnancy, but the majority of reports indicate that a further increase in growth occurs during the second half of pregnancy. Recurring pregnancies increase the amount of mammary gland growth up to a mature size. This is probably the reason that cows reach their maximum yield during the third and fourth lactations (80, 92, 96). The change in the amount of mammary gland growth during pregnancy, lactation, and involution is illustrated in Figure 4-6. The histological changes in the mammary gland during pregnancy and lactation are shown in Figure 4-7.

4-5   MAMMARY GROWTH
DURING LACTATION

Even though a large proportion of the secretory tissue is developed by the end of pregnancy, DNA measurements of mammary gland growth indicate that additional growth takes place during the first part of lactation. This work has been done primarily in the laboratory animals. In most species a wave of mitosis occurs shortly before or after parturition. A continuation of this growth occurs until the peak of lactation, when the mammary DNA content reaches a maximal value. Incorporation of ^{3}H-labeled thymidine in the nucleus (a measure of DNA synthesis in preparation for cell division) is seen after the first few days of lactation, but at a very low rate of activity in comparison to that during pregnancy or shortly after parturition. Similar results have also been obtained when colchicine was used to accumulate mitotic figures (8, 29, 81, 85).

Almost all of the mammary gland growth has taken place by the peak of lactation and very little cellular proliferation takes place thereafter. Cells that are destroyed and eliminated through the milk apparently are not replaced by mitosis during the declining phases of lactation.

4-6   HORMONAL CONTROL OF MAMMARY GLAND GROWTH

Historical Aspects

Some of the hormones responsible for mammary gland growth are the same as those involved in reproduction. This is especially true of the ovarian hormones. The development of the mammary gland is a by-product of reproduction, the mammary gland development being initiated for the purpose of nourishing the young. An extensive number of papers have been published on this subject. Lyons (44) states that deRothschild published a list of 10,000 references prior to 1900 with supplements added in 1901 and 1902. Since that time a large number of papers have been added. Reviews of the subject are found in Cowie (11), Folley (25, 26), Jacobsohn (35), Meites (51, 52, 53), and Norgren (63). Only the basic concepts and recent work in this area will be discussed.

The earliest observations on the mammary gland indicated that its development followed the process of reproduction. Ovariectomy caused a regression of the mammary gland, during either pregnancy or lactation. These results indicated that the hormones of the pituitary and ovaries are responsible for the development of the mammary gland. Early work also indicated that estrogen was primarily responsible for the duct development and progesterone was primarily responsible for lobulo-alveolar development. These general conclusions are still valid for most species.

Mammary Gland Measurements

One limiting factor in studying mammary gland development has been a lack of quantitative values by which to measure objectively the extent of growth. This problem has been overcome in part in the past 15 years. The most common method of determining growth was the gross observation of the intact gland, which included only the size and gross appearance of the gland. This was followed by the use of whole mounts, which are histological sections of entire mammary glands from laboratory animals. The secretory tissue was stained with specific dyes to show the extent of duct and lobulo-alveolar growth, giving a more objective measurement of the extent of growth, especially when a planimeter was used to measure the area of growth. This procedure applies only to mammary glands that occur in relatively flat sheets of tissue and gives no measure of the three-dimensional development of the mammary gland. The use of whole mounts was also accompanied by histological sections. These give only subjective values of mammary gland growth; they do, however, give an evaluation of the normality of the growth.

Total Alveolar Surface Area   A method used to measure total alveolar surface area of the lung was applied to mammary tissue by Richardson (69). This procedure involves the removal of a mammary gland, determining its weight and specific gravity, and measuring the number of alveoli in histological sections per length of line. It measures the total area of the secretory tissue lining the alveoli. Measurements of alveolar surface area are highly correlated with previous milk production but have been applied only to goats and cows in which the mammary glands are three dimensional. It has not been applied to glands that occur in relatively flat sheets of tissue.

Deoxyribonucleic Acid Content   The DNA procedure to evaluate mammary gland growth is based on the assumption that the DNA content per nucleus is constant; therefore, the total DNA in the mammary gland gives an index of the number of epithelial cells. This method gives the most quantitative measurement of mammary gland growth; however, it is valid only if the basic assumption is true. Some recent work (74, 81) questions this assumption. Even though a measure of DNA content cannot give an accurate index of the number of cells in the mammary gland, it can be used as a comparative measure of growth during the different physiological stages of the mammary gland and as a measure of growth due to various experimental treatments. The total DNA content does not measure the normality of the tissue unless histological sections are also obtained. The DNA content is expressed either as total mammary DNA content, or as DNA content per 100 g of body weight, or as mg DNA per g of fat-free mammary tissue or per 100 g of wet weight.

Other Methods of Mammary Gland Measurement   Cellular proliferation has also been determined by the injection of ^{3}H-labeled thymidine to measure the percentage or number of cells preparing for mitosis. Colchicine has been used to arrest mitotic figures. Another method is to measure the milk production of the animals after mammary growth and initiation of secretion have taken place. The initiation process and the hormonal and nutritional factors affecting lactation after its initiation interfere with this method to measure only gland growth.

Estrogen and Progesterone

Much of the research work on hormonal requirements of mammary growth has been done on intact or ovariectomized animals. Many reports deal with the use of estrogen and progesterone in various amounts, in various ratios, and for various lengths of time to induce mammary gland growth. In most cases a combination of estrogen and progesterone produces considerable growth. The results support the general conclusion that estrogen is primarily responsible for duct growth and progesterone is primarily responsible for lobulo-alveolar development. On the other hand, estrogen and progesterone injections usually do not produce as much growth as that resulting from pregnancy. In rats, however, the injection of 1 μg of estradiol benzoate and 2 mg of progesterone to mature ovariectomized rats for 19 days produces mammary gland growth comparable to that found during the 18th to 20th day of pregnancy. This is based upon the total DNA content of the 6 posterior mammary glands per 100 g of body weight. The amount of mammary gland growth in mice resulting from a combination of these two hormones is considerably less than that resulting from pregnancy. Combinations of estrogen and progesterone are required for mammary gland growth in rabbits and the guinea pig. Most reports indicate that estrogen and progesterone are required for mammary gland growth; it is impossible, however, to evaluate the completeness of the growth since in most cases the amount of development was not compared to that resulting from pregnancy (3, 6, 46, 58, 79, 100).

The development of full mammary gland growth and lactation by means of injected hormones in dairy animals would be of economic value because sterile animals could be brought into milk production. Administration of estrogen to ruminants causes extensive duct growth and considerable lobulo-alveolar growth; however, the lobulo-alveolar tissue has histological abnormalities, which include cystic alveoli, folded epithelium, and immature lobules in addition to a great deficiency of alveolar surface area (Figure 4-8). The administration of progesterone eliminates the histological abnormalities and increases the alveolar surface area. In general, progesterone increases the amount of mammary gland tissue and ensuing milk yields, but in most cases, the milk yield resulting from

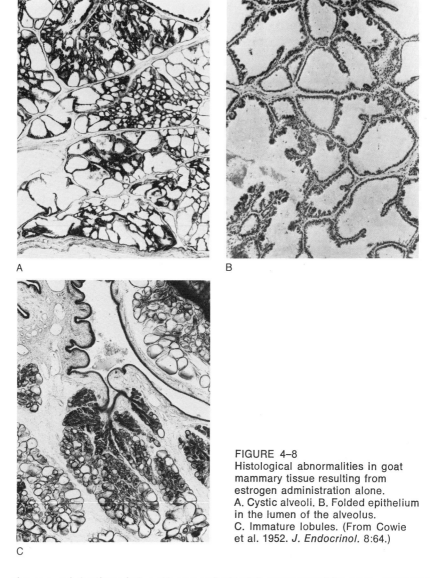

FIGURE 4-8
Histological abnormalities in goat
mammary tissue resulting from
estrogen administration alone.
A. Cystic alveoli. B. Folded epithelium
in the lumen of the alveolus.
C. Immature lobules. (From Cowie
et al. 1952. *J. Endocrinol.* 8:64.)

hormone injections is less than one-half of that expected from pregnancy
(4, 13, 72).

Two of the more successful attempts to induce milk secretion in nonpregnant animals have been reported by Reineke et al. (68) and Turner
(93). In the former experiment, estrogen and progesterone pellets were
implanted in five animals for various lengths of time. The best results

occurred in two Holstein cows that had had previous pregnancies. One of these produced over 11,000 lb of milk in the lactation. Three heifers with no previous pregnancies showed considerably less response. In the experiment by Turner (93), heifers were injected with 100 μg of estradiol and 100 mg of progesterone daily for 180 days; this was followed by additional 3-mg estradiol benzoate injections for another 14 days. Three freemartin heifers did not respond to the hormonal treatment, but the others showed increased mammary tissue growth. The mean daily milk production of the other heifers was stated to be 80–90% of that which would have been expected if the tissue growth was a result of pregnancy. The peak average milk production was only 22.7 lb, which is considerably less than the peak production expected from first-calf Jerseys.

Doubling the dose of estrogen and progesterone from that used in the trial by Turner (93) did not stimulate greater growth (98). Mammary glands become more responsive to injected hormones as the animals become more sexually mature. The best response to injected hormones occurs in animals that have had previous pregnancies (5, 33, 62).

On the basis of estrogen and progesterone injections to intact and ovariectomized animals, Folley (26) divided animals into three categories. One category includes the mouse, rat, rabbit, and cat, in which estrogen in physiological doses produces duct growth primarily, and the development of alveoli occurs only after prolonged administration of high levels of estrogen. The male gland has the same potential for growth as the female gland.

The second category includes the cow, goat, and guinea pig. In these animals, physiological doses of estrogen evoke extensive lobulo-alveolar growth in addition to the duct growth. The male mammary gland of the cow and goat does not have the same growth potential as that of the female of the species. The third category is one in which estrogen alone causes little or no mammary development, not even duct development. Included in this category is the bitch and possibly the ferret.

Mammary Growth in Hypophysectomized Animals

Estrogen and progesterone produce little, if any, mammary gland growth in the hypophysectomized animal. If it is produced, it is considerably reduced and abnormal. Anterior pituitary hormones are required in addition to estrogen and progesterone. The gonadal steroids may promote mammary growth by stimulating secretion of prolactin and somatotrophin (STH) by the anterior pituitary, by synergizing with the pituitary hormones, by sensitizing the mammary tissue to these hormones, or by directly stimulating mammary gland growth (53, 63).

One difficulty with the hypophysectomized animals is that the absence of the pituitary gland causes an upset in the general metabolism of the body. Restoration of the pituitary hormones or the hormones of its target organs does not indicate whether the hormone is directly responsible for mammary gland growth or involved in maintaining a normal metabolic state. Considerable work has been conducted on determining the role of the hormones concerned with metabolism on mammary gland development in the hypophysectomized animal. Specific hormones studied have been insulin, thyroxine, and cortisone. These papers have been reviewed by Cowie (11), Jacobsohn (34), and Norgren (63). Normal mammary gland growth cannot be produced in the hypophysectomized animal or the underfed animal. The lack of mammary gland growth in hypophysectomized animals is not due to a deficiency of nutrients, because no mammary gland growth results when hypophysectomized rats are force-fed and injected with estrogen. Rats injected with estrogen and progesterone and limited in feed to the amount consumed by hypophysectomized animals produce less mammary gland growth than that of normally fed rats. Injection of insulin with estrogen and progesterone in hypophysectomized rats results in some mammary gland growth; however, cortisone does not replace the effects of insulin but actually nullifies the beneficial effect of insulin. These studies indicate that adequate nutrition and a normal metabolic state are required for the mammary glands of an animal to respond to injected hormones.

The role of the anterior pituitary hormones in mammary gland growth was shown in some experiments by Lyons and coworkers (45). The hormone combination of estrogen, somatotrophin (STH), and deoxycorticosterone acetate produced mammary gland duct growth in the hypophysectomized-ovariectomized-adrenalectomized rat. Full lobulo-alveolar growth required the addition of protesterone and prolactin. These results were confirmed by Cowie and Lyons (15) in another strain of rats. The same hormones are also required for mammary gland growth in the hypophysectomized mouse (23, 60). In one strain of mice, bovine STH was found to be interchangeable with ovine prolactin (59, 61). Mammary gland development in the hypophysectomized goat requires estrogen, progesterone, prolactin, STH, and ACTH (16). From these experiments it is obvious that prolactin and STH are required for normal mammary growth. STH is primarily responsible for duct growth and prolactin plays a major role in lobulo-alveolar development. Adrenal corticoids increase the amount of mammary growth in the hypophysectomized rats injected with ovarian and pituitary hormones. It is impossible to determine whether they help to restore a normal metabolic state or whether they have a direct mammogenic effect. Both mineral corticoids and glucocorticoids, particularly large doses, stimulate mammary gland growth in rats and mice; however, they may merely mimic the action of the gonadal steroids (26, 51, 53).

Mammary Growth in Nonhypophysectomized Animals

The localized effect of prolactin was demonstrated in an experiment by Lyons (43) in which cellular proliferation occurred in the lobule of a pseudopregnant rabbit injected with prolactin. Somatotrophin and pro-lactin have been injected into intact and ovariectomized rats and mice concomitantly treated with estrogen and progesterone and into pregnant animals. In most cases, they produce additional mammary gland growth (22, 30, 36, 49, 56, 57).

Thyroxine has been injected into and fed to intact animals or ovari-ectomized animals treated with estrogen and progesterone to determine its effect on mammary gland growth. The results are conflicting. In some cases, thyroxine enhances mammary gland growth, whereas in other cases it depresses growth. Folley (26) indicated that hypothyroidism in the rat leads to an enhancement of the alveolar development; hypothy-roidism in the mouse inhibited mammary gland development. Recent evidence (73) indicates that thyroxine increases the amount of mammary gland growth in rats and mice above either that obtained with steroid hormone injections or that caused by pregnancy.

A negative response to an injected hormone in an animal with an intact pituitary cannot be interpreted to indicate that the hormone plays no role in mammary gland growth, since the level of the particular hormone may already be high enough for optimal mammary gland growth.

Are Estrogen and Progesterone Required?

The question of whether estrogen and progesterone play a direct role in mammogenesis is now being questioned. Clifton and Furth (9) trans-planted a pituitary mammotropic tumor into adrenalectomized-castrated rats and found that it caused considerable lobulo-alveolar development. The mammotropic graft secretes prolactin, STH, and ACTH, but none of the other pituitary trophic hormones. In this case lobulo-alveolar development occurred in the absence of any ovarian steroids. Lobulo-alveolar growth has been produced in the triple-operated rat with the injection of prolactin and STH (84). The implantation of a rat pituitary gland near or over one of the mammary glands of hypophysectomized-ovariectomized rats also caused localized lobulo-alveolar growth (17, 54). Regular twice-daily milking of three ovariectomized virgin goats resulted in some mammary growth and milk secretion. The goats reached peak yields of 0.8 to 2.0 liters per day. The response could not be brought about if the pituitary stalk was sectioned before milking started (14).

Meites (53) stated that the anterior pituitary hormones are the primary stimulators of mammary gland growth, even in normal physiological states. He stated that part or all of the effect of estrogen on mammary gland growth may be explained in its relationship to prolactin secretion, since it has been shown that estrogen stimulates prolactin secretion in the intact animal both by stimulating synthesis of the hormone in the pituitary and by acting on the hypothalamus to block release and synthesis of the prolactin-inhibiting factor.

The ovarian steroids cannot be completely ruled out as being involved in normal mammary gland growth, since estrogen and progesterone are required for full mammary gland growth in the hypophysectomized-ovariectomized rat (44). No quantitative measurements have been made on the amount of mammary gland growth when only anterior pituitary hormones have been administered. In order to rule out estrogen and progesterone completely, mammary gland growth comparable to that developed during pregnancy must be demonstrated to result from anterior pituitary hormones alone. Evidence against the concept that only STH and prolactin are directly involved in mammary gland growth is that some growth developed in hypophysectomized animals treated with estrogen, progesterone, and insulin (2). In addition, application of estrogens on the skin of the mammary gland of most mammals causes a localized mammary development whereas neighboring glands show no or very little response (24).

Organ Cultures

The hormonal requirements for organ cultures of mammary gland tissue are about the same as those for mammary gland growth in the triple-operated rat. Insulin and hydrocortisone are required for the survival and differentiation of the mammary gland tissue and prolactin is required for the histological development of the alveoli and the initiation of milk secretion. Epithelial cells must first divide in organ culture before they will synthesize casein in response to prolactin. Insulin is the only hormone required for cellular proliferation, but cells that proliferate in the absence of hydrocortisone are incapable of casein synthesis and histological development in the presence of prolactin. Insulin is required for the initiation of DNA synthesis. The addition of insulin or of STH to mammary gland cultures increases the rate at which epithelial cells initiate DNA synthesis, but does not alter the rate at which DNA is replicated. The rate of casein synthesis in cells grown *in vitro* is proportional to the rate of DNA synthesis during the preceding period. The initiation of DNA synthesis and the completion of DNA replication requires concurrent protein synthesis (19, 20, 42, 70, 82, 90).

In addition to initiation of DNA synthesis, insulin is also involved in protein synthesis in mammary gland explants by affecting ribonucleic acid (RNA) synthesis. Mammary gland explants grown in the absence of insulin incorporate adenine into RNA at a slowly decreasing rate so that the quantity of RNA in the tissue falls. Only with insulin is the RNA synthesis rapid enough to maintain its level in the tissue (47, 48). An early action of insulin is to increase the activity of transfer RNA methylases. The action of hydrocortisone in cell differentiation is associated with changes in methylase activity and the pattern of base methylation. Both hormones thus appear to affect RNA synthesis, which in turn affects protein synthesis (91).

Estrogen has not been shown to be necessary for growth in mammary gland organ cultures; however, progesterone produces some growth. Estrogen and progesterone together inhibit growth, but STH and prolactin stimulate it. These reports support the *in vivo* work in that STH and prolactin are stimulators of mammary gland growth and that progesterone is also involved. Estrogen probably is not involved in organ culture growth, since the amount of tissue grown is extremely small and very little duct growth would be expected in it (39, 65).

Specific Mammogens

Specific pituitary mammogens, in addition to the six known anterior pituitary hormones, have been proposed to cause mammary gland growth. This concept originated in Turner's laboratory and the first reports indicated that two specific mammogens were present in the anterior pituitary. Separate mammogens were proposed for duct and lobulo-alveolar growth (27, 28, 41, 55). Trentin and Turner (86) modified the two-mammogen theory to a single mammogen, which was associated with the protein fraction and caused both duct and lobulo-alveolar development. A mammogen has never been isolated as a chemically pure substance. Because of this and because of the work by Lyons et al. (45) showing that estrogen, progesterone, STH, and prolactin produced extensive mammary gland growth in the hypophysectomized-ovariectomized rats, little support has been given to the existence of a specific mammogen.

Placental Hormones

The role of the placenta in normal mammary gland development during pregnancy has never been fully elicited. Hormones possessing mammogenic, lactogenic, luteotrophic, and crop-sac-stimulating properties have been found in rat placenta tissue. Placental hormones apparently cause mammary gland development in mice, rats, and monkeys, since hypophysectomy during pregnancy does not result in a regression of mammary gland development (11). Regression occurs in the hypophysectomized nonpregnant animal with developed mammary glands. Placental hormones must therefore carry on the growth-promoting effects of the anterior pituitary hormones. The hormones of the placenta may also augment the effect of the ovarian steroids and pituitary hormones on mammary gland growth during pregnancy. Wrenn et al. (99) found that rats with an artificial deciduoma had more mammary gland growth than pseudopregnant rats, but it was considerably less than that resulting from pregnancy. This indicates that the placental hormones had some mammogenic effect in addition to the hormones involved in pseudopregnancy. Placental extracts induce some mammary gland growth when injected into mice and hypophysectomized-ovariectomized rats (7, 66).

Other Mammogenic Hormones
and Compounds

Other hormones and compounds have also been used to induce or augment mammary gland growth. Relaxin has been shown to stimulate mammary gland growth in rats and mice when given with estrogen or estrogen and progesterone. Relaxin administration to dairy goats for the last 30 days of an estrogen-progesterone injection regime resulted in a reduction in milk yields after lactation, apparently due to a decrease in mammary gland growth. The exact mechanism by which relaxin affects mammary gland growth is not known (12, 32, 78, 94, 95, 97).

The effect of androgens on mammary gland growth is difficult to evaluate. Testosterone stimulates mammary gland development in normal and castrated rats, but it is not effective in the absence of the pituitary or the pituitary hormones. The androgens may mimic the estrogens in the presence of the pituitary hormones since the steroids have similar structures. Testosterone may also exert its mammogenic effect through the release of prolactin from the pituitary in the intact animals (1, 18).

A series of drugs and nonspecific agents have been shown to stimulate mammary gland growth in the rat and rabbit—most of these trials occurring with intact animals primed with estrogen. Among the drugs that have been shown to be effective in the rat are reserpine, serotonin, epinephrine, acetylcholine, and chlorpromazine. Reserpine has been found to stimulate mammary lobulo-alveolar growth in estrogen-treated rabbits. These compounds can elicit ACTH and prolactin release from the pituitary and it is assumed that they exert their effect by causing the release of prolactin from the pituitary (50, 53).

The nervous system plays some role in mammary gland development, especially in rats. Pregnant rats prevented from licking their ventral body surfaces by neck collars had about one-half the mammary gland development of animals without collars. Neither the burden of wearing the collar nor stress occurring when formalin was injected into rats caused the depression in mammary gland growth. It is believed that the neural stimulus from licking probably caused a release of prolactin and other pituitary hormones from the pituitary gland (71).

4-7 SUMMARY

The fetal development of the mammary gland is similar in all animals. The first growth occurs in early fetal development and appears as a raised area of ectoderm on both sides of the midline in the areas where the mammary glands will develop. The ectoderm narrows into a raised line on each side of the midline. The raised line then congregates into mammary buds, which develop into the individual mammary glands. After the bud has developed into a small teat, a solid core of ectoderm cells arises from it and penetrates the underlying mesenchyme tissue and gives rise to the teat meatus, the teat and gland cisterns, and the duct system. This core of cells, the primary sprout, becomes canalized and then sends off secondary sprouts that become the major ducts of the mammary gland. At the same time the blood and lymphatic systems develop and lipid accumulates in the connective tissue. Most of the fetal development takes place during the first half of pregnancy. At 6 months of fetal age in the calf, the mammary gland consists of a small teat with a meatus, a teat cistern, a gland cistern, and a primitive duct system. Very little further development takes place before birth.

From birth to puberty there is a small amount of growth of the secretory tissue, but most of the growth is due to a deposition of adipose tissue. With each recurring estrous cycle after puberty, some further mammary gland development takes place. Estrogen produced during each estrous cycle is primarily responsible for duct growth and progesterone is primarily responsible for the development of the secretory tissue. When pregnancy occurs, a marked increase in mammary gland growth takes place. Most of the duct growth occurs during the first part of pregnancy and the lobulo-alveolar system takes form during the middle and latter parts of pregnancy.

A wave of mitosis occurs shortly before or after parturition. A slight amount of growth may continue until the peak of lactation, but after this no further growth takes place. The cells that are destroyed or eliminated after the peak of lactation apparently are not replaced during lactation.

The hormonal requirements for mammary gland growth are not well defined because of a lack of objective measures of mammary gland growth. No completely effective measure has been developed. The results to date indicate that estrogen, progesterone, prolactin, and somatotrophin (STH) are required for mammary gland development in the intact animal. Some recent evidence questions whether estrogen and progesterone are required; however, the injection of anterior pituitary hormones alone has not been shown to produce growth comparable to that occurring during pregnancy. The placenta may also influence mammary gland development during pregnancy. Hormones possessing mammogenic, lactogenic, luteotrophic, and crop-sac-stimulating properties have been found in rat placental tissue. In some animals, hypophysectomy during pregnancy does not result in a regression of mammary gland development, indicating that the placenta probably takes over the function of the anterior pituitary in producing mammary gland growth.

Other hormones, especially insulin and the adrenal corticoids, appear to be more directly involved in maintaining a normal metabolic state in the hypophysectomized animals, but they have direct effects on mammary gland proliferation and secretion in organ culture. Epithelial cells must first divide in organ culture before they will synthesize casein in response to prolactin. The cell division is under the influence of insulin; however, the cells must proliferate in the presence of hydrocortisone in order to produce casein in the presence of prolactin.

Other compounds and hormones have been shown to be involved in mammary gland growth, but it has not been determined whether these compounds or hormones play a role in the normal development. There is no conclusive evidence that specific mammogens are present in the anterior pituitary in addition to the six known anterior pituitary hormones.

REFERENCES

1. Ahren, K., and M. Etienne. 1959. *Acta Endocrinol.* 30:109.
2. Ahren, K., and D. Jacobsohn, 1956. *Acta Physiol. Scand.* 37:190.
3. Anderson, R. R., A. D. Brookreson, and C. W. Turner. 1961. *Proc. Soc. Exptl. Biol. Med.* 106:567.

4. Benson, G. K., A. T. Cowie, C. P. Cox, D. S. Flux, and S. J. Folley. 1955. *J. Endocrinol.* 13:46.
5. Benson, G. K., A. T. Cowie, C. P. Cox, S. J. Folley, and Z. D. Hosking. 1965. *J. Endocrinol.* 15:126.
6. Benson, G. K., A. T. Cowie, C. P. Cox, and S. A. Goldzveig. 1957. *J. Endocrinol.* 15:126.
7. Cerruti, R. A., and W. R. Lyons. 1960. *Endocrinology* 67:884.
8. Ciaccio, E. I. 1959. Oxidative phosphorylation in guinea pig mammary gland mitochondria during different functional states. Ph.D. Thesis, Cornell University.
9. Clifton, K. H., and J. Furth. 1960. *Endocrinology* 66:893.
10. Cowie, A. T. 1949. *J. Endocrinol.* 6:145.
11. Cowie, A. T. 1966. In G. W. Harris and B. T. Donovan, eds., *The Pituitary Gland*, Vol. 2. Berkeley: Univ. Calif. Press. Ch. 13.
12. Cowie, A. T., C. P. Cox, S. J. Folley, Z. D. Hosking, and J. S. Tindal. 1965. *J. Endocrinol.* 31:165.
13. Cowie, A. T., S. J. Folley, F. H. Malpress, and K. C. Richardson. 1952. *J. Endocrinol.* 8:64.
14. Cowie, A. T., G. S. Knaggs, J. S. Tindal, and A. Turvey. 1968. *J. Endocrinol.* 40:243.
15. Cowie, A. T., and W. R. Lyons. 1959. *J. Endocrinol.* 19:29.
16. Cowie, A. T., J. S. Tindal, and A. Yokoyama. 1966. *J. Endocrinol.* 34:185.
17. Dao, T. L., and D. Gawlak. 1963. *Endocrinology* 72:884.
18. Donovan, B. T., and D. Jacobsohn. 1960. *Acta Endocrinol.* 33:214.
19. Elias, J. J. 1957. *Science* 126:842.
20. Elias, J. J. 1959. *Proc. Soc. Exptl. Biol. Med.* 101:500.
21. Flux, D. S. 1954. *J. Endocrinol.* 11:223.
22. Flux, D. S. 1957. *J. Endocrinol.* 15:266.
23. Flux, D. S. 1958. *J. Endocrinol.* 17:300.
24. Folley, S. J. 1947. *Brit. Med. Bull.* 5:130.
25. Folley, S. J. 1952. In A. S. Parkes, ed., *Marshall's Physiology of Reproduction*, Vol. 2, 3rd ed. London: Longmans, Green and Co. Ch. 20.
26. Folley, S. J. 1956. *The Physiology and Biochemistry of Lactation.* Edinburgh: Oliver and Boyd.
27. Gomez, E. T., and C. W. Turner. 1937. *Mo. Agr. Expt. Sta. Res. Bull.* 259.
28. Gomez, E. T., and C. W. Turner. 1937-38. *Proc. Soc. Exptl. Biol. Med.* 37:607.
29. Greenbaum, A. L., and T. F. Slater. 1957. *Biochem. J.* 66:155.
30. Griffith, D. R., and C. W. Turner. 1963. *Proc. Soc. Exptl. Biol. Med.* 112:424.
31. Hammond, J. 1927. *The Physiology of Reproduction in the Cow.* London: Cambridge Univ. Press.
32. Hamolsky, M., and R. C. Sparrow. 1945. *Proc. Soc. Exptl. Biol. Med.* 60:8.
33. Hindery, G. A., and C. W. Turner. 1964. *J. Dairy Sci.* 47:1092.
34. Jacobsohn, D. 1958. *Proc. Royal Soc. (London), Ser. B*, 149:325.
35. Jacobsohn, D. 1961. In S. K. Kon and A. T. Cowie, eds., *Milk: The Mammary Gland and Its Secretion*, Vol. I. New York: Academic Press. Ch. 3.

36. Kumaresan, P., and C. W. Turner. 1966. *Endocrinology* 78:396.
37. Kwong, F. J. 1940. *J. Amer. Med. Assoc.* 96:36.
38. Laguchev, S. S. 1965. *Zh. Obshch. Biol.* 26:219.
39. Lasfargues, E. Y., and M. R. Murray. 1959. *Devel. Biol.* 1:413.
40. Legates, J. E., T. G. Martin, W. W. Swett, and R. W. Touchberry. 1960. *Purdue Agr. Expt. Sta. Res. Bull.* 692.
41. Lewis, A. A., and C. W. Turner. 1939. *Mo. Agr. Expt. Sta. Res. Bull.* 310.
42. Lockwood, D. H., F. E. Stockdale, and Y. J. Topper. 1967. *Science* 156, 945.
43. Lyons, W. R. 1942. *Proc. Soc. Exptl. Biol. Med.* 51:308.
44. Lyons, W. R. 1958. *Proc. Royal Soc. (London)*, *Ser. B*, 149:303.
45. Lyons, W. R., C. H. Li, and R. E. Johnson. 1958. *Recent Progr. Hormone Res.* 14:219.
46. Lyons, W. R., and D. A. McGinty. 1941. *Proc. Soc. Exptl. Biol. Med.* 48:83.
47. Mayne, R., and J. M. Barry. 1967. *Biochim. Biophys. Acta* 138:195.
48. Mayne, R., J. M. Barry, and E. M. Rivera. 1966. *Biochem. J.* 99:688.
49. McDonald, G. J., and R. P. Reece. 1963. *Proc. Soc. Exptl. Biol. Med.* 114:513.
50. Meites, J. 1957. *Proc. Soc. Exptl. Biol. Med.* 96:728.
51. Meites, J. 1959. In H. H. Cole and P. T. Cupps, eds., *Reproduction in Domestic Animals*, Vol. I. New York: Academic Press. Ch. 16.
52. Meites, J. 1961. In S. K. Kon and A. T. Cowie, eds., *Milk: The Mammary Gland and Its Secretion*, Vol. I. New York: Academic Press. Ch. 8.
53. Meites, J. 1966. In L. Martini and W. F. Ganong, eds., *Neuroendocrinology*, Vol. I. New York: Academic Press. Ch. 16.
54. Meites, J., and C. L. Kragt. 1964. *Endocrinology* 75:565.
55. Mixner, J. P., and C. W. Turner. 1943. *Mo. Agr. Expt. Sta. Res. Bull.* 378.
56. Moon, R. C. 1961. *Amer. J. Physiol.* 201:259.
57. Moon, R. C. 1965. *Proc. Soc. Exptl. Biol. Med.* 118:181.
58. Moon, R. C., D. R. Griffith, and C. W. Turner. 1959. *Proc. Soc. Exptl. Biol. Med.* 101:788.
59. Nandi, S. 1958. *Science* 128:772.
60. Nandi, S. 1959. *Univ. Calif. Publ. Zool.* 65:1.
61. Nandi, S. 1961. *Proc. Soc. Exptl. Biol. Med.* 108:1.
62. Nellor, J. E., and E. P. Reineke. 1958. *J. Dairy Sci.* 41:789.
63. Norgren, A. 1968. *Acta Univ. Lund. II.*, No. 4.
64. Paape, M. J., and H. A. Tucker. 1969. *J. Dairy Sci.* 52:518.
65. Prop, F. J. A. 1960. *Exptl. Cell Res.* 20:256.
66. Ray, E. W., S. C. Averill, W. R. Lyons, and R. E. Johnson. 1955. *Endocrinology* 56:359.
67. Raynaud, A. 1961. In S. K. Kon and A. T. Cowie, eds., *Milk: The Mammary Gland and Its Secretion*, Vol. I. New York: Academic Press. Ch. 1.
68. Reineke, E. P., J. Meites, C. F. Cairy, and C. F. Huffman. 1952. *Proc. 89th Mtg., Amer. Vet. Med. Assoc.*, p. 325.
69. Richardson, K. C. 1953. *J. Endocrinol.* 9:170.
70. Rivera, E. M., and H. A. Bern. 1961. *Endocrinology* 69:340.

71. Roth, L. L., and J. S. Rosenblatt. 1968. *J. Endocrinol.* 42:363.
72. Schmidt, G. H., and W. Hansel. 1961. *J. Dairy Sci.* 44:2259.
73. Schmidt, G. H., and W. H. Moger. 1967. *Endocrinology* 81:14.
74. Simpson, A. A., and G. H. Schmidt. 1969. *Proc. Soc. Exptl. Soc. Biol. Med.* 132:978.
75. Sinha, Y. N., and H. A. Tucker. 1966. *Amer. J. Physiol.* 210:601.
76. Sinha, Y. N., and H. A. Tucker. 1969. *Proc. Soc. Exptl. Biol. Med.* 131:908.
77. Sinha, Y. N., and H. A. Tucker. 1969. *J. Dairy Sci.* 52:507.
78. Smith, T. C. 1954. *Endocrinology* 54:59.
79. Smith, T. C., and B. Richterich. 1958. *Endocrinology* 63:89.
80. Sod-Moriah, U. A. 1966. Deoxyribonucleic acid content and proliferative pattern of the epithelial cells in the mammary glands of the Dutch-Belted rabbit. Ph.D. Thesis, Cornell University.
81. Sod-Moriah, U. A., and G. H. Schmidt. 1968. *Exptl. Cell Res.* 49:584.
82. Stockdale, F. E., W. G. Juegens, and Y. J. Topper. 1966. *Develop. Biol.* 13:266.
83. Swett, W. W., J. H. Book, C. A. Matthews, and M. H. Fohrman. 1955. *USDA Tech. Bull.* 1111.
84. Talwalker, P. K., and J. Meites. 1961. *Proc. Soc. Exptl. Biol. Med.* 107:880.
85. Traurig, H. H. 1967. *Anat. Rec.* 157:489.
86. Trentin, J. J., and C. W. Turner. 1948. *Mo. Agr. Expt. Sta. Res. Bull.* 418.
87. Tucker, H. A., and R. P. Reece. 1963. *Proc. Soc. Exptl. Biol. Med.* 112:370.
88. Tucker, H. A., and R. P. Reece. 1963. *Proc. Soc. Exptl. Biol. Med.* 112:409.
89. Tucker, H. A., and R. P. Reece. 1963. *Proc. Soc. Exptl. Biol. Med.* 112:1002.
90. Turkington, R. W. 1968. *Endocrinology* 82:540.
91. Turkington, R. W. 1969. *Federation Proc.* 28:724.
92. Turner, C. W. 1952. *The Mammary Gland.* Columbia, Mo.: Lucas Brothers.
93. Turner, C. W. 1959. *Mo. Agr. Expt. Sta. Res. Bull.* 697.
94. Wada, H., and C. W. Turner. 1958. *Proc. Soc. Exptl. Biol. Med.* 99:194.
95. Wada, H., and C. W. Turner. 1959. *Proc. Soc. Exptl. Biol. Med.* 101:707.
96. Wada, H., and C. W. Turner. 1959. *J. Dairy Sci.* 42:1198.
97. Wada, H., and C. W. Turner. 1959. *Proc. Soc. Exptl. Biol. Med.* 102:568.
98. Williams, R., and C. W. Turner. 1961. *J. Dairy Sci.* 44:524.
99. Wrenn, T. R., J. Bitman, W. R. DeLauder, and M. L. Mench. 1966. *J. Dairy Sci.* 49:183.
100. Yamamoto, H., and C. W. Turner. 1956. *Proc. Soc. Exptl. Biol. Med.* 92:130.

5

HORMONAL CONTROL
OF LACTATION

The development of the mammary gland after puberty is under hormonal control (Chapter 4). Hormones are further involved in lactation in that they are responsible for the initiation of milk secretion. They also play a vital role in the maintenance of milk secretion after it has been established.

The terminology used to describe the various aspects of lactation is often confused. In order to establish a common basis of understanding, the general descriptions reviewed by Cowie (18) will be followed. Milk secretion refers to the synthesis of milk by the epithelial cells and the passage of milk from the cytoplasm of the cells into the alveolar lumen. Milk removal includes the passive withdrawal of milk from the cisterns and sinuses and the ejection of milk from the alveolar lumina. Lactation refers to the combined processes of milk secretion and removal. Lacto-genesis is the initiation of milk secretion; mammogenesis describes the development of the mammary gland; and galactopoiesis refers to the enhancement of established lactation.

5-1 INITIATION OF MILK SECRETION

Most mammary gland growth takes place during pregnancy with some growth continuing until the peak of lactation. During the terminal phase of pregnancy, the epithelial cells begin to secrete. Lipid and protein granules form in the epithelial cells and accumulate in the lumen of the alveolus to form colostrum. The initiation of lactation is brought about by a sudden increase in the rate of secretory activity of the epithelial cells near the time of parturition. In the rat, lactose secretion appears absent until the time of parturition, and the sudden appearance of lactose appears to be an important aspect of the initiation of milk secretion (65). Part of the increased rate of secretion after parturition is due to the evacuation of secretory products and part is due to a hormonal stimulation.

Biochemical Changes

Biochemical changes occur in the mammary gland as it turns from a quiescent state to an active secretory one. There is a marked increase in the RNA level of the epithelial cells. This causes the ribonucleic acid (RNA):deoxyribonucleic acid (DNA) ratio, which is less than 1 during late pregnancy, to increase to over 2:1 during secretion. RNA is an index of protein secretion and DNA is an index of the cell numbers. The change in the ratio indicates a marked increase in the secretory status of the cell at the time of parturition. A large increase in the number of ribosomes occurs, as well as an increased incorporation of amino acids into soluble protein by mammary gland tissue slices (29, 30, 31, 92, 96).

Mammary gland tissue removed shortly after parturition also shows a marked increase in oxygen consumption, again indicating a marked increase in secretory function. The respiratory quotient (R.Q.) of mammary gland tissue during lactation is greater than 1; this indicates that carbohydrates and acetate are being converted to lipids. During pregnancy and involution, the R.Q. is less than 1 (36, 37, 92).

Histological Changes

The histological changes occurring during the initiation process are primarily associated with changes due to the accumulation of fluid in the alveolar lumen. This causes an increase in the size of the alveolus, a flattening of the epithelial cells, and a decrease in the number of cells per sight field. Changes in histological sections of rat mammary gland from the 18th day of pregnancy to the time of parturition are shown in Figure

4-7. The cells have a greater abundance of endoplasmic reticulum with attached ribosomes and a marked increase in number of mitochondria. The nucleoli also become more distinct during secretion (111).

Hormones Involved in Lactogenesis

Anterior Pituitary Hormones   The initiation of milk secretion is brought about in part by anterior pituitary hormones. It has long been recognized that hypophysectomy prevents the initiation of lactation and causes a cessation of established lactation. As early as 1928, Stricker and Grueter (113) indicated that the anterior pituitary contained a specific hormone or hormones capable of initiating lactation. They found that aqueous extracts of the anterior pituitary injected into ovariectomized pseudopregnant rabbits initiated lactation. Anterior pituitary extracts also initiate lactation in monkeys, cows, goats, sows, dogs, rabbits, and guinea pigs, if they have adequately developed mammary glands (35).

A few years after the work of Stricker and Grueter, Riddle et al. (102) demonstrated that a hormone of the anterior pituitary was responsible for enlargement and secretory activity of the pigeon crop sac. This compound is the same hormone, or at least one of the hormones, responsible for the initiation of milk secretion demonstrated by Stricker and Grueter. Riddle called the hormone prolactin and other workers have referred to it as galactin, mammotropin, lactogen, and lactogenic hormone. Prolactin will be the name used in this discussion.

The direct involvement of prolactin in the initiation of secretion was shown by the experiment of Lyons (71). The injection of prolactin into the mammary gland of a pseudopregnant rabbit caused a localized hyperplasia and initiated secretion in the injected duct and not in the other ducts. An example of this process is shown in Figure 5-1. The oxygen consumption of the gland injected with prolactin was higher than that of the control glands; however the R.Q. never reached unity (89).

Pituitary and Adrenal Cortical Hormones   Prolactin alone does not initiate secretion in hypophysectomized animals, except for the rabbit. Unfractionated anterior pituitary extracts, on the other hand, initiate milk secretion in hypophysectomized animals with adequate mammary gland development. It is now well established that prolactin and adrenal corticoid hormones are required for the initiation of lactation in the rat and guinea pig (22, 40, 49, 61, 73, 97, 98).

Somatotrophin (STH) and cortisol are as effective as prolactin and cortisol in initiating lactation in the $C_3H/Crgl$ strain of mice (93). The combination of STH, prolactin, and cortisol is more effective than the

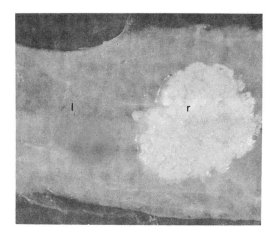

FIGURE 5–1
Localized initiation of milk secretion by prolactin
in the 16-day pseudopregnant rabbit. Twenty
units of prolactin were injected into the lobe on
the right (R). The lobe on the left (L) showed
little growth and no initiation of secretion.

combination of any two of the three hormones in most strains of mice
(94, 95). Lactation can be initiated in the hypophysectomized goat udder
half receiving a local injection of prolactin, after a systemic injection of
STH (26).

The adrenal corticoids apparently are not needed for the initiation of
lactation in the rabbit, since prolactin alone initiates milk secretion in the
hypophysectomized rabbit and in the adrenalectomized pseudopregnant
rabbit (28, 40, 61). On the other hand, ACTH injections into pseudopregnant rabbits cause the initiation of milk secretion (13).

Cortisol, cortisone, prolactin, and human placental lactogen (HPL)
given separately induce lactation in pregnant rabbits; however, a combination of an adrenal corticoid and prolactin or HPL increases the intensity
of lactation (41, 80). It thus appears that the adrenal corticoids either
synergize with the circulating prolactin or act independently to initiate
milk secretion.

Single Hormone or Lactogenic Complex? The question of whether a
single lactogenic hormone or a complex of lactogenic hormones is responsible for the initiation of lactation has not been resolved. The results
in the rabbit indicate that prolactin is the only hormone necessary for the
initiation of secretion; however, the adrenal corticoids may be important

in the normal animal. For the rat, mouse, goat, and guinea pig, a complex of hormones including the adrenal corticoids is necessary for the initiation of milk secretion. The exact role of STH in the initiation process can not be identified for the rat and goat, since its beneficial effect in the hypophysectomized animal may be to restore a normal metabolic state. STH does play a direct role in some strains of hypophysectomized mice.

In Vitro Results   The results on the initiation of milk secretion in the intact mouse have been largely confirmed by *in vitro* studies of mouse mammary gland tissue. Prolactin and STH added to the media containing insulin and cortisol (hydrocortisone) or aldosterone induce secretory activity. The concentrations of these hormones needed to produce secretory responses are four times greater for early prelactating tissue than for tissue taken during late pregnancy. This implies that tissue from the advanced stages of pregnancy is more sensitive to hormones than tissue from the earlier stage of pregnancy. Insulin and cortisol are the minimal hormonal requirements for the maintenance of mammary tissue explants (104, 120).

In order for mouse mammary gland tissue to synthesize casein *in vitro,* the cells must first divide. Casein-producing cells formed *in vivo* lose their ability to secrete casein *in vitro,* but they can still synthesize α-lactalbumin and β-lactoglobulin. An insulin-mediated cell proliferation in the presence of hydrocortisone produces a cell population that synthesizes casein in the presence of prolactin or human placental lactogen (HPL). Prevention of cell division by colchicine prevents casein synthesis in the presence of prolactin or HPL, but colchicine does not interfere with casein synthesis if it is present after the postmitotic period. The administration of actinomycin D, an inhibitor of ribonucleic acid synthesis, prevents the induction of casein synthesis of differentiated cells in the presence of prolactin or HPL. This suggests that the induction of milk protein synthesis requires new DNA-directed RNA synthesis (70, 117).

The naturally occurring corticoids of the mouse adrenal, corticosterone and aldosterone, are as effective in initiating secretion as cortisol in mouse tissue cultured in media containing insulin, prolactin, and STH; however, deoxycorticosterone is not effective. STH from bovine, ovine, and porcine sources are effective in initiating milk secretion in mammary gland explants from the $C_3H/Crgl$ mouse; however, they are only 20–50% as effective as ovine prolactin. Simian and human STH have equal or greater ability than ovine prolactin in initiating lactation in $C_3H/Crgl$ mouse mammary glands. Only one of three human growth hormone preparations studied is effective in initiating milk secretion in explants from the strain A mouse mammary gland tissues. These results demonstrate the differential response of mammary gland cultures due to genetic background of the tissues (103, 105).

Human STH is unique in comparison to nonprimate growth hormones in the fact that its lactogenic activity in the pseudopregnant rabbit mammary gland is as high as that of sheep prolactin. Human STH has only very slight crop-stimulating activity, but it possesses all of the other biological effects characteristic of animal prolactin. Human STH and prolactin are closely associated in man in their lactogenic and galactopoietic effects (18).

Other Lactogenic Hormones, Drugs, and Stimulants   Various hormones, tranquilizers, drugs, nonspecific stresses, and rat hypothalamic extracts initiate lactation in either the estrogen-primed rat or the pseudopregnant or pregnant rabbit. Compounds and procedures that have been shown to initiate lactation are acetylcholine, epinephrine, reserpine, electrical stimulation of the cervix, electrical stimulation of the head lumbar region, nasal mucosa and nipples, and rat hypothalamic tissue. Most of these agents act either through the central nervous system or directly stimulate the pituitary to release prolactin and ACTH (75, 76, 77, 81, 82, 85, 86).

Changes in the Blood Hormone Levels in Relation to Lactogenesis

Since the hormones required for the initiation of lactation appear to be the same as those required for the maintenance of milk secretion, a plausible concept for the initiation of secretion must also explain how milk secretion takes place during pregnancy, as is usual in the cow. It may be that the levels of hormones responsible for maintenance of milk secretion are high enough to overcome the inhibitory effects of the hormones primarily responsible for the maintenance of pregnancy. A definite antagonism exists between the hormones of pregnancy and the lactogenic hormones. Large doses of estrogen inhibit milk secretion; progesterone alone does not, but the combination of the two markedly inhibit secretion (83). Pregnancy, however, does not reduce the pituitary prolactin content (87). The amount of prolactin needed to initiate lactation in rabbits treated with estrogen and progesterone is much higher than that required after the two hormones are withdrawn (83, 84). In addition, the amount of prolactin and cortisol required to initiate lactation is much higher in the pregnant rabbit than in the nonpregnant one (80).

Theories   Prolactin and the adrenal corticoids are required to initiate lactation; therefore, the circulating blood levels of these must change at parturition or inhibitory levels of other substances, such as progesterone, must drop in order for lactation to occur. A number of theories have been put forward to explain the hormonal control of the initiation process. These have been summarized by Cowie (17) and Folley (36). Meites (79) summarized his latest explanation for the hormonal control of the initiation process in this way: During pregnancy there is an insufficient amount of prolactin or of the adrenal glucocorticoids, or of both, to initiate lactation. Estrogen and progesterone, which are secreted in large quantities during pregnancy, render the mammary gland relatively refractory to the stimulation of prolactin and glucocorticoid hormones. The higher levels of steroids are of lesser importance than the lack of adequate amounts of lactation-stimulating hormones. At the time of parturition a rise in circulating prolactin and glucocorticoids occurs with a concomitant fall in estrogen and progesterone levels. Even though estrogen is a potent stimulator of prolactin secretion, it does not appear to promote prolactin secretion during pregnancy, possibly because of the high levels of progesterone present during gestation.

The adrenal glucocorticoids may not exert their maximum biological activity during pregnancy, since some evidence exists that there is an increased binding of these hormones to the protein transcortin at this time. This is believed to inhibit biological activity of the glucocorticoids. Estrogens may increase the amount of transcortin (79). The corticosteroid-binding activity of blood serum rises during pregnancy in mice, rabbits, and guinea pigs and falls to virgin levels during lactation (44).

The theory put forward by Folley (36) is similar to the revised Meites theory except that Folley states that low circulating levels of estrogen activate the lactogenic function of the anterior pituitary while higher levels tend to inhibit lactation. Meites's concept does not relate to the higher level. The similarities of these two theories are more striking than their differences. Both authors relate to a lactogenic complex instead of a single lactogenic hormone. Both stress the importance of the estrogen-progesterone combinations in inhibiting milk secretion during pregnancy. This either blocks the production of the hormones by the pituitary or renders the mammary glands refractory to the lactogenic hormones. Both also emphasize the importance of the drop in progesterone at the time of parturition.

The exact events taking place at parturition have not been resolved. A definite rise in prolactin and ACTH secretion occurs at parturition. Meites (79) enumerates four possible ways in which the rise in these hormones is brought about and their relationship to the initiation process: (1) estrogen becomes predominant over progesterone at the end of gestation and causes an increase in prolactin secretion; (2) transcortin disappears from the circulation to increase the level of biologically active adrenal corticol hormones; (3) circulating levels of estrogen and progesterone decrease to make the mammary glands more responsive to the lactogenic hormones; and (4) neural stimuli from the reproductive tract, as a result of the fetus passing through the cervix and uterine contractions, increase the production or release of prolactin and ACTH via the hypothalamus.

Nandi and Bern (95) indicate that the increase in the effective glucocorticoid level rather than the prolactin level is the essential component for lactogenesis in mice. They reason that because prolactin and STH are both required for full lobulo-alveolar development and since the amount required for lobulo-alveolar development is about the same as that required for lactogenesis, the level of prolactin necessary for lactogenesis at parturition is already present. They conclude that there may be an increase in prolactin secretion at parturition, but this increase is not essential for the initiation of milk secretion. This concept is supported in part by the fact that the injection of glucocorticoids initiates lactation in the pregnant rat, mouse, rabbit, and cow; and large doses of prolactin do not initiate lactation in pregnant rats and mice (79). Accurate measurements of the changes in the blood hormone concentrations at the time of parturition will help to resolve the question of the role of the various hormones and their levels in the lactogenesis process.

In Vitro *Results*   A more definitive explanation of the hormonal control of the initiation of milk secretion is possible from results of mouse mammary gland organ cultures and studies of lactose synthesis. The lactose synthetase activity of rat mammary gland increases markedly on the last day of pregnancy from a near zero value and parallels the increase in tissue lactose concentration. This enzyme is exclusively concerned with lactose synthesis. It has been suggested that lactose synthetase is the rate-limiting enzyme for lactose biosynthesis (64). Lactose synthetase is composed of two proteins: the A protein, which is a galactosyltransferase, and the B protein, which is whey protein α-lactalbumin (119). During the latter half of pregnancy, the A protein activity of mouse mammary gland rises to nearly maximum values; however, the B protein values remain low and rise to maximum values after parturition (118). Prolactin induces the synthesis of both A and B proteins in mouse mammary gland organ cultures; progesterone, however, prevents the increase in activity of α-lactalbumin, but does not prevent the induction of galactosyltransferase activity. Progesterone injections into mice 1 or 2 days before parturition prevent the marked rise in α-lactalbumin concentration after parturition found in the noninjected animals. These results indicate that progesterone takes part in the control of lactose synthesis by repressing α-lactalbumin formation during pregnancy. When the plasma concentration of progesterone falls at parturition, there is an increase in the rate of synthesis of α-lactalbumin, which interacts with galactosyltransferase in the final step of lactose synthesis (119).

5-2 CONTROL OF PROLACTIN
SECRETION AND RELEASE

Prolactin plays a major role in the hormonal control of mammary gland growth, the initiation of lactation, and the maintenance of milk secretion. For this reason the control of prolactin release and production by the anterior pituitary will be reviewed briefly (for references, see Meites, 79).

The control of prolactin secretion and release from the pituitary occurs either by some direct effect on the pituitary or by a compound mediated via the hypothalamus. The hypothalamus produces a substance that has an inhibitory effect on the prolactin production or release by the pituitary. This compound is known as the prolactin inhibitory factor (PIF). The PIF compound has not been chemically defined; however, it appears in the acid extract of the hypothalamus and it is a small molecule. PIF is unique since it is the only inhibiting factor produced by the hypothalamus.

The presence of PIF has been shown in a number of ways. Pituitaries transplanted to other parts of the body have an increased secretion of prolactin, whereas they produce or release very little of the other trophic hormones. Lesions in certain areas of the hypothalamus cause an increase in prolactin secretion by the pituitary. Sectioning of the pituitary stalk increases the prolactin production by the pituitary. The administration of various central nervous system depressant drugs and certain stressful agents increase prolactin secretion. Anterior pituitary sections of all species tested, except the pigeon, release 10–16 times as much prolactin in organ culture during a 4-day culture than was originally present in the anterior pituitary. In contrast to this the release of ACTH, STH, and FSH, the follicle-stimulating hormone, by the rat pituitary gland ceases after 3–4 days in culture. When the pituitary cultures are incubated with hypothalamic extracts, they release less prolactin and retain less prolactin at the end of culture in contrast to pituitary pieces incubated with cerebral cortex tissue. The hypothalamic extract neither inactivates the prolactin nor inhibits its action when injected into pigeons. The hypothalamic extract also increases the STH release from human pituitary slices in organ culture.

The sucking stimulus, reserpine, and estradiol deplete the hypothalamus of the PIF compound. Epinephrine and acetylcholine reduce the amount of PIF in the hypothalamus. All of these compounds have been shown to initiate lactation. Several hormones act on the anterior pituitary directly to increase prolactin secretion or release. Thyroxine (T_4) and triiodothyronine (T_3) cause a significant increase in the prolactin release of pituitary glands in organ culture. Intrahypophysial implants of estrogen promote prolactin release and initiate mammary gland secretion.

5-3   MAINTENANCE OF MILK SECRETION

The knowledge of the hormonal requirements for the maintenance of milk secretion has been gained primarily from research in animals with their endocrine glands removed. When hormones are injected into intact animals and an increase in milk secretion results, it is difficult to determine whether the hormone had a direct effect on milk secretion or an indirect effect, such as the effect of thyroactive compounds on increasing the metabolic rate. The administration of hormones to intact animals will be discussed under galactopoeisis.

Suckling Stimulus

The maintenance of milk secretion is also dependent upon the milking or suckling stimulus, which is involved in the release of prolactin, ACTH, and oxytocin from the pituitary gland (77). In addition, the suckling or milking process removes the milk from the gland; removal is required for further milk synthesis to take place. The goat appears to be an exception to the group of animals that requires suckling or milking stimulus for the maintenance of milk secretion. Goats under anesthesia continued to secrete normal amounts of milk when they were milked. Rats treated in the same way and given oxytocin for milk ejection produced a subnormal amount of milk (121).

Failure to remove the milk causes pressure to build up within the gland, resulting in a cessation of secretion and the beginning of involution. The suckling stimulus can maintain the secretory activity of glands in which the milk is not removed because of ligated ducts (109). The suckling stimulus can also prolong lactation for long periods of time. Replacement of young foster litters on lactating dams can extend the lactation period for as long as 10–12 months in the rat (12).

Hypophysectomy

The removal of the pituitary gland during lactation results in a complete cessation of milk secretion (38). In the rat, hypophysectomy causes a cessation of milk secretion within 24 hours and the metabolic activity of the gland is changed within 4–8 hours after hypophysectomy. Mammary gland slices from hypophysectomized rats incubated *in vitro* use less glucose, produce more lactic acid, and have a much lower respiratory quotient than tissue from control rats (10). The decline in milk secretion after hypophysectomy in the goat is more gradual and several weeks elapse before the secretion process stops completely (26). Hypophysectomy of the lactating rabbit inhibits secretion within 3–7 days (20).

Replacement Therapy to Hypophysectomized Animals

Early experiments on the replacement value of hormones to maintain lactation in hypophysectomized rats have to be discounted because oxytocin was not given to induce milk ejection. The work by Gomez (47, 48) was the first to use injections of posterior pituitary extract to produce milk ejection in hypophysectomized animals. An aqueous suspension of anterior pituitary powder, an adrenal cortex extract, a glucose solution, and a posterior pituitary extract resulted in a partial maintenance of lactation in hypophysectomized rats; however, the average body weight of the young was considerably less than that of the control animals.

Complete restoration of milk secretion in lactating hypophysectomized rats has not been achieved. In a study by Cowie (15), large doses of prolactin plus oxytocin for milk ejection produced milk yields of about 25% of normal. Neither ACTH nor STH given alone had any replacement value, but the combination of the two had a slight replacement value. About 50% restoration of milk secretion was obtained in two rats receiving prolactin and ACTH. A 50% restoration value was also obtained in mice (8) and rats (25) with prolactin and ACTH. Fujii and Uerno (42) concluded that prolactin was necessary to maintain lactation and that ACTH or hydroxycortisone played a supplementary role.

Hypophysectomy of the lactating rat results in depressions in activities of glucose 6-phosphate dehydrogenase, phosphogluconic acid dehydrogenase, fatty acid synthetase, uridine diphosphate pyrophosphorylase, phosphoglucomutase, malic enzyme, and citrate cleavage enzyme in the mammary gland. All are key enzymes in the synthesis of milk components. Treatment with cortisol or prolactin alone partially maintains the activity of some of the enzymes, but treatment of hypophysectomized rats with both hormones maintains essentially normal enzyme levels (62). These results indicate that adrenal corticoids and prolactin appear to be essential components of the hormone complex needed to maintain lactation in hypophysectomized rats and mice. The complete complex and levels of hormones required will not be known until complete restoration of milk secretion has been demonstrated in the hypophysectomized animal.

Complete restoration of milk production in hypophysectomized goats was obtained when prolactin, bovine STH, triiodothyronine (T_3), insulin and corticosteroid injections were begun immediately after hypophysectomy (21). Complete restoration of lactation was achieved in one goat in which the milk yield had been allowed to drop to nearly zero before treatment was begun, but the level of prolactin necessary for this was twice as high as that required when the therapy was begun immediately after hypophysectomy. Complete restoration of milk secretion was not possible in two other goats in which the milk production had dropped to nearly zero. In the rabbit, the preoperative level of milk yield was restored after hypophysectomy with daily injections of either 50 or 100 IU of sheep prolactin or 2.5 or 5 mg of human growth hormone. Neither bovine growth hormone, ACTH, nor cortisol acetate when added to human growth hormone or sheep prolactin increased the yields above those obtained with the growth hormone or sheep prolactin alone (20).

Coagulation of the median eminence in the hypothalamus or sectioning of the pituitary stalk of the lactating goat caused a drop in milk yield to about 15–30% of the preoperative levels. Complete restoration of milk production occurred in the goats with coagulated median eminences after the administration of ACTH, STH, T_3, and insulin, and partial restoration of lactation in the pituitary stalk-sectioned goats took place after STH, T_3, insulin, and corticosteroid administration. Withdrawal of STH caused an immediate and marked drop in milk secretion. In both cases, prolactin was not necessary for the restoration of milk production. This further demonstrates that the pituitary gland can secrete considerable quantities of prolactin in the absence of hypothalamic control (19, 45, 46).

Adrenal Corticoids and ACTH

The administration of ACTH to hypophysectomized rats with pituitary grafts under the kidney capsules maintained milk secretion at 30% of normal value (27). This indicates that the graft is capable of secreting prolactin; these results give little information, however, on the hormones required for full replacement therapy. The impairment of lactation resulting from hypothalamic lesions is correlated with the degree of adrenal atrophy. In the rats with hypothalamic lesions, lactation can be restored to 70–80% of normal by injections of cortisol. Prolactin was not effective. In this case, the pituitary was probably secreting normal amounts of prolactin, and a deficiency of ACTH caused the impairment of lactation (27).

Further evidence on the role of the adrenal in maintaining milk secretion indicates that adrenalectomy causes an inhibition of milk secretion.
Restoration of milk secretion in the adrenalectomized rat and goat
requires both the mineral corticoids and glucocorticoids or compounds
such as 9- α-chlorohydrocortisone, which has properties like those of both
corticoids (1, 2, 3, 23, 24). It is impossible to assign a direct effect of the
adrenal corticoids on milk secretion since adrenalectomy impairs the
electrolyte balances in the body as well as protein and carbohydrate
metabolism. It may be that the adrenal corticoids maintain normal balances of these metabolic processes, balances that allow milk secretion to
occur.

Thyroid and Parathyroid Hormones

The role of the thyroid in normal lactation has been reviewed by Cowie
(17) and he concludes that the thyroid gland is not absolutely essential
for milk secretion, but in its absence the intensity and duration of milk
secretion is reduced. Thyroidectomy lowers the milk yield and shortens
the duration of lactation in the cow and goat. In these species, the surgical
procedure of thyroidectomy does not remove all of the parathyroid tissue.
   Removal of the thyroids in rats also removes the parathyroids. Destruction of the thyroid glands in rats with radioiodine does not inhibit lactation. This leaves the parathyroids intact. Removal of the parathyroids in
rats causes a marked inhibition of milk secretion (17). Restoration of
milk secretion in thyroparathyroidectomized rats is brought about by the
administration of thyroxine (T_4), oxytocin, and injected parathormone or
dihydrotachysterol given orally. Injected dihydrotachysterol given with
T_4 and oxytocin is not as effective in restoring milk secretion as the orally
administered dihydrotachysterol (5, 7, 33).
   Thyroparathyroidectomy of lactating cows caused a significant decrease
in serum calcium and a slight decrease in serum inorganic phosphate. A
drop in milk production also occurred, but not to the extent of that
occurring in rats after parathyroidectomy. It is suggested that the high
calcium to phosphorus content of the natural ration of the ruminant
allows the cow to maintain lactation to a certain extent without parathyroid glands (112).

5-4   GALACTOPOIESIS

Galactopoiesis will be restricted to a discussion of the response of lactating animals to exogeneous hormones. This type of experimentation
gives some indication of the hormones involved in the control of lactation;
however, a positive response to an injected hormone may be the result of

a direct stimulation of milk secretion or a response to an indirect effect, such as increasing the metabolic rate. A negative response to an injected hormone does not mean that the hormone plays no role in milk secretion, as the circulating levels of hormones may already be optimum for milk secretion.

Pituitary Extracts

Crude extracts of bovine pituitary glands gave a marked increase in milk production when injected into lactating cows (Table 5-1). Cows do not respond to injection of anterior pituitary extracts during the peak of lactation and it is effective only during declining phases of lactation (78).

TABLE 5-1
Mean increase in milk yield for 2 days after a single subcutaneous injection of the hormone, expressed as a percentage of the mean yield for the 2 days before treatment.

Treatment	Dose	No. of cows	Percentage increase in milk yield
Saline	—	12	− 1.9
Growth hormone	15 mg	4	2.8
Growth hormone	30 mg	12	6.3
Growth hormone	60 mg	8	3.4
Bovine anterior pituitary extract	5 ml	4	2.9
Bovine anterior pituitary extract	10 ml	7	6.6
Prolactin	40 mg	4	− 2.3
Prolactin and growth hormone	40 mg 30 mg	3	7.9
ACTH	7 mg	7	− 6.6
ACTH	28 mg	4	−10.1
ACTH and growth hormone	7 mg 30 mg	3	4.3

Source: Cotes et al. 1949. *Nature* (London), 164:992.

Prolactin

There is only a slight relationship between the galactopoietic activity of pituitary extracts in lactating cows and the prolactin content of the extracts as assayed by the pigeon crop method. Prolactin has little or no galactopoietic activity in lactating cows but does increase milk production of goats in late lactation (78).

Significant increases in litter weight gain have been reported in rats injected with prolactin. Rat mammary gland tissue that received locally administered prolactin had a higher rate of oxygen consumption than control mammary glands. Prolactin thus appears to play a galactopoietic role in the rat (60, 66, 89). In the rabbit, sheep prolactin was found to increase the milk yield, as well as the lactose percentage, in late lactation (16).

Somatotrophin

Most of the galctopoietic activity of anterior pituitary extracts administered to cows can be attributed to the STH present in the extract (see Table 5-1). Single injections of 15-mg and 30-mg doses of STH gave percentage increases in milk production for 2 days of 2.8% and 6.3%, respectively. Five ml and 10 ml of a crude pituitary extract gave percentage increases of 2.9% and 6.6%, respectively. The galactopoietic effect of STH in dairy cows, sheep, and goats has been substantiated by a large number of workers. A linear relationship exists between the percentage increase in milk production and the log dose of STH injected on a single injection basis. The mode of action of STH has not been established. It has been reported that STH increases the net efficiency of milk production and causes a marked increase in the size of the udder. The effect of STH on milk fat content has not definitely been established, since some workers have reported an increase, but others have not been able to confirm this (14, 58, 78).

In contrast to its galactopoietic activity in ruminants, STH does not have the same properties in the rat and mouse, but it increases dam weights during the period of injection (17, 74, 78). The injection of STH during lactation causes a significant increase in the amount of milk obtained by suckling young in one half-hour nursing after a 10-hour separation (6, 53, 90). In this procedure the animals are anesthetized and injected with oxytocin, after which the litters are allowed to nurse. Whether or not this increase in milk production applies during the entire lactation of the rat is difficult to assess because the litters of the STH-treated dams do not have a faster growth rate than the control animals. In addition, the 6 animals in the litter used to evacuate the milk may not challenge the dam in milk secretion or give a complete evacuation of the milk (67).

Adrenal Corticoids and ACTH

Even though the adrenal-pituitary mechanism is required for the maintenance of lactation, ACTH and cortisol injections into lactating cows cause a marked depression in the milk production (14, 17, 78). (See Table 5-1.) In rats, ACTH has been shown to increase the litter growth rate. Cortisone in large daily doses (10–20 mg) inhibits milk secretion in rats, whereas lower doses (0.5–1.0 mg) increase it, and a low dose (0.25 mg) has no effect. The cortisone effects in other species and the effects of other corticoids in laboratory animals are conflicting (17). Talwalker et al. (115) indicate that 0.5 mg of hydrocortisone acetate increases the litter growth rate when injected into the mothers, whereas 0.25 mg and 1.0 mg are not effective. Corticosterone is effective in increasing the milk obtained by young rats during a 30-minute suckling period after a 10-hour separation (55). The adrenal corticoids are thus essential for milk secretion, but excess amounts inhibit lactation.

Estrogen and Progesterone

In some trials, estrogen has been shown to have some galactopoietic activity in the cow; however, it is effective only within a very narrow dose range. This has been reviewed by Cowie (17) and Meites (78). Estrogens can initiate lactation and increase the pituitary prolactin content in a number of species. Large doses of estrogen to cows in advanced lactation inhibit milk production. In addition, estrogen and progesterone combinations have an inhibitory effect on lactation in the cow. In one trial (11), diethylstilbestrol feeding starting 60 days after parturition and continuing for 8 months resulted in an increase in 4% fat-corrected milk production and an increase in persistency of lactation. In another trial (59), it was found that single injections of 12.5 mg of estradiol monobenzoate into lactating cows caused significant increases in fat and solids-not-fat yields, but higher levels of the estrogenic compound caused a significant decline in milk yield. Most of the results indicate that the galactopoietic effect in dairy cows is dependent upon the dose level and stage of lactation. Most of the response is due to an increase in milk fat and solids-not-fat contents of the milk.

The injection of ovarian steroids into lactating rats has been summarized by Cowie (17) and further work has been reported (4, 43, 52). Ovarian extracts administered to laboratory animals cause a depressed rate of growth and an increased mortality rate of their young. When the lactating animals are treated with estrogens, removal of their ovaries decreases the depression in litter growth rate and litter mortality. Larger doses of estrogens are required to depress the growth rate of litters in the ovariectomized rat in contrast to the intact rat. The inhibition of milk secretion is much greater when estrogen and progesterone act together in contrast to either acting alone. Progesterone alone does not affect the litter growth rate in the rat. The inhibitory effect of estrogen and progesterone appears to render the mammary gland insensitive to prolactin.

Insulin

The injection of insulin into lactating dairy cows results in a decrease in milk production, milk lactose percentage, blood glucose levels, and an increase in the percentage composition of milk fat and protein. The increases in milk fat and protein percentages during insulin treatment cannot be explained entirely by a decrease in milk production (63, 106, 107).

Insulin *in vitro* enhances the incorporation of radioactive-labeled amino acids into isolated rat diaphragm, epididymal fat pad, liver slices, perfused heart, heart slices, and rat mammary gland. The increased amino acid incorporation brought about by insulin into diaphragm protein occurs in the absence of glucose or an oxidizable substrate (107).

Adding insulin *in vitro* to rat mammary gland slices incubated with glucose or glucose and acetate caused a marked increase in the respiratory quotient, an increase in oxygen consumption, and an increased acetate uptake when acetate was present as a substrate. Sheep mammary gland tissue was completely insensitive to the stimulatory action of insulin (39). The daily injection of insulin into lactating rats resulted in highly significant increases in milk yield when milk yield was measured during a one-half-hour nursing after a 10-hour separation from the dam. No significant increase in the litter weight gain occurred (68).

Thyroid Hormones

The first demonstration that thyroid hormone was galactopoietic in the cow was by Hertoghe (57). Graham (50, 51) rediscovered this phenomenon and demonstrated that injected thyroxine gave galactopoietic effects in cows as did the feeding of dried thyroid glands. The introduction of thyroprotein (iodinated casein) by Reineke and Turner (101) resulted in a readily made and inexpensive product. The commercial synthesis of L-thyroxine (T_4) in addition to the thyroprotein provided inexpensive thyroactive materials and resulted in a large number of experiments with dairy cows. The biological effects of thyroprotein are due to its thyroxine content. The use of thyroprotein and T_4 in stimulating milk production has been reviewed by Blaxter (9), Folley (36), Hansel (56), Meites (78), and Moore (91).

Another biologically active compound has been isolated from the thyroid gland. It is 3:5:5'-triiodo-L-thyronine (T_3) and it differs from thyroxine in that it contains three iodine molecules instead of four. Oral administration of T_3 to lactating cows produces no galactopoietic effect; however, its injection into lactating cows causes an increase in milk yield and milk fat percentage. T_3 is either rapidly broken down by rumen microorganisms or less rapidly absorbed from the intestinal tract of ruminants than is T_4 (36).

In most cases, the feeding of the thyroprotein to dairy cows in the declining phase of lactation results in a 15–20% increase in production for periods of 2–4 months. The beneficial effect of its feeding over a longer period of time is dependent upon the nutrition of the animal. If extra energy is fed along with the thyroprotein and if this regime is started after the peak of lactation, an increase in lactation production usually results in comparison to control animals fed according to their requirements. This kind of comparison measures both the effect of the thyroprotein and the extra energy. A valid comparison of the thyroprotein effect is to maintain similar energy intakes between the control and experimental cows. When this is done, the thyroprotein-fed cows produce more milk for a period of 60–120 days, but after this their production drops below the level of the controls and results in equal or only slightly higher lactation milk yields. This results in spite of increasing the energy intake to 125% of the requirements of the control group (91).

When thyroprotein is withdrawn, a marked decline in production occurs. In many cases, the decrease in milk production after thyroprotein withdrawal is equal to the increased production during its feeding. Gradual withdrawal has been shown to prevent the precipitous drop in production resulting from abrupt withdrawal; however, this procedure is not always beneficial. Turning cows out to pasture at the time of withdrawal helps to prevent the marked drop in production. It is generally recommended that the feeding of thyroprotein should start 60 or more days after parturition because thyroxine injections are less effective in stimulating milk production during the peak and end of lactation in comparison to midlactation (99).

The feeding of thyroprotein for successive lactations has received some study. Thomas and Moore (116) found that cows receiving thyroprotein for three lactations produced less milk during the second and third lactations than during the first. One limitation of this study is the small number of control cows and experimental cows that finished the trial. Similar results were obtained by Swanson (114). Leech and Bailey (69) conducted a large field trial with more than 2,000 cows. Either thyroprotein or T_4 was fed for 11 weeks of each lactation for three successive lactations. The cows receiving the thyroactive compounds out-produced the control cows by 51, 197, and 442 lb of milk for the first, second, and third lactations, respectively.

There is some relationship between the amount of thyroprotein fed daily and the response of the dairy cows. The feeding of 5 g daily produces no significant increase in milk production. The feeding of 10 g daily increases the milk production somewhat, whereas 15 g shows a further increase in production. Higher doses have been tried, but extremely high doses cause an increase in milk yield accompanied by severe losses in body weight and elevated rectal temperatures (78).

The fat content of milk is increased by 0.2–0.4% with the short-term feeding of thyroprotein. It is questionable whether the extended feeding of thyroprotein increases it (56, 78). In an extensive study by Leach and Bailey (69), thyroprotein-fed cows averaged 3.74% and control cows averaged 3.76% milk fat. No other changes in milk composition occur with the feeding of thyroactive substances.

The question of the efficiency of milk production during thyroprotein feeding is related to the length of feeding and whether the changes in body weight are considered. The short-term thyroprotein feeding does not lower the efficiency of production even when body weight changes are considered. The long-term feeding of thyroprotein does result in a decrease in efficiency of conversion of feed energy into milk when the body weight changes are considered. When they are disregarded the efficiency of production of thyroprotein-fed animals appears to be about the same as that of the control animals. This is particularly true in the first lactation (56).

Losses in body weight invariably result during thyroprotein feeding and cows gain body weight after it is withdrawn. The loss in body weight can be partially, but not completely, offset by giving extra feed during thyroprotein feeding. The loss in body weight due to thyroprotein is accompanied by changes in paunch girth and gastrointestinal fill. The changes in gastrointestinal fill account for a major portion of the weight losses; however, decreases in body tissue weight also occur. The amount of body weight loss is partially dependent on the dose of thyroprotein, since the higher doses result in greater weight losses (56, 78).

The feeding of thyroprotein causes an increase in the heart and respiration rates, indicators of increased metabolic rates. Part of the increase in heart and respiration rates may be due to an increase in the feeding of extra nutrients (56). In most cases, the general health of the animals is not adversely affected by thyroprotein feeding; however, the mortality rate of calves from thyroprotein-fed cows appeared higher in one study (116). In a recent paper (34), it was found that T_3 implants increased either the severity or the incidence of ketosis symptoms in comparison to control animals. Over two-thirds of the cows displaying clinical symptoms of ketosis did not have other diseases or elevated temperatures.

Other reported physiological effects of thyroxine include: an increase in blood glucose level, decrease in the blood fat, and a greater uptake of glucose and fatty acids by the mammary glands. It increases the rate of work by the whole body and its sole action may be to increase the general metabolic rate of the animal (78).

In general, the benefits of thyroprotein feeding to a herd of cows has not been economical. It may be of importance in special market situations or where cows receive the material for short periods of time before drying off or being turned out to pasture. In all cases it appears that thyroprotein feeding should be done on an individual cow basis, and not on a herd basis.

Feeding high levels of T_3 and T_4 inhibits milk secretion in the lactating rat and increases the young mortality rate (108). Low doses of injected T_4 increase the milk production of lactating rats and the growth rate of their young (6, 32, 54). These results indicate that low supplemental levels of thyroactive materials enhance lactation and high levels have an inhibitory effect.

Nutrition

It is a common observation that increasing the nutrient intake of dairy cows usually results in an increase in milk production. Starvation of the mother rat from the 10th to the 14th days postpartum results in a decrease in pituitary lactogen content and a cessation of milk secretion (88). Neither anterior pituitary powders, STH, T_4, cortisol acetate, nor prolactin will increase the milk production of underfed rats, again indicating the importance of nutrition in the milk secretion process (100). Lactating rats on a severe protein-deficient diet have markedly impaired growth of their litters (10). Hormonal regimes including prolactin or the lactogenic corticoid (Prednisolone) do improve the lactation performance on a protein-free diet (72).

5-5 SUMMARY

Initiation of Secretion

Prior to parturition lipid and protein granules form in the epithelial cells and accumulate in the lumen of the alveolus as colostrum. In the rat, lactose does not appear in the milk until the time of parturition. The initiation of milk secretion is characterized by an increase in the RNA:DNA ratio, an increase in the number of ribosomes, a marked increase in the endoplasmic reticulum, and an increase in the number of mitochondria per cell. The histological changes that occur are primarily associated with the changes due to milk accumulation within the lumen of the alveolus.

Hypophysectomy prevents the initiation of lactation. The anterior pituitary contains specific hormones responsible for the initiation of lactation, of which prolactin appears to be the important hormone. Prolactin causes a localized initiation of milk secretion when injected into the rabbit mammary gland. In addition to prolactin, adrenal corticoid hormones are required for the initiation of lactation in most animals. In one strain of mouse, somatotrophin (STH) can replace prolactin in the initiation process. In the rabbit, prolactin alone can initiate lactation in the hypophysectomized animals.

Insulin and cortisol are the minimal hormone requirements for maintaining viable mammary gland tissue explants *in vitro*. In order for these cells to synthesize casein, the cells must first divide. The cell division must take place in the presence of insulin and cortisone in order for the cells to synthesize casein in response to prolactin or human placental lactogen.

The hormonal control of the initiation of lactation has not been fully explained. The theories used to explain the initiation process center on either a rise in the blood levels of prolactin and adrenal glucocorticoids at the time of parturition or a drop in the level of compounds that have an inhibitory effect on the milk secretion process, namely progesterone and transcortin. Transcortin binds the adrenal corticoids and inhibits their biological activity. Recent evidence from mouse tissue culture work indicates that progesterone inhibits the activity of α-lactalbumin during pregnancy; α-lactalbumin is one of the two proteins that make up lactose synthetase. Lactose synthetase is postulated to be the rate-limiting enzyme for lactose biosynthesis. It is thus postulated that initiation of milk secretion is brought about by a drop in blood progesterone levels, which allows an increase in α-lactalbumin activity to produce sufficient lactose synthetase for the synthesis of lactose.

Control of Prolactin Production   The prolactin secretion and/or release by the pituitary gland is controlled by the hypothalamus and by a direct action of compounds on the pituitary gland. The hypothalamus produces a chemical compound, PIF, which inhibits the prolactin production and/or release from the pituitary. Pituitaries transplanted to other parts of the body or grown in organ culture without the hypothalamic extract increase the release of prolactin. Compounds, such as reserpine, epinephrine, and acetylcholine, and the suckling stimulus exert their effect by decreasing the hypothalamic content of PIF. Estradiol appears to work in the same way, as well as having a direct stimulatory effect on the pituitary gland. Triiodothyronine (T_3) and thyroxine (T_4) appear to have a direct effect on prolactin release from the pituitary.

Maintenance of Milk Secretion

The maintenance of milk secretion is dependent upon the removal of the milk and a suckling or milking stimulus in most animals. The goat appears to be an exception in that it does not seem to require a milking stimulus to maintain secretion. The suckling stimulus is involved in the release of prolactin, ACTH, and oxytocin from the pituitary gland.

Hypophysectomy causes a cessation of milk secretion. In the rat the cessation of secretion occurs within hours, whereas several weeks may elapse before the secretion process stops completely in the goat. Replacement therapy to maintain lactation in hypophysectomized animals requires the injection of oxytocin for milk ejection. Replacement therapy to hypophysectomized lactating rats has not been very successful. From the limited work it appears that prolactin and the adrenal corticoids are the essential components, however other factors must be involved since only 25–50% restoration has been attained. Complete restoration of milk production has been obtained in hypophysectomized goats with the injection of prolactin, bovine STH, T_3, insulin, and corticosteroid. Prolactin alone restores lactation to preoperative levels in the hypophysectomized rabbit.

Galactopoiesis

Much work has been done on the feeding and injection of hormones to intact animals, especially the ruminant animals. Anterior pituitary extracts have been found to increase production in the dairy cow. Most of this increase is due to the STH content. Prolactin has very little effect on increasing the milk production of lactating cows but causes a slight increase in milk production in goats in late lactation. Prolactin injections into lactating rats increase the growth rate of their young. Prolactin injections into lactating rabbits during late lactation increases milk yields and the percentage of lactose.

Somatotrophin injections cause a marked increase in the milk production of lactating cows. The long-term effect of STH injections has not been assessed because of the high cost of the hormone. STH does not have a galactopoietic activity in the rat or mouse since the litter weight gains are not increased; the dam, however, increases its weight after the injection. Large doses of ACTH or adrenal corticoids inhibit lactation in the rats and ruminants. Cortisone and hydrocortisone increase the litter weight gains in rats when injected over a narrow dose range; however, high levels tend to inhibit milk secretion and lower doses have no effect. The feeding of thyroprotein and T_4 and the injection of T_3 cause an increase in milk production in lactating cows. The feeding of thyroprotein increases milk production for periods of 2–4 months and also results in a transitory increase in milk fat percentage. Thyroprotein has been used on commercial dairy farms to increase milk production; however, information on the beneficial effects over complete lactations is still lacking. The feeding of thyroprotein causes an increased need for nutrients, a loss in body weight, and increases in heart rate, respiration rate, and body temperature.

REFERENCES

1. Anderson, R. R., and C. W. Turner. 1962. *Proc. Soc. Exptl. Biol. Med.* 110:349.
2. Anderson, R. R., and C. W. Turner. 1963. *Amer. J. Physiol.* 205:1077.
3. Anderson, R. R., and C. W. Turner. 1963. *Proc. Soc. Exptl. Biol. Med.* 112:997.
4. Ben-David, M. H., H. Roderig, K. Khazen, and F. G. Sulman. 1965. *Proc. Soc. Exptl. Biol. Med.* 120:620.
5. Berswordt-Wallrabe, R. von, and C. W. Turner. 1960. *Proc. Soc. Exptl. Biol. Med.* 104:113.
6. Berswordt-Wallrabe, R. von, R. C. Moon, and C. W. Turner. 1960. *Proc. Soc. Exptl. Biol. Med.* 104:530.
7. Berswordt-Wallrabe, R. von, and C. W. Turner. 1960. *J. Dairy Sci.* 43:1838.
8. Bintarningsih, W. R. Lyons, R. E. Johnson, and C. H. Li. 1958. *Endocrinology* 63:540.
9. Blaxter, K. L. 1952. *Vitamins and Hormones* 10:218.
10. Bradley, T. R., and A. T. Cowie. 1956. *J. Endocrinol.* 14:8.
11. Browning, C. B., F. C. Fountaine, G. B. Marion, and F. W. Atkeson. 1957. *J. Dairy Sci.* 40:1590.
12. Bruce, H. M. 1961. *J. Reprod. Fertil.* 2:17.
13. Chadwick, A., and S. J. Folley. 1962. *J. Endocrinol.* 24:xi.
14. Cotes, P. M., J. A. Crichton, S. J. Folley, and F. G. Young. 1949. *Nature* (London) 164:992.
15. Cowie, A. T. 1957. *J. Endocrinol.* 16:135.
16. Cowie, A. T. 1969. *J. Endocrinol.* 44:437.
17. Cowie, A. T. 1961. In S. K. Kon and A. T. Cowie, eds., *Milk: The Mammary Gland and Its Secretion*, Vol. I, New York: Academic Press. Ch. 4.

18. Cowie, A. T. 1966. In G. W. Harris, and B. T. Donovan, eds., *The Pituitary Gland.* London: Butterworths Scientific Publ. Ch. 13.
19. Cowie, A. T., P. M. Daniel, G. S. Knaggs, M. M. L. Pritchard, and J. S. Tindal. 1964. *J. Endocrinol.* 28:253.
20. Cowie, A. T., P. E. Hartmann, and A. Turvey. 1969. *J. Endocrinol.* 43:651.
21. Cowie, A. T., G. S. Knaggs, and J. S. Tindal. 1964. *J. Endocrinol.* 28:267.
22. Cowie, A. T., and W. R. Lyons. 1959. *J. Endocrinol.* 19:29.
23. Cowie, A. T., and J. S. Tindal. 1955. *Endocrinology* 56:612.
24. Cowie, A. T., and J. S. Tindal. 1958. *J. Endocrinol.* 16:403.
25. Cowie, A. T., and J. S. Tindal. 1961. *J. Endocrinol.* 22:403.
26. Cowie, A. T., and J. S. Tindal. 1961. *J. Endocrinol.* 23:79.
27. Cowie, A. T., J. S. Tindal, and G. K. Benson. 1960. *J. Endocrinol*, 21:115.
28. Cowie, A. T., and S. C. Watson. 1966. *J. Endocrinol.* 35:213.
29. Davis, J. W., T. M. Y. Liu, and C. L. Eddington. 1966. *Federation Proc.* 25:348.
30. Denamur, R. 1961. *Ann. Endocrinol.* 22:767.
31. Denamur, R. 1963. *C. R. Acad. Sci.* 256:4748.
32. Desclin, L. 1949. *C. R. Soc. Biol.* (Paris) 143:1156.
33. Djojosoebagio, S., and C. W. Turner. 1964. *Proc. Soc. Exptl. Biol. Med.* 116:909.
34. Emery, R. S., and J. A. Williams. 1964. *J. Dairy Sci.* 47:879.
35. Folley, S. J. 1952. In A. S. Parkes, ed., *Marshall's Physiology of Reproduction*, 3rd ed. London: Longmans, Green and Co. Ch. 20.
36. Folley, S. J. 1956. *The Physiology and Biochemistry of Lactation.* Edinburgh: Oliver and Boyd.
37. Folley, S. J., and T. H. French. 1949. *Biochem. J.* 45:270.
38. Folley, S. J., and F. H. Malpress. 1948. In G. Pincus and K. V. Thimann, eds., *The Hormones*, Vol. I. New York: Academic Press. Ch. 15.
39. Folley, S. J., and M. L. McNaught. 1958. *Brit. Med. Bull.* 14:207.
40. Fredrikson, H. 1939. *Acta Obstet. Gynec. Scand.* 19, Suppl. 1.
41. Friesen, H. G. 1966. *Endocrinology* 72:212.
42. Fujii, K., and S. Uerno. 1958. *Bull. Tokyo Med. Dent Univ.* 5:479.
43. Gala, R. R., and R. P. Reece. 1962. *J. Dairy Sci.* 45:681.
44. Gala, R. R., and U. Westphal. 1967. *Acta Endocrinol.*, Copenhagen, 55:47.
45. Gale, C. C. 1963. *Acta Physiol. Scand.* 59:269.
46. Gale, C. C. 1964. *Acta Physiol. Scand.* 61:228.
47. Gomez, E. T. 1939. *J. Dairy Sci.* 22:488.
48. Gomez, E. T. 1940. *J. Dairy Sci.* 23:537.
49. Gomez, E. T., and C. W. Turner. 1936. *Proc. Soc. Exptl. Biol. Med.* 34:404.
50. Graham, W. R. Jr. 1934. *Biochem. J.* 28:1368.
51. Graham, W. R. Jr. 1934. *J. Nutr.* 7:407.
52. Griffith, D. R., and C. W. Turner. 1962. *Proc. Soc. Exptl. Biol. Med.* 110:862.
53. Grosvenor, C. E., and C. W. Turner. 1959. *Proc. Soc. Exptl. Biol. Med.* 100:158.

54. Grosvenor, C. E., and C. W. Turner. 1959. *Proc. Soc. Exptl. Biol. Med.* 100:162.
55. Hahn, D. W., and C. W. Turner. 1966. *Proc. Soc. Exptl. Biol. Med.* 121:1056.
56. Hansel, W. 1957. *Proc. Cornell Nutr. Conf.*, p. 72.
57. Hertoghe, E. 1896. *Bull. Acad. Med. Belg.* 10:381.
58. Hutton, J. B. 1957. *J. Endocrinol.* 16:115.
59. Hutton, J. B. 1958. *J. Endocrinol.* 17:121.
60. Johnson, R. M., and B. V. Alfredson. 1958. *Federation Proc.* 17:81.
61. Kilpatrick, R., D. T. Armstrong, and R. O. Greep. 1964. *Endocrinology* 74:453.
62. Korsrud, G. O., and R. L. Baldwin. 1969. *Federation Proc.* 28:273.
63. Kronfeld, D. S., G. P. Mayer, J. M. Robertson, and F. Raggi. 1963. *J. Dairy Sci.* 46:559.
64. Kuhn, N. J. 1968. *Biochem. J.* 106:743.
65. Kuhn, N. J., and J. M. Lowenstein. 1967. *Biochem J.* 105:995.
66. Kumaresan, P., R. R. Anderson, and C. W. Turner. 1966. *Proc. Soc. Exptl. Biol. Med.* 123:581
67. Kumaresan, P., R. R. Anderson, and C. W. Turner. 1967. *Proc. Soc. Exptl. Biol. Med.* 126:41
68. Kumaresan, P., and C. W. Turner. 1965. *Proc. Soc. Exptl. Biol. Med.* 119:415.
69. Leech, F. B., and G. L. Bailey. 1953. *J. Agr. Sci.* 43:236.
70. Lockwood, D. H., F. E. Stockdale, and Y. J. Topper. 1967. *Science* 156:945.
71. Lyons, W. R. 1942. *Proc. Soc. Exptl. Biol. Med.* 51:308.
72. Lyons, W. R. 1966. *Endocrinology* 78:575.
73. Lyons, W. R., C. H. Li, and R. E. Johnson. 1958. *Recent Progr. Hormone Res.* 14:219.
74. MacDonald, G. J., and R. P. Reece. 1961. *J. Animal Sci.* 20:196.
75. Maqsood, M., and J. Meites. 1961. *Proc. Soc. Exptl. Biol. Med.* 106:104.
76. Meites, J. 1957. *Proc. Soc. Exptl. Biol. Med.* 96:728.
77. Meites, J. 1959. *Proc. Soc. Exptl. Biol. Med.* 100:750.
78. Meites, J. 1961. In S. K. Kon and A. T. Cowie, eds., *Milk: The Mammary Gland and Its Secretion*, Vol. I. New York: Academic Press. Ch. 8.
79. Meites, J. 1966. *Neuroendocrinology*, Vol. I. New York: Academic Press.
80. Meites, J., T. F. Hopkins, and P. K. Talwalker. 1963. *Endocrinology* 73:261.
81. Meites, J., C. S. Nicoll, and P. K. Talwalker. 1959. *Proc. Soc. Exptl. Biol. Med.* 101:563.
82. Meites, J., C. S. Nicoll, and P. K. Talwalker. 1959. *Proc. Soc. Exptl. Biol. Med.* 102:127.
83. Meites, J., and J. T. Sgouris. 1953. *Endocrinology* 53:17.
84. Meites, J., and J. T. Sgouris. 1954. *Endocrinology* 55:530.
85. Meites, J., P. K. Talwalker, and C. S. Nicoll. 1960. *Proc. Soc. Exptl. Biol. Med.* 103:298.

86. Meites, J., P. K. Talwalker, and C. S. Nicoll. 1960. *Proc. Soc. Exptl. Biol. Med.* 104:192.
87. Meites, J., and C. W. Turner. 1948. *Mo. Agr. Exp. Sta. Res. Bull.* 415.
88. Meites, J., and C. W. Turner. 1948. *Mo. Agr. Exp. Sta. Res. Bull.* 416.
89. Mizuno, H., and M. Naito. 1959. *Endocrinol. Jap.* 6:93.
90. Moon, R. C. 1965. *Proc. Soc. Exptl. Biol. Med.* 118:181.
91. Moore, L. A. 1958. *J. Dairy Sci.* 41:452.
92. Nagasawa, H. 1962. *Jap. J. Zootech. Sci.* 33:350.
93. Nandi, S. 1958. *J. Nat. Cancer Inst.* 21:1039.
94. Nandi, S., and H. A. Bern. 1960. *J. Nat. Cancer Inst.* 24:907.
95. Nandi, S., and H. A. Bern. 1961. *Gen. Comp. Endocrinol.* 1:195.
96. Nelson, W. L., P. G. Heytler, and E. I. Ciaccio. 1962. *Proc. Soc. Exptl. Biol. Med.* 109:373.
97. Nelson, W. O., and R. Gaunt. 1936. *Proc. Soc. Exptl. Biol. Med.* 34:671.
98. Nelson, W. O., R. Gaunt, and M. Schweizer. 1943. *Endocrinology* 33:325.
99. Ralston, N. P., W. C. Cowsert, A. C. Ragsdale, H. A. Herman, and C. W. Turner. 1940. *Mo. Agr. Exptl. Sta. Res. Bull.* 317.
100. Ratner, A., and J. Meites. 1963. *Amer. J. Physiol.* 204:268.
101. Reineke, E. P., and C. W. Turner. 1942. *Mo. Agr. Exptl. Sta. Res. Bull.* 355.
102. Riddle, O., R. W. Bates, and S. W. Dykshorn. 1933. *Am. J. Physiol.* 105:191.
103. Rivera, E. M. 1964. *Proc. Soc. Exptl. Biol. Med.* 116:568.
104. Rivera, E. M., and H. A. Bern. 1961. *Endocrinology* 69:340.
105. Rivera, E. M., I. A. Forsyth, and S. J. Folley. 1967. *Proc. Soc. Exptl. Biol. Med.* 124:859.
106. Rook, J. A. F., J. E. Storry, and J. V. Wheelock. 1965. *J. Dairy Sci.* 48:745.
107. Schmidt, G. H. 1966. *J. Dairy Sci.* 49:381.
108. Schmidt, G. H., and W. H. Moger. 1967. *Endocrinology* 81:14.
109. Selye, H., J. B. Collip, and D. L. Thomson. 1934. *Endocrinology* 18:237.
110. Stanley, D. E., and R. P. Reece. 1967. *J. Dairy Sci.* 50:972.
111. Stockdale, F. E., W. G. Juergens, and Y. J. Topper. 1966. *Develop. Biol.* 13:266.
112. Stott, G. H., and V. R. Smith. 1957. *J. Dairy Sci.* 40:897.
113. Stricker, P., and F. Grueter. 1928. *C. R. Soc. Biol.* (Paris) 99:1978.
114. Swanson, E. W. 1951. *J. Dairy Sci.* 34:1014.
115. Talwalker, P. K., J. Meites, C. S. Nicoll. 1960. *Amer. J. Physiol.* 199:1070.
116. Thomas, J. W., and L. A. Moore. 1953. *J. Dairy Sci.* 36:657.
117. Turkington, R. W. 1968. *Endocrinology* 82:575.
118. Turkington, R. W., L. Brew, T. C. Vanaman, and R. L. Hill. 1968. *J. Biol. Chem.* 243:3382.
119. Turkington, R. W., and R. L. Hill. 1969. *Science* 163:1458.
120. Wellings, S. R., R. A. Cooper, and E. M. Rivera. 1966. *J. Nat Cancer Inst.* 36:657.
121. Yokoyama, A., and K. Ota. 1965. *J. Endocrinol.* 33:341.

6

NEURAL CONTROL OF LACTATION

The maintenance of lactation in most species is dependent upon a milking or suckling stimulus and the removal of milk from the mammary glands. The nervous system plays a role in both areas. It also controls the blood flow through the mammary gland, thereby regulating the supply of hormones and milk precursors to the gland.

6-1 THE ROLE OF THE MILKING AND SUCKLING STIMULUS IN SECRETION

Mammary gland function is under the hormonal control of the pituitary gland. The central nervous system regulates the activity of the hypothalamo-hypophysial system, which in turn controls the anterior pituitary hormone output. The role of the suckling stimulus in the release of prolactin was first demonstrated by Selye (50), who showed that the suckling stimulus prevented the involution of mammary glands with ligated galactophores. In rats, the periodic replacement of the young with foster litters can provide a continued suckling stimulus that also prolongs lactation. Stimulation of the nipples causes release of prolactin and ACTH by the pituitary gland. Both hormones are involved in milk secretion. The suckling stimulus increases food and water intake, which can also be mediated by electrical stimulation of the appetite and water intake centers in the hypothalamus (12, 38, 39).

The suckling stimulus is required for the maintenance of milk secretion in the rat, but not in all species. In the rabbit, deep anesthesia inhibits efferent stimulus during suckling, but does not inhibit milk secretion if oxytocin is given to induce milk ejection (52).

The nervous connections between the mammary gland and the central nervous system are not necessary for the maintenance of milk secretion in the sheep and goat. This was first demonstrated by Eckard (17), who cut the main nerve supply to one-half of the lactating goat udder and showed that it did not result in a decrease in milk production in comparison to the intact half udder. The isolation of whole or half udders of goats and sheep from the central nervous system has no great effect on lactational performance. Transplantation of mammary glands to other parts of the body does not have a significant effect on milk production. Goats with denervated glands and in which no milk ejection process is observed still produce normal amounts of milk. Goats under deep anesthesia do not require oxytocin injections to produce normal milk yields. Thus the normal milk ejection brought about by oxytocin as a result of afferent nervous stimuli is not necessary for lactation in the goat. The normal milk-ejection reflex in the goat is of importance only in aiding complete emptying of the glands (22, 37, 59).

Cowie and Tindal (8) reviewed the theories to explain how milk secretion is maintained in animals that do not require nervous stimuli from the suckling or milking process. One theory states that the secreting mammary gland consumes prolactin and the decrease in the prolactin content of the blood exerts a feedback effect on the hypothalamo-hypophysial axis independent of the suckling stimulus. A second theory states that the mammary gland secretes a humoral agent into the blood that exerts its effect on the hypothalamus to induce prolactin secretion. A third theory is that oxytocin acts directly on the anterior pituitary gland to induce prolactin release. Another theory is that the anterior pituitary function is influenced through the sympathetic innervation of the pituitary. This means that a nervous stimulation of the pituitary instead of a humoral one induces it to secrete prolactin. An additional theory states that environmental stimuli, such as visual, olfactory, or tactile stimuli, induce the release of pituitary hormones. The evidence for all these theories is limited. Cowie and Tindal propose their own theory, which is that the uptake of milk precursors from the bloodstream by the lactating mammary gland results in a stimulation of the appetite centers in the hypothalamus. The activation of the appetite center or the inhibition of the satiety center may favor the secretion of pituitary hormones that are concerned in the maintenance of lactation. The appetite control centers are located close to the median eminence and the origin of the pituitary portal system.

The nervous system also affects lactation in several other ways: the suckling stimulus is involved in nipple erection; the supply of blood to the glands is influenced by vasomotor nerves; and nervous centers in the brain control appetite and regulate the secretion of anterior pituitary hormones and milk-ejection hormones from the posterior pituitary gland (12).

6-2 NERVOUS INNERVATION OF THE MAMMARY GLAND

Efferent Innervation

The mammary gland develops entirely from cutaneous sources and, because of this, has only somatic sensory and sympathetic motor fibers. Parasympathetic fibers are absent in the general skin areas of the body. Since the perineal nerve arises from the sacral vertebra, some authors have suggested that the mammary glands receive parasympathetic innervation. Cross (12) summarized these results and concluded that recent investigations failed to substantiate the presence of parasympathetic nerve endings in the mammary gland. Stimulation of the perineal nerve causes vasoconstriction of the blood vessels, which can be blocked by sympathetic blocking agents. These results also indicate that the perineal nerves leading to the mammary gland are sympathetic nerve fibers (36).

The study of nerve endings in the mammary gland has received considerable attention over the years. There is a profuse innervation of the teats; however, the data for the innervation of the parenchyma are inconclusive. Russian workers have described an extensive system of both myelinated and unmyelinated fibers within the lobes and lobules, with the nerve endings actually piercing the alveolar membrane. Other nerve fibers also supply blood vessels, the ducts, and the smooth muscle fibers in the mammary gland. Other workers have obtained different results: they state that nerve fibers enter the mammary gland and innervate the muscle fibers within the connective tissues surrounding the lobes and the lobules, the blood vessels, and the adventitial layers of the duct, but that the fibers do not pierce the alveoli. If there is an innervation of the parenchyma, it is not profuse. The evidence for the secretomotor innervation of the mammary gland is not convincing. There is abundant evidence that milk secretion proceeds independently of motor innervation of the mammary glands (1, 12, 20).

Stimulation of the nerves leading to the mammary gland causes a vasoconstriction of the blood vessels. This has a prejudicial effect on milk secretion, because it decreases the blood flow to the mammary gland. The smooth muscles located within the mammary gland are innervated by the sympathetic nervous system. Smooth muscles are very prevalent within the teat and especially around the streak canal as circular muscle fibers. The innervation of the smooth muscles surrounding the teat meatus is important in keeping the meatus closed between milkings. There are also some longitudinal muscles in this area. Abundant smooth muscle fibers are also located in the walls of the teat around the teat cistern, but they become scarcer as the distance from the teat increases. Denervation of the mammary gland causes a dilation of the ducts and relaxation of the smooth muscles. The efferent innervation thus has some control over the duct diameter and teat meatus (12, 20).

Afferent Innervation

The sensory nerve fibers are most common in the teat and are involved in producing the afferent stimuli that initiate milk ejection in most mammals. The sensory stimuli arising from milking or suckling also cause nipple erection, increased food intake, initiation of rumination in goats, and changes in the blood pressure and respiration rate of animals. Receptors responsive to changes in intramammary pressure have been demonstrated. These few receptors are thought to be part of the normal dermal innervation but became enmeshed in the glandular tissue during development. It appears that these receptors are not sufficiently activated by the changes in intramammary pressure within the physiological range to act as the afferent limb of the reflex arcs, even though gross changes from distension to emptiness can probably cause an effect. The existence of chemoreceptors has been postulated, but the evidence for these is far from conclusive (12, 20).

6-3 MILK EJECTION

An integral part of lactation is the milk-removal process, which includes the passive withdrawal of milk from the cisterns and ducts of the mammary gland and the ejection of milk from the alveolar lumen into the ducts. The ejection process involves a neurohormonal reflex.

The neurohormonal reflex theory of milk ejection was first proposed by Ely and Petersen (18). This theory was based upon their work and an evaluation of previous research work. The theory, generally accepted today, is that a nervous stimulus resulting from palpation of the teat, suckling, or other stimuli that a mammal associates with the milking act reaches the central nervous system and causes the posterior lobe of the pituitary to release oxytocin into the blood (Figure 6-1). The oxytocin travels to the mammary gland and contracts the myoepithelial cells, thus forcing the milk from the alveoli into small ductules. This is shown diagrammatically in Figure 6-2. Inhibition of milk ejection is attributed to the presence of adrenalin in the blood.

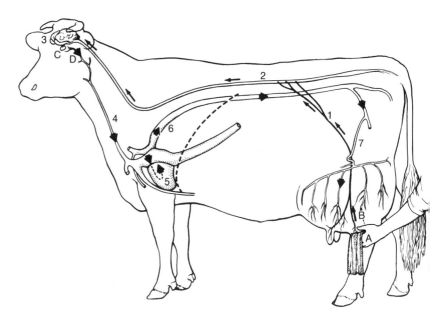

FIGURE 6–1
The neurohormonal reflex of milk ejection. The stimulus (A) that a cow associates with milking causes a nerve impulse (B) to travel via the inguinal nerve (1) to the spinal cord (2) and the brain (3). The brain causes the release of oxytocin (D) from the posterior pituitary (C). Oxytocin is released into a branch of the jugular vein (4) and travels to the heart (5) and is then transported to all parts of the body by the arterial blood. The oxytocin reaching the udder leaves the heart by the aorta (6) and enters the udder through the external pudendal arteries (7). In the udder, it causes the myoepithelial cells to contract, resulting in milk ejection from the alveoli.

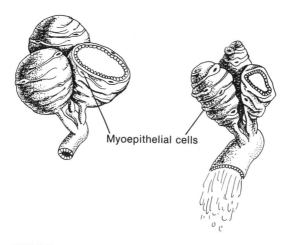

FIGURE 6–2
Milk ejection—the contraction of the myoepithelial
cells surrounding the alveolus forces milk
out of the lumen into the ducts.

Ely and Petersen (18) showed that denervating half of a cow's udder did not cause a decrease in milk production, which indicated that milk ejection was not under the direct control of the central nervous system. Injection of oxytocin after a normal milking caused a more complete evacuation of milk from the udder. Fright and intrajugular injections of adrenalin resulted in the cessation of milk ejection. Further work showed that blood taken from a cow in which milk ejection had occurred caused milk ejection when it was perfused through an isolated bovine udder. Blood from unstimulated cows did not induce milk ejection (45).

Historical Aspects

As early as 1910, Ott and Scott (43) reported that posterior pituitary extracts injected into lactating goats caused milk to flow from cannulated teats. They interpreted this response as a stimulation of milk secretion. In 1915, Gaines (25) showed that the injection of posterior pituitary extracts into goats caused a response similar to that occurring during the milking process. He also showed that anesthesia of a lactating bitch prevented the removal of milk by suckling pups. Milk removal was restored by injecting a posterior pituitary extract. He interpreted his results as a pharmacological result instead of a physiological one. In 1939, Gomez (27, 28) showed that hypophysectomized rats required the injection of a posterior pituitary extract in order for their litters to survive.

Sensory Stimuli

The afferent part of the neurohormonal reflex is a neural one. A considerable amount of work has been done to trace the afferent system through the central nervous system. Only recently has the afferent path been traced through the brain of the guinea pig and rabbit (53, 55). The milk-ejection reflex is a part of a group of neuroendocrine mechanisms that originate as stimuli from the mammary gland receptors and affect the hypothalamus and the anterior pituitary. Among these are a rumination reflex, stimulation of the appetite and thirst centers, variation in the arterial pressures, and influence of the respiratory rhythm. Total section of the spinal cord interrupts the milk-ejection reflex in the rabbit, rat, goat, and cat (16).

The afferent pathway to the hypothalamus passes through the brain stem reticular formation and the nonspecific thalamic nuclei with the exception of the olfactory paths. It is postulated that the afferent impulses of mammary origin are analyzed, integrated, and modulated at several levels before they reach the supraoptic and paraventricular nuclei in the hypothalamus. These levels are the brain stem reticular formation, the limbic system midbrain circuit, and the thalamo-cortical apparatus. These systems condition the ejection reflex that is seen in the lactating humans and animals (16).

The milk-ejection reflex can be modified and/or conditioned. The higher nerve centers apparently condition the release of the milk-ejection hormone as shown in the anticipation of suckling by women, cows, and other lactating females. In the cow the stimuli that produce the milk-ejection reflex are ranked in the following order of importance: (1) showing calf to its mother, (2) washing the udder, (3) combined washing with showing calf to the mother, and (4) suckling by the young. Conditioned afferent stimuli for milk ejection in cows include rattling of milk buckets, washing udders, placing of the feed before the cows, nuzzling of the calves, and approach of the milker. The ejection reflex can be conditioned in women by the sound of a crying baby or by such unrelated stimuli as drinking a glass of liquid. Milk ejection is also brought about by vaginal distension in the ewe and by stimulation of the seminal vesicles and ampullae of the ram when its blood circulation is connected to a ewe (3, 7, 14, 15, 18, 41, 44).

Milk ejection, however, is not necessary for the evacuation of milk from the mammary gland in the goat and the ewe. It has been suggested that the anatomical structure of the mammary gland of the goat and ewe facilitate the drainage of the alveoli into the larger ducts and cisterns. This is because of the large storage area in the ducts, cisterns, and teats and the efficiency of the mechanical massage in emptying the udder. In addition, it is possible that the myoepithelial cells are stimulated by the mechanical massage during the mechanical milking process (8, 16, 37, 59).

Sites of Oxytocin Secretion

The posterior pituitary (neurohypophysis) is entirely nervous in origin and consists of nerve fibers and neurological elements. Nerve fibers reach the posterior pituitary lobe via the hypothalamo-hypophysial tracts from cells in the hypothalamic nuclei (Figure 6-3). The most conspicuous supply of fibers comes from the supraoptic and paraventricular nuclei of the hypothalamus. Up to 90% of the cells in these nuclei disappear if the hypothalamo-hypophysial tract is sectioned. The hormones found in the

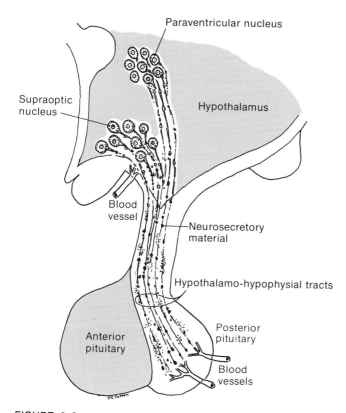

FIGURE 6-3
Hypothalamus and pituitary showing the hypothalamo-hypophysial tracts. (From Hansel. 1961. *Internat. J. Fertil.* 6:241.)

neurohypophysis are transported down the axons. The neurosecretory material can be traced along the axons from the paraventricular and supraoptic nuclei into the neurohypophysis. Sectioning of the pituitary stalk causes an accumulation of the neurosecretory material at the cut ends (12, 49).

Further evidence that the oxytocin is produced in the hypothalamus was obtained by Benson and Cowie (2) who found that oxytocin injections were necessary for normal growth of suckling rats whose dams had their posterior pituitaries removed. The rats were allowed to become pregnant again and during the second lactation they raised their litters without exogeneous oxytocin. Apparently enough regrowth of the neural stalk had taken place to release adequate levels of oxytocin for normal litter growth rate. The mother rats exhibited a mild polyuria, indicating that they still had a deficiency of antidiuretic hormone. The results also indicate that the oxytocin secretion and release are probably independent of vasopressin production and release.

A series of experiments has shown the involvement of the hypothalamo-neurohypophysial system in the secretion of oxytocin and vasopressin. Inhibition of lactation is brought about by either the removal of the posterior pituitary gland, electrolytic lesions placed in the pituitary stalk, sectioning of the pituitary stalk, or electrolytic lesions placed in the supraoptical-hypophysial tract. The milk-ejection reflex can be initiated by the electrical stimulation of the supraoptical-hypophysial tract, stimulation of the supraoptic and paraventricular nuclei in the rabbit, stimulation of the anterior hypothalamus in the conscious sheep and goats despite spinal anesthesia or denervation of the udder, and stimulation of the pituitary stalk or the posterior pituitary in the rabbit. Injection of hypertonic saline solutions into the carotid artery also induces milk ejection in the sheep and goat (3, 12, 16).

Sufficient evidence has been accumulated to indicate that the posterior pituitary hormones are produced by the paraventricular and supraoptic nuclei of the hypothalamus. Some recent evidence indicates that the paraventricular nuclei are especially concerned with oxytocin production; however, the evidence does not provide a decisive argument in favor of a specialization of the hypothalamic nuclei for the secretion of a particular hormone (2, 16, 32).

The mechanism by which nervous stimuli cause a release of the neurohypophysial hormones is not known. The liberation of these hormones is preceded by an increased electrical activity in the supraoptic nuclei, activity which travels to the axonal terminations of the neurohypophysis. Electronmicroscope studies of the neurohypophysis indicate that the liberation of the hormones coincides with a disappearance of the dense material located in the neurosecretory vessels of the cells. Three theories have been proposed to explain how the nerve impulses traveling along the hypothalamo-neurohypophysial tract provide liberation of the hormones. One hypothesis is that acetylcholine, which is secreted at the axonal terminations in the neurohypophysis, is involved in the liberation of oxytocin. The second hypothesis states that the nerve impulse acts on the pituicytes to cause the liberation of the posterior pituitary hormones. A third is that the nervous impulse produces a depolarization of the axonal terminations of the neurohypophysis and permits the entrance of calcium ions. The calcium ions modify the intracellular environment to bring about the release of the hormones (16).

Posterior Pituitary Hormones

The two hormones produced in the hypothalamus and stored in the neurohypophysis are oxytocin and vasopressin. The latter has vasoconstrictor and antidiuretic properties. Oxytocin is a polypeptide hormone containing eight amino acids with a molecular weight of approximately 1,000. It has a cyclic structure as a result of a disulfide bridge between the two cystine molecules. The oxytocin molecule was first synthesized by duVigneaud and associates (58).

Vasopressin also has some milk-ejection capabilities, but oxytocin is about five to six times more active than vasopressin. The milk-ejection stimulus also causes a preferential release of oxytocin, as indicated by the fact that the suckling stimulus in the rabbit causes a release of approximately 100 times more oxytocin than vasopressin. Also, stimulation of the afferent path of the milk-ejection reflex in the midbrain and hypothalamus in the guinea pig causes the release of oxytocin without detectable release of vasopressin. It is unlikely that vasopressin plays any part in the normal milk-ejection process. A number of analogues have been synthesized and have been shown to have some milk-ejection properties; they are less active, however, than the natural hormone in the contraction of myoepithelial cells. It is questionable whether these are involved in the normal milk-ejection process (11, 12, 16, 54).

Blood Oxytocin Levels

Assay Methods   The amount of oxytocin in the bloodstream after milk ejection has been estimated in two ways. In one method, oxytocin is injected to increase intramammary pressure or to allow suckling young to obtain normal amounts of milk from anesthetized dams. The amount of oxytocin required is dependent upon the route of administration, i.e., intramuscular, intraperitoneal, or intravenous, the stage of lactation, and the species. On the basis of body weight, the rat liberates approximately three times as much oxytocin from the posterior pituitary as the rabbit and the goat, 15 times as much as the sow, and approximately 50 times as much as the cow and dog (16).

The second method involves the measurement of the blood oxytocin concentrations by removing blood samples and testing them in a biological assay. The biological systems that have been used are contraction of isolated rat uteri, mammary gland pressure measurements in rabbit, rat, and guinea pig after arterial injection of the compound, and ejection of milk from isolated pieces of lactating rat mammary gland tissue and strips of rabbit and rat mammary gland tissue (4, 16, 23, 33, 56, 57).

Oxytocin Levels   Numerous papers report the measurements of oxytocin levels in the blood of animals during milk ejection and parturition. Most of these reports suffer from a lack of sensitive assay methods. In many assays, the oxytocin must be extracted and purified, but these procedures do not produce a chemically pure product. A recent assay reported by Van Dongen and Hays (57) shows much promise as an assay for measuring blood oxytocin concentrations. It is sensitive in a range of 10^{-2} through 10^{-10} IU/ml of solution. One problem in the assay procedures is the fact that a very small amount of oxytocin induces milk ejection, indicating the high potency of the hormone. At little as 0.002 μg of oxytocin induces milk ejection in rabbits (12).

Measurements of blood oxytocin levels have shown that milking or suckling causes a marked increase in the blood oxytocin concentration in the ewe, cow, goat, and sow. The amount of oxytocin liberated during suckling of the rabbit depends upon the intensity of the stimulus, since the amount released by the doe increases as the young become more mature. The amount of oxytocin released is also related to the size of the litter, but is independent of the amount of milk present in the mammary gland (7, 21, 23, 24, 31, 40, 46).

The amount of oxytocin in the blood is also dependent upon the time interval after the release from the neurohypophysis. This is an important aspect in dairy cattle management since the milking machine is applied after the milk-ejection process has been induced. The decline in the oxytocin level is due to either an elimination of the oxytocin from the bloodstream or a destruction of the oxytocin in the body. Oxytocinase has been demonstrated in lactating women, but is absent from the blood of the lactating rat, rabbit, dog, ewe, and cow (16).

Momongan and Schmidt (40) measured the blood oxytocin concentrations of Holstein cows with and without udder washing and foremilking. The blood levels of oxytocin of cows whose udders were washed reached peak concentrations one minute after application of the milking machine (Figure 6-4). Thereafter, the concentration fell rapidly to undetectable amounts at 5 minutes after teat cup application. When cows were milked without udder preparation, the application of the teat cups acted as the stimulus for milk ejection and the peak oxytocin concentrations occurred 1 to 2 minutes after teat cup application. Cows not stimulated for milk ejection gave the same amount of milk as those with normal udder preparation. There were no significant differences in peak levels of oxytocin between the cows with udder preparation and those with no preparation.

Half-life of Oxytocin   The half-life of oxytocin in the blood has been measured by various workers (Table 6-1). Oxytocin is eliminated from the blood by the kidneys and liver in the rat, rabbit, cow, and ewe. In the rat, the half-life of oxytocin was found to increase from 1.65 to 2.12 minutes after the splanchnic vascular area was tied off. Removal of the kidneys resulted in an increase in the half-life to 2.95 minutes. In lactating rats with kidneys removed and the splanchnic vascular tied off, the oxytocin continued to disappear from the blood; this was attributed to its uptake by the mammary gland. In nonpregnant animals with kidneys removed and the splanchnic vascular beds tied off, the oxytocin concen-

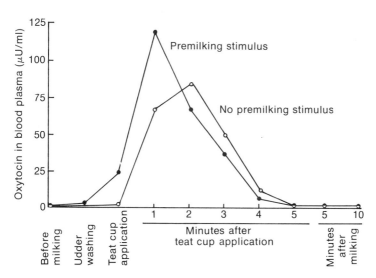

FIGURE 6-4
Blood plasma oxytocin (microunits/ml) of Holstein cows before, during, and after milking when they were milked with and without a premilking stimulus. (From Momongan and Schmidt. 1970. *J. Dairy Sci.* 53:747.)

tration in the blood fell for the first 10 minutes and then reached equilibrium. The initial decrease was thought to be due to the oxytocin reaching an equilibrium with the extravascular spaces. The uterine muscle also metabolizes oxytocin during the last third of gestation. Elimination of oxytocin in the milk does not appear to represent an important path for the elimination of oxytocin in the cow or goat (16, 26, 42, 48).

TABLE 6-1
Half-life (in minutes) of oxytocin
in the bloodstream.

Species and condition	Half-life
Female rat	
In estrous	1.73
Lactating	1.19
Pregnant	2.01
Male rat	1.65
Female rabbit	3.30
Female cat	8.50
Female goat	1.23
Cow	1.08–1.58
Ewe	<1.0

Source: Denamur. 1965. *Dairy Sci. Abstr.* 27:193.

Myoepithelial Cells

The final component of the neurohormonal milk-ejection reflex is the myoepithelial cells in the mammary gland. Ely and Petersen (18) speculated on the existence of the specialized musculature surrounding the alveoli and small ductules, but the presence of myoepithelial cells was first demonstrated by Richardson (47) in 1949. He used a special silver impregnation technique and demonstrated that the myoepithelial cells were abundant in the mammary gland and in close relationship to the alveoli, interlobular ducts, and cisterns. The smooth muscles were shown to be too sparsely located throughout the mammary gland to bring about milk ejection. He postulated that the myoepithelial cells were the contractile units within the mammary gland; this was not proven, however, until Linzell (35) showed that the mammary alveoli contracted in the living mouse in direct response to the topic application of oxytocin.

The presence of myoepithelial cells in the mammary gland of many species has been confirmed by a number of workers using the silver impregnation technique as well as histochemical methods to show the alkaline phosphatase in the myoepithelial cells. The activation of the myoepithelial cells causes contraction of the alveoli, which is accompanied by a widening of the ducts. There is little doubt that the myoepithelial cells are the contractile units within the mammary gland. There is no unequivical evidence about the innervation of the myoepithelial cells, but the compelling experimental evidence is against the view that the myoepithelial cells are under direct efferent control. It appears that myoepithelial cells are under hormonal control and that the motor innervation of the mammary gland plays no part in normal milk ejection (1, 3, 12, 13, 20, 34, 51).

The mode of action of oxytocin on the myoepithelial cells is not known. Denamur (16) suggests that the first stage of hormone action is the formation of a disulphide bond between the oxytocin molecule and the protein of the specific receptors, i.e., the myoepithelial cells. Little is known about the effect beyond this particular stage.

The myoepithelial cells in mice, rats, and goats are also sensitive to mechanical stimulation. The milk-ejection response can be produced by mechanical stimulation in the presence of general anesthesia, local mammary gland anesthesia, and intense vasoconstriction of the mammary gland blood vessels. During active suckling, both the mechanical and oxytocic stimulation of the myoepithelial cells appear to contract the alveoli and increase the diameter of the ducts to produce a high rate of milk flow to the exterior of the gland (9, 19, 20).

Inhibition of Milk Ejection

From the work of Ely and Petersen (18) and the many observations in lactating dairy animals and humans, it is known that fright and stress interfere with the milk-ejection process. Fright and stress activate the neuroadrenal system and cause the release of adrenalin. Fright induced by the exploding of paper bags or placing a cat on the cow's back inhibit the milk-ejection reflex. Injection of adrenalin was found to interfere with the milk ejection in the same manner as fright. Emotional disturbance in lactating women, such as embarrassment, pain, or discomfort also blocks milk ejection (41).

The inhibitory effect of adrenalin on milk ejection occurs both centrally in the brain and in the mammary gland. Adrenalin and noradrenalin intervene at several points of the central nervous system, such as the synaptic transmission of the supraoptic nuclei, the posterior hypothalamus, and at the level of the mesencephalic reticulum. The peripheral inhibitory effect is twofold. One inhibition is brought about by the vasoconstriction of the blood vessels leading to the mammary gland; this prevents the oxytocin from reaching the myoepithelial cells. The second is a direct inhibitory effect on the myoepithelial cells in which adrenalin acts as a physiological antagonist to oxytocin. Adrenalin injections to lactating animals before oxytocin injections causes vasoconstriction of the blood vessels by its actions on the α-receptors, probably located in the mammary blood vessels. When oxytocin and adrenalin are injected simultaneously, the inhibitory effect on milk ejection is mediated through the β-receptors, which are most likely situated in the myoepithelial cells. When agents blocking β-receptors are injected with adrenalin and oxytocin, a normal milk ejection occurs. On the other hand, adrenalin neither prevents contraction of the myoepithelial cells in living mouse mammary gland tissue when the oxytocin is applied topically nor inhibits the milk-ejection response to mechanical tap stimuli applied to the mammary gland (5, 12, 16, 35).

Stimulation of the sympathetic nerves to the mammary gland causes the same inhibitory effect on milk ejection as the intravenous injection of adrenalin. Placing rabbits and guinea pigs on their backs prevents the milk-ejection process, even though the young are allowed to suckle. Other environmental factors that interfere with milk ejection are the odor of oil of peppermint, intermittent bright light, and intermittent low intensity sounds in rats (6, 10, 29, 35).

6-4 SUMMARY

The maintenance of lactation in most species requires a milking or suckling stimulus and the removal of milk from the mammary glands. The nervous system plays a role in both factors. The suckling stimulus is involved in release of prolactin and ACTH from the pituitary gland. Both hormones are involved in milk secretion. The suckling stimulus also increases food and water intake of the animal and is involved in nipple erection in some species. The nervous connections between the mammary gland and the central nervous system are not necessary for the maintenance of milk secretion in the sheep and goat. Mammary glands that have been denervated or transplanted to other parts of the body are capable of producing normal amounts of milk.

Innervation of the Mammary Gland

The efferent innervation of the mammary gland is entirely sympathetic in origin. Stimulation of the nerves leading to the mammary gland causes a vasoconstriction of the blood vessels, which has a prejudicial effect on milk secretion because the blood flow to the mammary gland is decreased. The preponderance of evidence indicates that the efferent nerve fibers innervate the muscle fibers within the connective tissue surrounding the lobes and lobules, the blood vessels, the adventitial layers of the duct, but the fibers do not pierce the alveoli. The efferent fibers apparently play an important role in innervating the smooth muscles within the teat and especially those around the teat meatus to keep it closed between milkings.

The afferent innervation arises primarily from the sensory nerve fibers in the teat and skin and are involved in the initiation of the milk-ejection process. Even though receptors responsive to changes in intramammary pressure have been demonstrated, they are not sufficiently activated by changes in mammary gland pressure within the physiological range to act as the stimulus for milk ejection.

Milk Ejection

The removal of milk from the mammary gland of most species is dependent upon the neurohormonal reflex process of milk ejection. This results from a nervous stimulus that an animal associates with the milking or suckling process, such as palpation of the teats or suckling of the young. This stimulus reaches the central nervous system and causes the posterior lobe of the pituitary to release oxytocin. The oxytocin travels via the blood to the mammary gland and there contracts the myoepithelial cell. The contraction process forces the milk from the alveoli into the duct system, through which it flows to the gland and teat cisterns. Adrenalin inhibits the process.

The posterior pituitary hormones are produced in the hypothalamus and travel to the posterior pituitary, where they are stored until they are released. The paraventricular nuclei are especially concerned with oxytocin production, but the supraoptic nuclei may also be involved. The two hormones produced in the hypothalamus are oxytocin and vasopressin. Oxytocin contains eight amino acids and has a molecular weight of approximately 1,000. Vasopressin is a similar molecule and has some oxytocic properties; oxytocin, however, appears to be five to six times more active in milk ejection. During milk ejection, considerably more oxytocin is released than vasopressin.

The measurement of oxytocin levels in the bloodstream has been of limited success because of a lack of sensitive bioassay methods. Recent evidence does indicate that the milking or suckling stimulus causes a marked increase in the blood oxytocin concentrations in mammals. The amount of oxytocin in the bloodstream disappears quite rapidly after it has been released. This is brought about either by the destruction of the oxytocin in the body or by the elimination of the oxytocin from the blood. The kidneys, liver, and mammary gland are mainly involved in removing the oxytocin from the bloodstream.

The contractile tissue within the mammary gland is the myoepithelial cell. Myoepithelial cells surround the alveoli, the interlobular ducts, and the cisterns. The myoepithelial cells contract in response to oxytocin. The contraction is accompanied by an increase in the diameter of the ducts in order to produce a high rate of milk flow to the exterior of the gland. The preponderance of evidence indicates that the myoepithelial cells are under direct hormonal control and the motor innervation of the cells plays no part in normal milk ejection. The smooth muscles are too sparsely located throughout the mammary gland to be important in the normal milk-ejection process.

The milk-ejection process is inhibited by the release of adrenalin, which can be brought about by fright and emotional disturbances. The inhibitory effect of adrenalin can occur both centrally in the brain and in the mammary gland. Adrenalin intervenes at several points of the central nervous system to prevent the release of oxytocin. Adrenalin also causes vasoconstriction of the blood vessels leading to the mammary gland, thus preventing the oxytocin from reaching the myoepithelial cells. In addition, adrenalin can act as an antagonist to oxytocin, probably by its effect on the β-receptors that are most likely located in the myoepithelial cells.

REFERENCES

1. Ballantyne, B., and G. A. Bunch. 1966. *J. Comp. Neurol.* 127:471.
2. Benson, G. K., and A. T. Cowie. 1956. *J. Endocrinol.* 14:54.
3. Benson, G. K., and R. J. Fitzpatrick. 1966. In G. W. Harris and B. T. Donovan, eds., *The Pituitary Gland,* Vol. 3. Berkeley: Univ. Calif. Press. Ch. 15.
4. Bisset, G. W., B. J. Clark, J. Haldar, M. C. Harris, G. P. Lewis, and M. Rocha e Silva, Jr. 1967. *Brit. J. Pharmacol. Chemother.* 31:537.
5. Bisset, G. W., B. J. Clark, and G. P. Lewis. 1967. *Brit. J. Pharmacol. Chemother.* 31:550
6. Chaudhury, R. R., M. R. Chaudhury, and F. C. Lu. 1961. *Brit. J. Pharmacol.* 17:305.
7. Cleverley, J. D. 1968. *J. Endocrinol.* 40:ii.

8. Cowie, A. T., and J. S. Tindal. 1964. *Proc. 2nd Intern. Congr. Endocrinol.,* pp. 646–654.

9. Cross, B. A. 1954. *Nature* (London) 173:450.

10. Cross, B. A. 1955. *J. Endocrinol.* 12:29.

11. Cross, B. A. 1955. *Brit. Med. Bull.* 11:151.

12. Cross, B. A. 1961. In S. K. Kon and A. T. Cowie, eds., *Milk: The Mammary Gland and Its Secretion.* Vol. I. New York: Academic Press. Ch. 6.

13. Cross, B. A., R. F. W. Goodwin, and I. A. Silver. 1958. *J. Endocrinol.* 17:63.

14. Debackere, M., and G. Peeters. 1960. *Naturwissenschaften* 47:189.

15. Debackere, M., and G. Peeters. 1960. *Naturwissenschaften* 47:329.

16. Denamur, R. 1965. *Dairy Sci. Abstr.* 27:193, 263.

17. Eckard, C. 1858. *Beitr. Anat. Physiol.* 1:1.

18. Ely, F., and W. E. Petersen. 1941. *J. Dairy Sci.* 24:211.

19. Findlay, A. L. R., and C. E. Grosvenor. 1967. *Proc. Soc. Exptl. Biol. Med.* 126:637.

20. Findlay, A. L. R., and C. E. Grosvenor. 1969. *Dairy Sci. Abstr.* 31:109.

21. Fitzpatrick, R. J. 1961. In R. Caldeyro-Barcia and H. Heller, eds., *Oxytocin.* Oxford: Pergamon Press. pp. 358–379.

22. Folley, S. J. 1961. *Dairy Sci. Abstr.* 23:511.

23. Folley, S. J., and G. S. Knaggs. 1966. *J. Endocrinol.* 34:197.

24. Fuchs, A.-R., and G. Wagner. 1963. *Acta Endocrinol.* 44:581.

25. Gaines, W. L. 1915. *Amer. J. Physiol.* 38:285.

26. Ginsburg, M., and M. W. Smith. 1959. *Brit. J. Pharmacol.* 14:327.

27. Gomez, E. T. 1939. *J. Dairy Sci.* 22:488.

28. Gomez, E. T. 1940. *J. Dairy Sci.* 23:237.

29. Grosvenor, C. E., and F. Mena. 1967. *Endocrinology* 80:840.

30. Hansel, W. 1961. *Intern. J. Fertil.* 6:241.

31. Hawker, R. W., and V. S. Roberts. 1957. *Brit. Vet. J.* 113:459.

32. Heller, H. 1966. *Brit. Med. Bull.* 22:227.

33. Holton, P. 1948. *Brit. J. Pharmacol.* 3:328.

34. Linzell, J. L. 1952. *J. Anat.* 86:49.

35. Linzell, J. L. 1955. *J. Physiol.* 130:257.

36. Linzell, J. L. 1959. *Quart. J. Exptl. Physiol.* 44:160.

37. Linzell, J. L. 1963. *Quart. J. Exptl. Physiol.* 48:34.

38. Meites, J. 1959. In H. H. Cole and P. T. Cupps, eds., *Reproduction in Domestic Animals,* Vol. I. New York: Academic Press. Ch. 16.

39. Meites, J. 1966. *Neuroendocrinology,* Vol. I. New York. Academic Press.

40. Momongan, V. G., and G. H. Schmidt. 1970. *J. Dairy Sci.* 53:747.

41. Newton, M. 1961. In S. K. Kon and A. T. Cowie, eds., *Milk: The Mammary Gland and Its Secretion,* Vol. I. New York: Academic Press. Ch. 7.

42. Noddle, B. A. 1962. *Intern. Congr. Physiol. Sci.,* Leiden, 2:523.

43. Ott, I., and J. C. Scott. 1910. *Proc. Soc. Exptl. Biol. Med.* N. Y., 8:48.

44. Peeters, G., H. Stormorken, and F. Vanschoubroek. 1960. *J. Endocrinol.* 20:163.

45. Petersen, W. E., and T. M. Ludwick. 1942. *Federation Proc.* 1.66.

46. Pritchard, D. E., and R. L. Hays. 1966. *J. Dairy Sci.* 49:736.

47. Richardson, K. C. 1949. *Proc. Royal Soc.* (London), Ser. B, 136:30.

48. Sawyer, W. H. 1954. *Proc. Soc. Exptl. Biol. Med.* 87:463.

49. Scharrer, E., and B. Scharrer. 1954. *Recent Progr. Hormones Res.* 10: 183.
50. Selye, H. 1934. *Amer. J. Physiol.* 107:535.
51. Silver, I. A. 1954. *J. Physiol.* 125:8p.
52. Tindal, J. S., C. Beyer, and C. H. Sawyer. 1963. *Endocrinology* 72:720.
53. Tindal, J. S., G. S. Knaggs, and A. Turvey. 1967. *J. Endocrinol.* 38:337.
54. Tindal, J. S., G. S. Knaggs, and A. Turvey. 1968. *J. Endocrinol.* 40:205.
55. Tindal, J. S., G. S. Knaggs, and A. Turvey. 1969. *J. Endocrinol.* 43:663.
56. Tindal, J. S., and A. Yokoyama. 1962. *Endocrinology* 71:196.
57. Van Dongen, C. G., and R. L. Hays. 1966. *Endocrinology* 78:1.
58. Vigneaud, V. du, C. Ressler. J. M. Swan, C. W. Roberts, P. G. Katsoyannis, and S. Gordon. 1953. *J. Amer. Chem. Soc.* 75:4879.
59. Yokoyama, A., and K. Ôta. 1965. *J. Endocrinol.* 33:341.

7

MAMMARY GLAND INVOLUTION

After the peak yield in milk secretion, which usually occurs within a few days or weeks after parturition in most species, a decrease in milk secretion takes place. This decrease is primarily due to the involution of the mammary gland tissue. Involution results in a decrease in the number of secretory cells in the mammary gland tissue. Part of the reduction in milk yield after peak lactation may also be due to a reduction in secretion rate for each remaining cell.

An almost complete involution of secretory tissue takes place after the cessation of milking or the suckling of young. This induced involution is a much more drastic form of involution than the process that takes place during lactation. After the cessation of milking or suckling of young, there is a very rapid disappearance of the secretory cells and a degeneration of the alveolar and lobular structures.

If hormonal, nutritional, environmental, or other factors could be found to eliminate or reduce the involutional process in animals kept for milk production purposes, it would greatly affect the efficiency of milk production and change the dairy industry. Under most dairy farm conditions, cows are bred to calve at approximately yearly intervals in order to take advantage of the high milk yields in early lactation. If this high milk yield could be retained for longer periods of time, it would markedly increase the milk production per cow and would result in longer lactation periods and fewer dry periods.

7-1 HISTOLOGICAL CHANGES

Mammary gland involution in the cow results in a progressive regression of tissue from the periphery of the gland towards the gland cisterns. Entire lobes and lobules degenerate at a time, instead of a degeneration of individual epithelial cells. Histological sections of cow, goat, and guinea pig mammary tissue show that involution is characterized by a decrease in the size of the alveoli, a decrease in the number of alveoli per lobule, a decrease in the total number of alveoli and lobular volume, a decrease in the number of cells per alveolus, and an increase in the height of the alveolar cells. The connective tissue either proliferates or becomes more obvious, the alveoli appear collapsed and folded, and complete lobules appear to disintegrate in parts of the udder (19, 35, 45).

The involuted bovine mammary gland is characterized by lobules that are reduced to a few branching ductules with loose but highly vascular intralobular connective tissue. The essential lobular structure of the gland is still recognizable; it is not so in the virgin gland (22). A photograph of involuted tissue is shown in Figure 7-1. Figure 7-2 shows lobules of involuted tissue (b) next to several lobules of tissue that are still secreting milk (a).

Changes in alveolar surface area of goat mammary glands are related to the decrease in milk production with advancing lactation (35). A high correlation exists between the alveolar surface area of goat udders during lactation and the milk production of the udders prior to their removal. The decrease in the amount of secretory tissue therefore plays a major role in determining the level of milk production after the peak of lactation. The amount of DNA in the mammary gland during various stages of lactation has been measured in the guinea pig, rabbit, rat, and mouse, and in all cases, a decrease in the total DNA content occurs after the peak of lactation, indicating a decrease in the number of cells (7, 9, 12, 15, 16, 29, 30, 31, 33, 41).

The decrease in the number of epithelial cells after the peak of lactation is not the only factor causing involution, because the hormones somatotrophin and thyroxine stimulate milk secretion during the declining phase of lactation. This indicates that the rate of activity of the cells can be

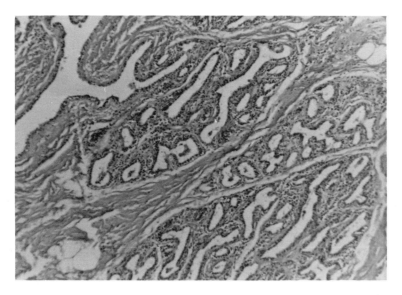

FIGURE 7–1
Mammary gland tissue from an involuted goat udder.

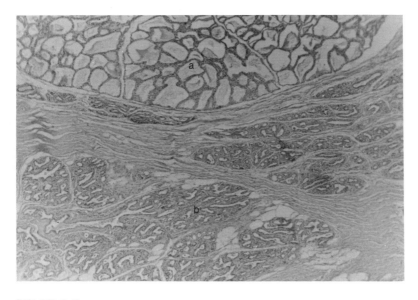

FIGURE 7–2
Lobules of secretory tissue (a) still secreting milk next to lobules
that have involuted (b) in the goat udder.

stimulated, since the response occurs before an appreciable number of new cells can be formed. The amount of milk secreted per gram of mammary tissue decreases with advancing lactation. The RNA:DNA ratio in rat mammary tissue decreases after the 21st day of lactation. The declining ratio indicates a decrease in protein synthesis per cell (21, 41, 42).

The cause of the decrease in the epithelial cell numbers in the mammary gland during involution is not known. A decrease in the hormonal stimulus for milk production after peak lactation is a possible explanation. Another is that the accumulation of milk in the gland leads to a degeneration of some of the cells. When the young become mature enough to eat solid feed, less milk is consumed and it begins to accumulate in the gland. This explanation does not apply to the dairy cow in which the milk removal is not dependent upon the nursing of the calf.

No possible way has yet been found to increase the number of cells in the mammary gland after the peak of lactation or to maintain the number of epithelial cells. If ways could be found to either prevent the degeneration of existing epithelial cells or cause a marked mitosis after the peak of lactation, a decline in milk production could probably be prevented.

The involution occurring after the cessation of milking or suckling is much more abrupt and is brought about in part by the accumulation of milk in the alveoli and ducts. The accumulation of secretory products increases the pressure in the cells and causes a degeneration of the secretory tissue. The degenerated secretory cells are sloughed off into the milk. The involution continues until the gland is similar to that of the virgin animal; however, it does not completely regress to the virgin state.

Definite changes in the mammary gland epithelium of rats occur after the teats have been ligated. Acute mammary engorgement causes an enlargement of alveoli and deformation of the epithelial cells. Irreversible changes take place in the cytoplasm with regression of the epithelium. The damage is attributable to an interference with the blood supply to the gland epithelium. Increasing pressure in the alveoli causes rupture of the cytoplasm and damage to the basal membrane. This in turn allows the secretion to move into the interstitial tissue where phagocytosis and breakdown of milk components take place. Resorption of the secretion brings about cytolysis. These changes are similar to the changes that occur during physiological involution following lactation. Similar results have been observed in the pig in which alveolar collapse and solidification occur within 24 hours after occlusion of one teat. By 48 hours the alveolar lumina were largely obscured by degenerated epithelial cells swollen with fat (2, 10).

Light and electron microscopy of mouse, rat, and rabbit mammary gland tissue shortly after the cessation of suckling reveals a decrease in the amount of epithelial tissue, an increase in the stromal adipose tissue, accumulation of fat and protein droplets in the epithelial cells, and vacuolization of the cells. The reduction in epithelial tissue is caused by a decrease in cellular volume and localized degeneration of cells without rupture of the duct system. The myoepithelial cells do not undergo degeneration and play an important role in bridging the gap where necrotic cells have been eliminated to hold the surviving cells together. The stored secretory materials are digested without participation of the lysosomes. The decrease in the cellular volume in surviving cells and the degeneration of the dying cells involve the participation of the lyosomes. The amount of endoplasmic reticulum and Golgi apparatus disappears rapidly and free ribosomes appear. The dying cells become vacuolated and are either eliminated as colostrum bodies into the alveolar lumina or lysed and eliminated in the interstitial tissue. By the 5th day of involution in the mouse, nuclei, mitochondria, fat droplets, and other structures are released into the alveoli and ducts. By the 15th day of involution, only small ducts with intact cells are present (17, 47, 49).

The onset of induced involution is also characterized by a drop in the RNA content and a reduction in the RNA:DNA ratio, which soon returns to the ratio of the virgin state. The DNA content of the mammary glands continues to decrease and at 5 days following weaning in mice, the level has decreased 53% in comparison to 20-day lactating mice (1, 11, 37, 43).

7-2 BIOCHEMICAL CHANGES

Biochemical alterations of the mammary gland occur within hours after the cessation of suckling or milking. The metabolic activity of the mammary gland begins to decrease within 8–12 hours after the young are removed. This is shown by a decrease in the respiratory quotient and an accumulation of lactic acid in the mammary gland tissues. Shortly after weaning, there is a considerable increase in mammary gland weight, lactose content, and DNA content. The increased DNA content appears to be correlated with an increase in the leucocyte content of the involuting gland. An increase in the free ribonuclease and B-glucoronidase contents during early induced involution also occurs, which may be due to the bursting of lysomal particles during early involution (28, 37, 38, 51).

Ligated mammary glands lose their ability to incorporate fatty acids, acetate, and glucose into lipids even though the remaining mammary glands are suckled. This is also accompanied by a reduction in the oxidation of glucose. Dephosphorylation of the nucleotides, especially adenosine diphosphate (ADP) and adenosine triphosphate (ATP), takes place within 12 hours after weaning of rats (20, 23, 48).

The oxidative phosphorylation of guinea pig mitochondria is uncoupled within 12–24 hours after the young are removed. The coupling of oxidation of compounds with the phosphorylation of ADP is the method used by the cell to convert the chemical energy of substrates into a form of energy that can be used for the energy-requiring reactions carried on by the cell. The uncoupling process is complete at 25 hours after the last suckling. Mitochondrial and microsomal fractions from involuting mammary glands completely uncouple phosphorylation of mitochondria obtained from rat liver. The upcoupling of oxidative phosphorylation of nonlactating mammary gland mitochondria is due to long-chain unesterified fatty acids, with oleic acid being the most effective uncoupler. The regression of the mammary gland tissue is associated with an irreversible alteration of the respiratory chain. A three-fold increase in the activity of oleic-acid-activating enzyme is present in lactating tissue as compared to involuted tissue. It may be that part of the process of preventing involution is that of preventing the accumulation of oleic acid or other fatty acids in the mammary gland tissue (8, 32).

7-3 RELATION OF THE SUCKLING STIMULUS TO INVOLUTION

The suckling stimulus plays an important role in the maintenance of lactation. This was first demonstrated by Selye (36) who ligated some of the teats of the rat and allowed the young to suckle the remaining teats. The secretory state of the ligated mammary glands was maintained. He postulated that these effects were due to the release of prolactin from the anterior pituitary gland. Nonstimulated mammary glands showed complete involution. Similar results have been shown in the dairy goat (46). The involution of unsuckled lactating mammary glands can be retarded by the administration of prolactin (18, 50).

The suckling stimulus is also involved in the maintenance of the nucleic acid content of the lactating rat mammary gland. The amount of DNA in the mammary gland on the 21st day of lactation increases with the number of suckling young. Maintaining a strong suckling stimulus through the use of foster litters maintains the mammary gland DNA content through 61 days and the integrity of the lobulo-alveolar system through 70 days postpartum, but the protein synthetic activity, as measured by the RNA:DNA ratio, declines after 21 days postpartum. These results indicate that the involution process is a result of reduced cell numbers as well as a reduced functional activity of the cells (39, 40, 42). The suckling stimulus without milk removal neither prevents cellular loss nor maintains the protein synthetic activity of the mammary gland. Ligated abdominal inguinal mammary glands of rats show a decrease in DNA and RNA contents and a decrease in the RNA:DNA ratio in comparison to the contralateral nonligated glands of the normal lactating rats. These results show that the nursing stimulus is necessary for the maintenance of the secretory activity, presumably through prolactin release, and the removal of secretory products is necessary to maintain the biochemical integrity of the gland (30, 44).

7-4 RETARDATION OF INVOLUTION

The involution of rat mammary glands that normally occurs after the cessation of milking is markedly retarded by oxytocin injections (Table 7-1). The retardation of involution does not occur in the absence of the pituitary. An extract of the natural hormone, synthetic oxytocin, and a synthetic analogue (valyl oxytocin) are all effective in retarding involution. Vasopressin gives a less well-marked effect. The evidence was interpreted to indicate that oxytocin evokes the release of prolactin from the anterior pituitary (4, 5, 6). A number of papers have reported similar

TABLE 7-1
Effect of pituitary hormone treatment for 9 days on the percentage parenchyma of mammary glands of lactating rats after the removal of litters.

Treatment	Daily dose	Percentage parenchyma
Controls	—	18.8
Oxytocin	4.5 IU	46.7
Oxytocin	3.0 IU	40.0
Oxytocin	0.75 IU	43.8
Prolactin	100 IU	48.1
STH	1.00 mg	27.7
STH and Prolactin	1.0 mg 100 IU	78.1
Vasopressin	3.0 IU	36.1

Source: Benson and Folley, 1957. *J. Endocrinol.* 16:189.

results, but the authors did not support the hypothesis. Another interpretation of the data is that the oxytocin causes a direct release of milk from
the alveoli into the ducts and stromal tissue, where it can be absorbed.
This permits more milk to be synthesized and helps to maintain the structural integrity of the tissue (25, 26).

Biochemical evidence also rejects the prolactin-release hypothesis. Rats
whose litters had been removed were injected with oxytocin and prolactin
(Table 7-2). Oxytocin preserved the structural integrity of the mammary
tissue as indicated by the DNA content and persistent alveolar structure
but failed to maintain the functional state of the tissue. Prolactin prevented the degeneration of the tissue structure as well as maintaining the
functional activity of the gland as measured by the RNA content and the
RNA:DNA ratio. Similar results have been obtained in rabbits; however,
the RNA:DNA ratio of prolactin-treated rabbits was considerably higher
than the oxytocin-treated ones, but somewhat below those of rabbits that
were continued to be suckled. Mammary gland slices of rats treated with
oxytocin and prolactin after the removal of litters consume less oxygen
and produce more lactic acid than slices from lactating rats (13, 34, 51).

TABLE 7-2
Effect of oxytocin and prolactin administration for 3 days on the nucleic acid
content of mammary glands after the removal of litters.

Daily hormone treatment	DNA (mg/gland)	RNA (mg/gland)	RNA/DNA
Lactating controls	0.86	3.08	3.67
Controls (litters removed)	0.38	0.42	1.13
Oxytocin (3 IU)	0.48	0.54	1.16
Oxytocin (6 IU)	0.52	0.42	0.82
Prolactin (0.1 IU)	0.45	0.41	0.99
Prolactin (1.0 IU)	0.39	0.57	1.51
Prolactin (10 IU)	0.55	0.96	1.76
Prolactin (50 IU)	0.59	0.94	1.69
Prolactin (100 IU)	0.83	1.16	1.39

Source: Ôta et al. 1965. *Endocrinology* 76:1.

Reserpine, acetylcholine, serotonin, and epinephrine also prevent
involution of mammary gland tissue after the cessation of suckling. These
compounds are believed to have their effect through the hypothalamus
and cause an increased prolactin secretion by the pituitary gland (3, 24,
27). Reserpine also prevents the decline in DNA levels that normally

occurs during the first 24 hours after the cessation of suckling. This decline is prevented for 4 days; however, reserpine does not maintain the gland in a normal functional state. Reserpine may also stimulate ACTH secretion, which increases the amount of adrenal corticoids, which are also essential for milk secretion (3, 11, 14).

7-5 SUMMARY

Involution of the mammary gland takes place after the peak of lactation and after the cessation of the milking process or the suckling of the young. The cessation of milk removal has a more drastic effect on the involution process than that due to natural involution after the peak of lactation. Involution is due to a combination of decreases in cell numbers and the secretion rate of the remaining cells.

The histological changes during involution in the cow, goat, and guinea pig are characterized by a decrease in the size of the alveoli, a decrease in the number of alveoli per lobule, a decrease in the total number of alveoli and lobular volume, and a decrease in the number of cells per alveolus. Complete lobules also disintegrate in parts of the mammary gland during advancing involution. At the end of involution, the gland takes on the appearance of that of the virgin animal, but the essential lobular structure of the gland is still recognizable (it is not recognizable in the virgin state).

The engorgement of the mammary gland after the cessation of milking or suckling causes irreversible changes to take place in the cytoplasm of the epithelial cells. The changes are due to the interference with the blood supply to the gland epithelium. The accumulated milk products cause the alveoli to rupture and damage the basal membrane, damage which allows the secretion to move into the interstitial tissue. Here phagocytosis causes the breakdown of milk components. The cellular components degenerate with the participation of the lysosomes of the cell. The myoepithelial cells apparently do not undergo degeneration and are important in bridging the gap to hold the surviving cells together after the necrotic cells are eliminated. Similar changes also occur in the involution process during normal lactation, but the changes are not as abrupt.

In addition to the loss of epithelial cells, a decrease in the rate of activity per cell also occurs. Biochemical alterations occur within hours after the cessation of milking or suckling. These are a decrease in the respiratory quotient, a decrease in oxygen consumption and an accumulation of lactic acid in the mammary gland tissue. The oxidative phosphorylation of the mitochondria of the mammary gland is uncoupled within 12–24 hours after the young have been removed.

The suckling stimulus plays an important role in the maintenance of lactation, for it has been shown that the regression process is retarded by the suckling of ligated mammary glands. Prolactin injections also retard the involution process. The suckling stimulus also maintains the nucleic acid content of the lactating mammary gland. The suckling stimulus without milk removal, however, neither prevents a decrease in the cell loss nor maintains the protein synthesis activity of the gland. The maintenance of lactation thus requires the release of the hormones involved in milk secretion and the removal of the secretory products.

Oxytocin injections retard the involution process of rat mammary glands after the cessation of milking. Some investigators interpreted these results to indicate that oxytocin was involved in the release of prolactin by the anterior pituitary; however, other workers attribute this effect to a periodic milk ejection caused by oxytocin, which releases milk from the alveoli into the ducts and stromal tissue where it can be reabsorbed and allow further milk synthesis to occur. Prolactin injections prevent the involution process and maintain the biochemical integrity of the mammary gland to a greater extent than oxytocin injections; however, prolactin will not maintain full biochemical integrity of the tissue unless the secretory products are removed. Several drugs and hormones, such as reserpine, acetylcholine, serotonin, and epinephrine, also prevent involution of the mammary gland after the cessation of suckling. It appears that these compounds exert their effect by causing prolactin secretion by the pituitary gland.

REFERENCES

1. Anderson, R. R., and C. W. Turner. 1963. *Proc. Soc. Exptl. Biol. Med.* 113:333.
2. Bassler, R. 1961. *Frankfurt Z. Path.* 71:398.
3. Benson, G. K. 1958. *Proc. Soc. Exptl. Soc. Biol. Med.* 99:550.
4. Benson, G. K., and R. J. Fitzpatrick. 1966. In G. W. Harris and B. T. Donovan, eds., *The Pituitary Gland,* Vol. 3. Berkeley: Univ. Calif. Press. Ch. 15.
5. Benson, G. K., and S. J. Folley. 1957. *J. Endocrinol.* 16:189.
6. Benson, G. K., S. J. Folley, J. S. Tindal 1960. *J. Endocrinol.* 20:106.
7. Brookreson, A. D., and C. W. Turner. 1959. *Proc. Soc. Exptl. Biol. Med.* 102:744.
8. Butow, R. A. 1963. The role of fatty acids as metabolic regulating agents in the guinea pig mammary gland. Ph.D. Thesis, Cornell University.

9. Chikamune, T. 1963. *Jap. J. Zootech. Sci.* 34:387.
10. Cross, B. A., R. F. W. Goodwin, and I. A. Silver. 1958. *J. Endocrinol.* 17:63.
11. Darby, F. J., D. Y. Wang, and A. L. Greenbaum. 1964. *J. Endocrinol.* 28:329.
12. Denamur, R. 1961. *Ann. Endocrinol.* 22:767.
13. Denamur, R. 1962. *C. R. Acad. Sci.* 255:1786.
14. Gaunt, R., A. A. Renzi, N. Antonchap, G. J. Miller, and M. Gillian. 1954. *Ann. N. Y. Acad. Sci.* 59:22.
15. Griffith, D. R., and C. W. Turner. 1959. *Proc. Soc. Exptl. Biol. Med.* 102:619.
16. Griffith, D. R., and C. W. Turner. 1961. *Proc. Soc. Exptl. Biol. Med.* 107:668.
17. Hollman, K. H., and J. M. Verley. 1967. *Z. Zellforsch.* 82:222.
18. Hooker, C. W., and W. F. Williams. 1941. *Endocrinology* 28:42.
19. Lenfers, P. 1907. *Z. Fleisch. Milchhygiene* 17:340.
20. Levy, H. R. 1963. *Federation Proc.* 22:363.
21. Linzell, J. L. 1960. *J. Physiol.* 153:492.
22. McFarlane, D., J. C. Rennie, and P. S. Blackburn. 1949. Cited by C. W. Turner, 1952, in *The Mammary Gland.* Columbia, Mo.: Lucas Brothers. Ch. 10.
23. McLean, P. 1964. *Biochem. J.* 90:271.
24. Meites, J. 1959. *Proc. Soc. Exptl. Biol. Med.* 100:750.
25. Meites, J., and T. F. Hopkins. 1961. *J. Endocrinol.* 22:207.
26. Meites, J., and C. S. Nicoll.1959. *Endocrinology.* 65:572.
27. Meites, J., C. S. Nicoll, and P. K. Talwalker. 1959. *Proc. Soc. Exptl. Biol. Med.* 101:563.
28. Mizuno, H., and T. Chikamune. 1958. *Endocrinol. Jap.* 5:265.
29. Moon, R. C. 1962. *Amer. J. Physiol.* 203:939.
30. Moon, R. C. 1965. *Proc. Soc. Exptl. Biol. Med.* 119:501.
31. Munford, R. E. 1963. *J. Endocrinol.* 28:17.
32. Nelson, W. L., R. A. Butow, and E. I. Ciaccio. 1962. *Arch. Biochem. Biophys.* 96:500.
33. Nelson, W. L., P. G. Heytler, and E. I. Ciaccio. 1962. *Proc. Soc. Exptl. Biol. Med.* 109:373.
34. Ôta, K., Y. Shinde, and A. Yokoyama. 1965. *Endocrinology* 76:1.
35. Schmidt, G. H., R. T. Chatterton, Jr., and W. Hansel. 1962. *J. Dairy Sci.* 45:1380.
36. Selye, H. 1934. *Amer. J. Physiol.* 107:535.
37. Slater, T. F. 1962. *Arch. Int. Physiol Biochim.* 75:167.
38. Slater, T. F., A. L. Greenbaum, and D. Y. Wang. 1963. *Lysosomes.* Ciba Foundation Symposium. London: J. and A. Churchill. p. 311.
39. Thatcher, W. W., and H. A. Tucker. 1966. *J. Animal Sci.* 25:932.
40. Tucker, H. A. 1964. *Proc. Soc. Exptl. Biol. Med.* 116:218.
41. Tucker, H. A., and R. P. Reece. 1963. *Proc. Soc. Exptl. Biol. Med.* 112:409.
42. Tucker, H. A., and R. P. Reece. 1963. *Proc. Soc. Exptl. Biol. Med.* 112:688.
43. Tucker, H. A., and R. P. Reece. 1963. *Proc. Soc. Exptl. Biol. Med.* 112:1002.

44. Tucker, H. A., and R. P. Reece. 1963. *Proc. Soc. Exptl. Biol. Med.* 113: 717.
45. Turner, C. W. 1952. *The Mammary Gland.* Columbia, Mo.: Lucas Brothers.
46. Turner, C. W., and E. P. Reineke. 1936. *Mo. Agr. Exptl. Sta. Res. Bull.* 235.
47. Verley, J. M., and K. H. Hollman. 1967. *Z. Zellforsch.* 82:212.
48. Wang, D. Y. 1960. *Nature.* 118:1109.
49. Wellings, S. R., and K. B. DeOme. 1963. *J. Nat. Cancer Inst.* 30:241.
50. Williams, W. L. 1945. *Anat. Rec.* 93:171.
51. Yokoyama, A., and K. Ôta. 1959. *Endocrinol. Jap.* 6:259.

8

MILK SECRETION RATE

The daily milk yield of mammals is dependent upon the amount of secretory tissue in the mammary gland and the rate of secretion per unit of tissue. The secretion rate is controlled in part by the pressure in the alveolar lumina due to the accumulation of milk. As milk is secreted into the lumen of the alveolus, part of it oozes into the ducts and teat and gland cisterns. The accumulation of milk builds up pressure in the lumen of the alveolus. After the pressure increases to a certain level, the milk secretion rate decreases. If sufficient pressure occurs, milk secretion stops and the milk in the alveoli and ducts is resorbed by the blood.

8-1 UDDER PRESSURE

Instruments are not available to measure the pressure within the alveolus; consequently, pressures are measured in the cannulated teat of the dairy cow and goat. It is assumed that the pressures within the teat cisterns reflect those within the lumina of the alveoli. Measurement of pressures in the teat cisterns at various intervals after milking indicates that three

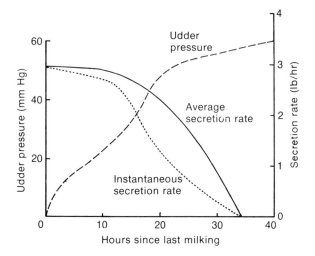

FIGURE 8–1
Relationship of udder pressure to secretion rates of
dairy cows. (Adapted from references 25, 40, 43.)

distinct phases occur in the milk pressure curve. Within one hour after
milking, a marked increase in pressure to approximately 8 mm Hg occurs
in the teat cistern (Figure 8-1). This hydrostatic pressure is caused by the
residual milk moving from the alveoli and smaller ducts into the cisterns.
This is followed by a slower increase in pressure due to the accumulation
of milk in the secretory tissue and its further oozing into the teat and
gland cisterns. This is followed by an accelerated rate of pressure increase
and constitutes the third phase of the pressure curve (25).

8-2   RESIDUAL MILK

The residual milk is the amount of milk left in the udder after a normal
milking. It can be obtained only after the injection of oxytocin and remilk-
ing the animal. The amount of residual milk is proportional to the amount
of milk present in the udder at the beginning of the milking (44, 46). The
percentages of residual milk are shown in Table 8-1. The percentage of
residual milk stays the same throughout lactation, thus the stage of lactation *per se* has no effect on the percentage. Older cows have higher percentages of residual milk than first-calf heifers, and cows with high
percentages of residual milk have a lower persistency of lactation. The
percentage residual milk is also higher in lower producers than higher

producers. The percentage residual milk is an inherited characteristic with a heritability estimate of .34. The repeatability of the trait has been estimated to be 0.77 (1, 16, 24).

TABLE 8-1
Percentage of milk present in the udder at the beginning of milking that remains as residual milk after milking. The values were obtained from different experiments under a variety of conditions.

Conditions under which measurements were made	Percentage residual milk	Reference
Milking intervals		
4, 6, 8, 10, 12, 14, 16 hours	9.6	16
6, 12, 18, 24 hours	9.8	31
10, 14, 24 hours	15.7	44
24 hours	13.9	46
10 and 14 hours	17.8	47
Lactation number		
First	10.0	23
Second and third	15.2	23
Fourth and later	17.9	23
Machine stripping		
Machine-stripped cows	12.8	20
Nonmachine-stripped cows	14.0	20
Cows receiving oxytocin subcutaneously	16.8	1
62 cows measured for 1 year	12.2	27
8 Shorthorn cows measured weekly for 16 weeks	22.1	11

8-3 UDDER PRESSURE AND SECRETION RATE

Udder Pressure

The pressure required to stop the secretion process has not been definitely determined and it probably varies from cow to cow. Petersen and Rigor (36) inflated the udder with air and determined that a pressure of 25 mm Hg caused a complete cessation of milk secretion. This does not include the hydrostatic pressure of about 8 mm Hg found by Korkman (25) to occur within one hour after milking. Korkman (25) found pressures higher than 25 mm Hg in the udder. It appears that the pressure at which milk secretion stops is somewhat higher than 25 mm Hg and probably even greater than 35 mm Hg. Tucker et al. (43) obtained udder pressure of 51 mm Hg 24 hours after the last milking when residual milk was removed after each milking. This pressure is considerably higher than that obtained by the earlier workers. In contrast to the divergence of experimental evidence on the relationship between udder pressure and milk secretion rate, there is rather good agreement that the secretion process stops about 35 hours after the last milking (43, 45). The general relationship between udder pressure and the rate of milk secretion is shown in Figure 8-1.

Korkman (25) studied the udder pressure of cows at various stages of lactation and with varying milk yields. The increase in pressure per unit of secreted milk is an individually inherited characteristic. The absolute increase in udder pressure is the same for high- and low-yielding cows, thus the increase in pressure per unit of secreted milk is smaller for high-producing cows.

Secretion Rate

When cows are milked at unequal intervals, an inverse relationship exists between the milk yield and fat percentage. This is usually explained by the fact that fat particles are less easily released into the lumen of the alveolus as pressure increases in the alveolus. In contrast to this explanation, Korkman (25) found that the higher udder pressure does not inhibit fat secretion as much as the secretion of the other milk constituents. The most probable explanation of the inverse relationship between milk yield and fat percentage when cows are milked at unequal intervals is a carry-over of residual milk. The amount of milk left in the udder after milking following a long interval is higher than that left after a shorter interval. Residual milk has a high milk fat percentage. Therefore the larger volume of milk left after a long interval with its high fat content is diluted with the milk secreted during the shorter interval. This gives the milk obtained after a shorter interval a higher milk fat percentage than the milk obtained after a long interval, which is composed of the milk secreted during the longer interval and the smaller amount of residual milk left over from the previous shorter interval. The solids-not-fat percentage is not affected by milking intervals.

The important questions on the relationship between udder pressure and milk secretion rate are: At what point does the udder pressure inhibit milk secretion and what is the rate of inhibition after it starts? Even if inhibition starts shortly after milking, it may have a very small effect on secretion rate if the rate of inhibition is small. An early experiment (38) indicated that cows should be milked at equal intervals in order to obtain maximum milk production. In that experiment, cows were milked at intervals of from 1 to 36 hours. The decline in milk secretion rate was approximately 5% per hour. Two limitations were present in the experiment. It took approximately three months to complete the experiment, and the longer intervals were used during the later part of the experiment. Thus the decrease in milk secretion rate during the longer intervals could have been due to the advanced stage of lactation. In addition, the periods preceding the experimental intervals were not standardized and they could have affected the milk secretion rate during the experimental intervals. Garrison and Turner (19) re-examined the data and concluded that the milk secretion rate did not decline until at least 14 hours after the last milking.

Other evidence was used to substantiate the recommendation that cows should be milked at equal intervals (5, 13). These data were obtained from milk production of cows milked at unequal intervals. Milk yields during unequal intervals were divided by the number of hours since the last milking. These results indicated that the secretion rate was higher during the shorter intervals. These workers did not consider the influence of residual milk on the rate of secretion. The importance of this was pointed out by Turner (44).

The amount of milk secreted during an interval is equal to the amount of milk obtained at the end of the milking interval plus the residual milk remaining in the udder minus the residual milk that was present in the udder at the beginning of the milking interval (44). Turner (44) used this principle to recalculate the data of Edwards (13) and concluded that there were no differences in the actual secretion rates during unequal milking intervals.

An example of the above concept is as follows: Cows milked at 10- and 14-hour intervals yielded 20 and 25 lb of milk at the end of each interval, respectively. The apparent secretion rate is obtained by dividing the milk yield by the number of hours since the last milking; this gives values of 2.0 and 1.79 lb per hour for the two intervals. If 15.7% of the milk is left in the udder as residual milk (44), then 23.7 lb of milk are present in the udder at the end of the 10-hour interval. At milking, 20 lb are obtained and 3.7 lb are left in the udder as residual milk. The actual secretion rate for the 10-hour interval is equal to milk yield at the end of the interval plus the residual milk left in the udder minus the residual milk at the beginning of the interval divided by the number of hours in the interval, i.e. $(20 + 3.7 - 4.7)/10 = 1.90$ lb/hr. The actual secretion rate during the 14-hour interval $= (25 + 4.7 - 3.7)/14 = 1.86$ lb/hr. The actual secretion rate during the two intervals is more nearly alike than the apparent secretion rates. This shows the erroneous results obtained when the residual milk effect is not considered.

The milk secretion rate has been measured during various milking intervals. Results from earlier work (4) indicated that the milk and fat secretion rates declined with increasing milking intervals with a greater rate of decline for milk than for fat. The fat percentage tended to increase with longer milking intervals. A long preceding interval had a detrimental effect on secretion rate. Part of the decrease in milk secretion rate after 12 hours could have been due to the effects of long preceding intervals. These workers did not remove the residual milk prior to each milking interval.

More recent experiments were designed to remove residual milk and to eliminate the previous interval effect. Turner (45) concluded that there was no significant inhibition of milk secretion for about 20 hours after the last milking. Elliott (15) found that the milk and solids-not-fat secretion rates were linear with milking intervals up to 16 hours. A study with high-producing Holstein and Brown Swiss cows (40) showed that there was no significant decrease in the milk secretion rate with intervals up to 12 hours when residual milk was removed. A significant decrease in milk secretion rate occurred during 16- and 20-hour intervals. High-producing cows were less adversely affected by the longer intervals than the lower-producing cows. Lower-producing cows have less secretory tissue in their udders, consequently the increase in udder pressure per unit of milk is greater in the younger and lower-producing cows than in higher-producing ones (25). This supports the concept that short milking intervals are of greater importance for young cows.

A previous long interval has a detrimental effect on the milk and fat secretion rates during the succeeding normal interval. The milk secretion rate during an interval is substantially influenced by one preceding interval, whereas fat secretion is affected by two or three preceding intervals (3, 18, 40, 44).

The general relationship between milk secretion rate and udder pressure is shown in Figure 8-1. The values up to 24 hours after the last milking are available in the literature; however, the values after 24 hours have been extrapolated to the time when the secretion process stops at about 35 hours after the last milking. The average secretion rate starts to drop about 10–12 hours after the last milking, but the instantaneous secretion rate starts to drop before this time (43), The instantaneous secretion rate is a measure of the secretion rate at a given time, whereas the average secretion rate is obtained by dividing the total yield by the time in that interval.

The milk secretion rates of rats have been determined using intervals of 3, 6, 9, and 12 hours. The milk secretion rate was measured by weighing the young and dams before and after a one-hour nursing after the various intervals. The milk secretion rate decreased with longer intervals since the last nursing (39).

The results of these studies indicate that residual milk plays an important part in the milk secretion rate and must be taken into consideration when actual secretion rates are calculated. A decline in the milk secretion rate takes place with longer intervals; however, the exact time when the decrease takes places has not been determined. Most studies indicate that the decline is not great until 16 hours after the last milking. The differences among the studies may be due to the production level of the animals, the breeds used, and possible stage of lactation effects.

8-4 MILKING INTERVALS AND FREQUENCIES

Unequal Intervals

An important consideration of the milk secretion rate is the effect of unequal milking intervals on the lactation milk production of dairy cows. Because of its practical importance, a number of experiments have been conducted to measure the effect of unequal milking intervals on milk production. These are summarized in Table 8-2. Some of the earlier studies were done with low-producing cows; however, the last two studies in the table include high-producing cows. Small but nonsignificant decreases in the milk yield occurred at the unequal intervals. Hansson et al. (21) found a 1.8% decrease in milk production of cows milked at 15- and 9-hour intervals and a 3.4% decrease for cows milked at 16- and 8-hour intervals, in comparison with cows milked at equal intervals. Schmidt

TABLE 8-2
Effect of unequal milking intervals on milk and fat production.

Intervals (hr)	No. of cows	Length of record	Milk (lb)	Fat (lb)	Reference
11 and 13	5	16 wk	2,448	—	47
16 and 8	5	16 wk	2,642	—	47
12 and 12	7	232 da	5,628	252	32
16 and 8	7	232 da	5,461	246	32
12 and 12	11	264 da	6,438	316	32
16 and 8	11	264 da	6,555	321	32
12 and 12	7	Lactations	5,543	211	26
14 and 10	7	Lactations	5,648	214	26
12 and 12	11	280 da	7,062	284	21
15 and 9	11	280 da	6,934	282	21
12 and 12	17	280 da	7,922	316	21
16 and 8	17	280 da	7,649	313	21
12 and 12	35	305 da	13,760	520	42
14 and 10	35	305 da	13,716	536	42
16 and 18	35	305 da	13,582	525	42
12.5—11.5	82	266 da	10,824	409	34
14.5— 9.5	82	266 da	10,584	398	34

and Trimberger (42) found percentage production decreases of 0.3 at 14- and 10-hour intervals and 1.3 at 16- and 8-hour intervals in comparison to equal intervals. Ormiston et al. (34) found a slightly higher reduction, 3.5%, in milk production due to the unequal intervals. No significant effects on milk fat percentages occur as a result of unequal milking intervals.

Frequency of Milking

The rate of milk secretion during an interval is also important in evaluating the additional milk produced when cows are milked more frequently than twice daily. Evidence for the evaluation of three-times or four-times-daily milking comes from three sources. The earlier studies involved the comparison of cows milked three times daily on Advanced Registry and Herd Improvement Registry testing programs. This work has been reviewed by Elliott (14). She concludes that the average increase in milk production of cows milked three times daily versus twice daily is 20%. Part of this increase is due to the fact that the cows milked more frequently usually receive more favorable feeding and management. In addition, cows on official testing programs milked three times daily usually have a higher milk production potential than those remaining on twice-daily milking. Dodd (9) concluded that 5–10% of the increase in milk production during three-times-daily milking was the result of decreased udder pressures and the remaining 10–15% was due to better feeding and management.

Another method of comparing three-times- versus twice-daily milking is the use of half udders. In one trial (30), half udders milked three times a day produced 16% more milk than the remaining half udders milked twice daily. In another trial (6), half udders milked three times a day throughout lactation were reported to produce 32% more milk than the halves milked twice daily; however the level of milk production was not reported. The half-udder milking procedure may have either a detrimental or a beneficial effect on the milk secretion rate of the udder milked twice daily. The udder half milked twice daily is subjected to at least one milk ejection without milk removal. This may stimulate more milk production or it may interfere with the milk-ejection process during the milking when the milk is removed. The importance of these two factors has not been determined.

A third method to determine the effect of more frequent milkings is to use different frequencies when the management and feed intake are standardized. In experiments of this kind, three-times-daily milking results in a 5–10% increase in production over twice-daily milking, which supports the earlier conclusion that decreased udder pressure accounts for only a part of the increase due to more frequent milkings (9, 14).

Milking cows four times daily gives a 5–10% increase in production over cows milked three times daily. Most of these reports are also based on comparison of cows on official test (9). In two controlled experiments, cows milked four times daily produced 7.9% and 8.1% more milk than cows milked twice daily. In an attempt to determine whether the beneficial effect of 4-times-a-day milking was due to the additional release of oxytocin, milk production of cows milked twice daily plus two udder stimulations between milkings were compared to those of cows milked and massaged twice a day. The massaging of the udders between milkings caused a 1.0–1.5% increase in production (28, 37).

Regular Milking Intervals

Regular milking has some importance for maximum milk production, regardless of the intervals used. In an early experiment, Woodward (49) compared the milk production of cows milked at three 8-hour intervals to those milked at unequal intervals of 6, 7, and 11 hours each day. Cows milked at regular intervals produced 3.9% more milk and 5.2% more milk fat than those milked at unequal intervals. In another trial (33), cows milked at 12-hour daily intervals produced 1.8% more milk than cows milked at 12- and 12-hour and 15- and 9-hour intervals on alternate days. Cows producing less than 30.8 lb of milk per day dropped 0.13 lb of milk per day and those producing over 30.8 lb of milk per day dropped 1.08 lb during the irregular milking intervals in comparison to the regular intervals.

Less Than Two Milkings Per Day

The effect of decreasing the number of milkings per day from twice-daily milking has also been compared. Hesseltine et al. (22) found that five cows milked once a day during the last 9 weeks of their lactation produced 38% less milk than cows milked twice daily. The milk fat test increased from 5.0% to 5.3%. Parker (35) divided 16 pairs of identical twin cows that had been lactating for about 6 months into two groups. One group was milked twice a day and the other group was milked once a day for the remainder of their lactations. Cows milked once a day produced 35% less milk during the experimental period and 12% less milk during the entire lactation than those milked twice daily. The average length of the lactation period of the cows milked once a day was reduced by 12 days. Milking cows once daily for complete lactations resulted in a 50%

reduction in milk production for first-calf heifers and a 40% reduction in second-lactation and older cows in comparison to twice-daily milking (8).

The average rate of milk secretion during a 24-hour milking interval is 15% less than that occurring during a 12-hour interval. A further reduction in milk production occurs during the interval following a long interval because of the detrimental effect of a preceding long interval on the milk secretion rate. After this, the milk secretion rate quickly returns to that occurring during normal twice-daily milking (46).

Cows milked 13 times a week produced 89.2% and 95.4% as much milk in the first and second lactations, respectively, as their identical twin mates that were milked 14 times a week (7). Cows milked at 3 intervals of 18, 18, and 12 hours for two days in each week for 8 weeks produced 93.5% as much milk for two days as when they were milked regularly twice a day (48). In a recent study, Autrey et al. (2) found that the elimination of one milking a week for 6 weeks did not result in any decrease in milk production. The elimination of two consecutive milkings per week caused a 16% reduction in milk production.

8-5   INCOMPLETE MILKING

Another facet of the residual milk aspect is that of incomplete milking, or incomplete stripping. Dodd et al. (12) subjected two groups of first-calf heifers to 4- or 8-minute milking durations for entire lactations. Half of the cows milked for 4 minutes were incompletely milked out, which resulted in reduction in production, especially during early lactation. Cows milked for 4 minutes produced 10% less milk during the lactation than those milked 8 minutes. Bailey et al. (4) machine-milked a group of cows without machine stripping. One-half of the udder was hand-stripped and the other half was not. Hand stripping yielded about one pound of milk for each half udder, which resulted in a 10% increase in milk production over the 54-day experimental period. The nonstripped halves did not recover the production attained by the stripped halves during a 15-day recovery period.

Dodd and Clough (10) removed either 60, 75, or 90% of the milk at four consecutive milkings in comparison to an initial control period. All of these resulted in a 5% permanent depression in milk production. In a second experiment, they removed only 75% of the yields for periods of 4, 8, and 20 days. They concluded that the permanent reduction in yield was more affected by the duration of the incomplete milking than the degree of incomplete milking. In contrast to this, Schmidt et al. (41) found that leaving 4 lb of milk in the udder at each milking, in addition to the residual milk for a 10-day period, resulted in a greater permanent reduction in milk yield than did leaving 2 lb of milk in the udder at each milking for a 10-day period. These results show that incomplete milking causes a permanent reduction in milk production.

8-6 MACHINE STRIPPING

Whether machine stripping is absolutely essential for high milk production has not yet been resolved. In one experiment (20), it was found that the elimination of machine stripping did not have a detrimental effect on milk production. Cows that were machine-stripped during 28-day experimental periods averaged 42.2 lb of milk and those not stripped averaged 42.1 lb. In a similar experiment (29), cows not stripped produced 44.3 lb of milk per day and those that were machine-stripped produced 44.6 lb per day. Cows that were machine-stripped had machine-on times 36 seconds longer than the nonstripped cows. In most cases, machine stripping is started before the milk flow stops. If the results from these two experiments are substantiated in larger trials, it would indicate that the milking machine does remove almost all of the available milk without machine stripping and that little or no incomplete milking results. In order to fully answer the question of the necessity of machine stripping, the elimination of machine stripping would have to be done for complete lactations on a relatively large number of cows and their milk production compared to cows that were machine-stripped.

8-7 SUMMARY

The rate of milk secretion is of more than academic importance to the dairyman. The secretion rate influences the required frequency of milking cows and the acceptable intervals between milkings. The milk secretion rate is dependent in part upon the pressure that accumulates within the mammary gland. As milk is secreted, pressure is built up in the alveolar lumina. The epithelial cells must then secrete against a higher pressure. After the pressure reaches a certain point, the rate of milk secretion decreases. If milk is allowed to accumulate within the mammary gland for a long enough period of time, the pressure is built up to a sufficient level to inhibit secretion and the milk is resorbed by the blood. Secretion stops at about 35 hours after the last milking.

Measurements of pressure in the udder at various time intervals after milking indicate that a marked increase in the udder pressure occurs within one hour after milking. This is due to the residual milk moving from the alveoli into the teat and gland cisterns. Thereafter, a gradual increase in the pressure occurs due to the oozing of milk from the alveoli to the teat and gland cisterns. After a period of hours, sufficient udder pressure has built up to cause a decrease in the milk secretion rate.

From a number of experiments, it appears that the rate of milk secretion is linear for about 10–12 hours after the last milking. After this time the rate decreases slightly. The rate continues to decrease until it finally reaches zero at about 35 hours after the last milking.

Part of the initial increase in udder pressure is due to the residual milk that is left in the udder after a normal milking. The amount of residual milk is approximately 15% of the milk present in the udder at the beginning of milking. The percentage of residual milk is higher in low-producing cows than high-producing cows. Cows with low persistence of lactation also have a high amount of residual milk. Earlier experiments failed to account for the residual milk effect on the milk secretion rate of cows milked at unequal intervals and the results indicated that cows should be milked at equal milking intervals. A re-evaluation of the data and of experiments designed to measure the effect of unequal milking intervals indicates that cows milked at 10- and 14-hour daily intervals produce from 0–1% less milk per lactation than cows milked at equal intervals. Cows milked at either 9- and 15-hour or 8- and 16-hour daily intervals produce 1–3% less milk than cows milked at equal intervals. Increasing the frequency of milking to three or four times daily increases the level of milk production. Three-times-a-day milking versus twice-a-day milking increases the milk production by 15–25%, but only about 5-10% of this is due to decreased udder pressure and the remaining 10–20% is due to better feeding and management. Most of the increase in four-times-a-day milking over three-times-a-day milking is due to the better feeding and management of the cows.

Decreasing the number of milkings per day from two causes a marked reduction in milk secretion. Skipping one milking a week results in a 5–11% drop in milk production in comparison to cows milked twice daily. Milking cows once a day results in a 50% reduction in milk production of first-calf heifers and a 40% reduction of older cows. Neither of these milking regimes seems practical for the average dairy farmer.

Incomplete milking for a short period of time causes a permanent depression in milk production. Cows completely milked out after incomplete milkings do not regain their normal milk production. Preliminary work on the necessity of machine stripping indicates that its elimination does not have a detrimental effect on milk production or the incidence of mastitis. Apparently the milking machine that is left on until milk flow stops removes almost all of the milk present in the udder and leaves very little milk in the udder in addition to the residual milk. Further work is necessary before it can be eliminated as a recommended routine management practice.

REFERENCES

1. Anderson, R. R., G. A. Hindery, V. Parkash, and C. W. Turner. 1968. *J. Dairy Sci.* 51:601.
2. Autrey, K. M., G. H. Rollins, and R. Y. Cannon. 1963. *J. Dairy Sci.* 46:626.
3. Bailey, G. L., P. A. Clough, and F. H. Dodd. 1955. *J. Dairy Res.* 22:22.
4. Bailey, G. L., P. A. Clough, F. H. Dodd, A. S. Foot, and S. J. Rowland. 1953. *Proc. 13th Intern. Dairy Congr.* 2:76.
5. Bartlett, S. 1929. *J. Agric. Sci.* 19:36.
6. Cash, J. G., and W. W. Yapp. 1950. *J Dairy Sci.* 33:382.
7. Claesson, O. 1962. *Dairy Fmr.,* Ipswich, 9:36 (*Dairy Sci. Abstr.* 25:28, 1963).
8. Claesson, O., A. Hansson, N. Gustafsson, and E. Brännäng. 1959. *Acta Agr. Scand.* 9:38.
9. Dodd, F. H. 1957. In J. Hammond, ed., *Progress in the Physiology of Farm Animals,* Vol. 3. London: Butterworths Scientific Publ. Ch. 20.
10. Dodd, F. H., and P. A. Clough. 1962. *Proc. 16th Internat. Dairy Congr.* 1:89.
11. Dodd, F. H., and A. S. Foot. 1948. *J. Minist. Agric.* 55:238.
12. Dodd, F. H., E. Henriques, A. S. Foot, and F. H. Neave. 1950. *J. Dairy Res.* 17:107.
13. Edwards, J. 1950. *J. Agric. Sci.* 40:100.
14. Elliott, G. M. 1959. *Dairy Sci. Abstr.* 21:435 and 481.
15. Elliott, G. M. 1960. *J. Dairy Res.* 27:293.
16. Elliott, G. M. 1961. *J. Dairy Res.* 28:123.
17. Elliott, G. M. 1961. *J. Dairy Res.* 28:209.
18. Elliott, G. M., F. H. Dodd, and P. J. Brumby. 1960. *J. Dairy Res.* 27:293.
19. Garrison, E. R, and C. W. Turner. 1936. *Mo. Agr. Expt. Sta. Res. Bull.* 234.
20. Goff, K. R., and G. H. Schmidt. 1967. *J. Dairy Sci.* 50:1787.
21. Hansson, A., O. Claesson, E. Brännäng, and N. Gustafsson. 1958. *Acta Agr. Scand.* 8:3.
22. Hesseltine, W. R., R. D. Mochrie, H. D. Eaton, F. I. Elliott, and G. Beall. 1953. *Conn. Agr. Expt. Sta. Bull.* 304.
23. Johansson, I. 1949. *Proc. 12th Intern. Dairy Congr.* 1:171.

24. Kashyap, T. S., J. D. Donker, R. E. Comstock, and W. E. Petersen. 1967. *J. Dairy Sci.* 50:722.
25. Korkman, N. 1953. *Kgl. Lantbr. Hosgk. Ann.* 20:303.
26. Koshi, J. H., and W. E. Petersen. 1954. *J. Dairy Sci.* 37:673.
27. Koshi, J. H., and W. E. Petersen. 1955. *J. Dairy Sci.* 38:788.
28. Linnerud, A. C., E. V. Caruolo, G. E. Miller, G. D. Marx, and J. D. Donker. 1966. *J. Dairy Sci.* 49:1529.
29. Little, J. A. 1968. *J. Dairy Sci.* 51:629.
30. Ludwick, L. M., A. Spielman, and W. E. Petersen. 1941. *J. Dairy Sci.* 24:505.
31. Marx, G. D., A. C. Linnerud, G. E. Miller, E. V. Caruolo, and J. D. Donker. 1963. *J. Dairy Sci.* 46:626.
32. McMeekan, C. P., and P. J. Brumby. 1956. *Nature,* London, 178:799.
33. Moore, C. L. 1968. *J. Dairy Sci.* 51:967.
34. Ormiston, E. E., S. L. Spahr, R. W. Touchberry, and J. L. Albright. 1967. *J. Dairy Sci.* 50:1597.
35. Parker, O. F. 1965. *Proc. Ruakura Fmrs. Conf. Week,* pp. 236-240.
36. Petersen, W. E., and T. V. Rigor. 1932. *Proc. Soc. Exptl. Biol. Med.* 31:254.
37. Porter, R. M., H. R. Conrad, and L. O. Gilmore. 1966. *J. Dairy Sci.* 49:1064.
38. Ragsdale, A. C., C. W. Turner, and S. Brody. 1924. *J. Dairy Sci.* 7:249.
39. Reddy, R. R., J. D. Donker, and A. C. Linnerud. 1964. *J. Dairy Sci.* 47:554.
40. Schmidt, G. H. 1960. *J. Dairy Sci.* 43:213.
41. Schmidt, G. H., R. S. Guthrie, and R. W. Guest. 1964. *J. Dairy Sci.* 47:152.
42. Schmidt, G. H., and G. W. Trimberger. 1963. *J. Dairy Sci.* 46:19.
43. Tucker, H. A., R. P. Reece, and R. E. Mather. 1961. *J. Dairy Sci.* 44:1725.
44. Turner, H. G. 1953. *Australian J. Agr. Res.* 4:118.
45. Turner, H. G. 1955. *Australian J. Agr. Res.* 6:145.
46. Turner, H. G. 1955. *Australian J. Agr. Res.* 6:514.
47. Turner, H. G. 1955. *Australian J. Agr. Res.* 6:530.
48. Witt, M., and B. Senft. 1963. *Mitt. dtn. LandwGes* 78:551 (*Dairy Sci. Abstr.* 28:405, 1966).
49. Woodward, T. E. 1931. *USDA Circ.* 180.

9

MILKING RATE OF DAIRY COWS

The milking rate of dairy cows is an important economic consideration of the dairy farmer. It determines the speed with which cows can be milked, which in turn has an effect on the number of cows that can be milked by the dairyman in an hour's time. This is extremely important with the increasing cost of farm labor. The milking rate of dairy cows is dependent upon the physiological factors of the dairy cow and the physical factors of the milking machine. Both of these will be discussed.

9-1 MILK FLOW MEASUREMENTS

A series of measurements has been used to determine milk flow rates. The two common measurements are the maximum rate (peak flow rate) and the average rate of milk flow. The maximum rate is the highest yield during any interval of the milking process and is usually measured in one-minute intervals. Two measures of average rate are used. One is obtained by dividing the yield before stripping by the milking time prior to machine stripping and the second is obtained by dividing the entire yield including strippings by the total milking time. The rate before machine stripping is a more valid measurement of average flow rate because it does not include the variations in the machine stripping rate and yield. The maximum rate of flow, however, is the best measure of the inherited milking rate (16).

Machine stripping time and yield are defined as the time and yield after the milk flow rate drops to a certain arbitrary level. This level is usually about 0.30 lb of milk per 15-second interval. This measurement of machine stripping almost always results in some machine stripping time and yield. A better measure would be the stripping time and yield after milk flow stops; however, under farm conditions machine stripping is usually started before milk flow stops. High correlations exist between the average and maximum rates of milk flow. A high correlation also exists between the maximum rate of milk flow and the yield or percentage yield for the first 2 minutes of milking (4, 12, 16, 34, 36, 37, 44).

The total duration of milking is dependent upon the average rate of flow, the milk yield, and the machine stripping time. The duration of milking is influenced more by the peak flow rate than by changes in the milk yield or changes in the yield of strippings (12).

9-2 PHYSIOLOGICAL FACTORS AFFECTING MILKING RATE

Teat Orifice

The most important physiological factor determining the rate of milk flow is the teat opening. This involves both the diameter of the teat meatus and the tautness of the sphincter muscles surrounding the meatus. This was demonstrated by Baxter et al. (3), who determined the milk flow rates on eight quarters of cows at three vacuum levels. These quarters were remilked with a cannula to give all teats a uniform size of teat meatus. The peak milk flow rates ranged from 1.12 to 2.85 lb/min with an average of 1.99 when the cows were milked at a vacuum level of 15.9 inches of mercury (Hg) without cannulae (Figure 9-1). When the cows were milked with cannulae, the peak flow rates ranged from 2.60 to 2.90 lb/min with an average of 2.74. Similar reductions in variation in milk flow rates of cows milked with cannulae in comparison to no cannulae occurred where the quarters were milked at 10.6 and 20.4 inches Hg. These results suggest that the teat orifice plays a major role in controlling the rate of milk flow. These results do not determine whether the size of the teat orifice or the tautness of the sphincter muscles surrounding the orifice is the most important factor. Significant positive correlations

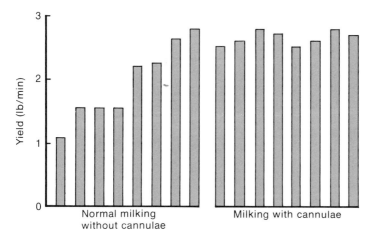

FIGURE 9–1
Milking rate of 8 quarters milked with and without a cannula at
15.9 inches Hg. vacuum. (From Baxter et al. 1950.
J. Dairy Res. 17:117.)

between the size of the teat orifice and the maximum milking rate have
been reported (23, 24). Johansson and Malven (19) conclude that the
size of the teat orifice is the main factor controlling the maximum rate
of milk flow during the first half of lactation.

In an attempt to determine the relative importance of the tonus of the
sphincter muscles and the size of the teat orifice, Naito et al. (22, 23)
determined partial correlations between the maximum rate of milk flow,
the tonus of the sphincter muscle, and the size of the teat orifice of Holstein and Jersey cows. The tonus of the sphincter muscles was more
closely related to the maximum rate of milk flow than was the size of the
orifice. The partial correlation coefficient between tonus of the sphincter
muscle and the maximum rate of milk flow of Holstein cows was −.735
when the size of the teat orifice was held constant. The partial correlation
coefficient between size of the teat orifice and maximum rate of flow was
only +.300 when the tonus was held constant. They concluded that the
most important characteristic determining the rate of milking is the tonus
of the sphincter muscle. Further support for this conclusion was obtained
by Buhr (6), who found that anesthesia of the teat increased the rate
of milk flow. The anesthesia apparently blocked the sympathetic nerves
that control the tonus of the sphincter muscle. Both tonus of the sphincter
muscle and size of the teat orifice must be involved under normal milking
conditions. The size of the orifice determines the rate of passage of a
liquid through it and the tonus of the sphincter muscle affects the size of
the opening.

A number of studies have indicated a negative relationship between the length of the teat and the maximum or average rate of milk flow (15, 19, 28, 33). The physiological reason for this is not known.

Internal Udder Pressure

A second factor that affects the rate of milk flow is the internal udder pressure due to the accumulation of milk within the mammary gland. This internal udder pressure may be equivalent to 2–3 inches Hg; however, it has a relatively small influence in comparison to changes in the milking machine, especially vacuum level (3, 12).

Age

Several workers have reported that the maximum and average rates of milk flow increase with lactations after the first lactation; however, age has no effect on either the maximum or average rates of flow when yield is held constant. The increase in the maximum and average flow rates with age is probably due to the fact that second-lactation cows and older cows have higher milk yields, and, consequently, higher flow rates than first-calf heifers. The duration of milking including machine stripping increases slightly each lactation, because the machine stripping yield increases as the cow ages (1, 12, 29, 36).

Inheritance and Breed Differences

The milking rate of the dairy cow is an inherited characteristic. The heritability estimates of average and maximum rates of flow range from 0.25 to 0.98. It is impossible to estimate an average heritability value for these traits because of the large variation in the observations, the different methods used to measure the milking rate, and the different procedures to measure heritability. In one study (36), it was found that Holstein cows had faster average and maximum milk flow rates, independent of milk yield, than did the Ayrshire or Brown Swiss cows used in the study. The repeatability of the maximum milk flow rates and flow rate curves is high and estimates range from 0.77 to 0.92 (4, 5, 15, 21, 29, 37, 44).

9-3   MILKING RATE AND YIELD

A number of measurements have been made to relate the milking rate of the cow to her daily and lactation milk yields. There is a high correlation between the daily milk yield and the average and maximum rates of flow. Cows with high lactation yields also have a higher rate of milk flow than the lower-producing cows. For each pound per minute increase in maximum milking rate, the lactation yield increases between 400 and 700 lb of milk. With yield at milking held constant, the partial correlation between the maximum rate of milk flow and lactation yield is not significant, which indicates that the higher maximum milking rate is a result of, and not a cause of, high lactation yields (6, 9, 11, 14, 15, 19, 30, 31, 32, 43, 44).

The relationship between maximum rate of milk flow and lactation length has not been fully resolved. Dodd and Foot (14) found that the lactation length was increased by 8 days and the persistency index by 10 days for each pound per minute increase in the maximum milk flow rate of first-calf heifers. In contrast to this, Desvignes and Poutous (11) found a negative correlation between the lactation length and the maximum rate of milk flow; whereas Johansson and Malven (19) found that the partial correlation between peak flow and persistency was not significant.

9-4 MACHINE FACTORS AFFECTING MILKING RATE

Principles of Milking Machine Operation

The basic principles of the operation of the milking machine have been reviewed by Guest and Spencer (17), Hall (18), Maffey (20) and Thiel (38). The milking machine, as we know it today, was first put together by Alexander Gillies from Australia, in 1903. He added a teat cup and liner to a machine that had been manufactured in Britain. This was the first machine to employ all of the principles of the modern milking machine. The essential components of the machine are: a source of vacuum, a receptacle for the collection of milk, a pulsator, and a teat cup and liner for each teat. In addition, hoses are necessary to attach the teat cups to the pulsator and milk receptacle and to attach the machine to a vacuum source. A claw is present in some milking machines. The claw serves as a collecting vessel before the milk moves to the milk receptacle.

All milking machines operate by vacuum. A partial vacuum is created when air is removed from a confined space. The atmosphere constantly exerts a pressure on all surfaces of approximately 14.7 lb/in^2 at sea level. This value decreases slightly with increasing elevation above sea level. The atmospheric pressure is measured by a barometer and is usually measured in inches or centimeters of mercury. If a tube closed on one end is filled with mercury, inverted, and placed in a bowl of mercury, the level in the tube will remain at a height above the level of mercury in an open vessel. This is shown in part A, Figure 9-2. A pressure of 14.7 lb/in² is exerted on the mercury in the bowl and raises the mercury in the column to a height of approximately 30 inches, which is the barometric height.

When the atmospheric pressure is reduced, the column of mercury falls and the extent of the drop is the level of vacuum. In part B, Figure 9-2, the atmospheric pressure has been reduced by one-half, which causes the column of mercury to drop to 15 inches. The difference between 30 and 15 inches Hg is the partial vacuum, 15 inches Hg. This is usually read on a vacuum gauge.

Milk is removed from the udder by a vacuum applied to the end of the teat. When the udder is filled with milk, a positive pressure exists within the udder. The pressure within the udder varies between 40 and 100 mm Hg after milk ejection. When the milking machine is applied, the pressure below the teat is reduced to the vacuum level of the milking machine. This creates a pressure difference across the teat orifice and causes it to open and milk to flow. This is shown in part A, Figure 9-3. The rate of milk removal is influenced by the pressure difference across the teat meatus. Machines operating at higher vacuum levels usually increase the rate of milk flow from the teat, because they create a larger pressure difference across the teat opening.

A constant rate of milk flow occurs when the vacuum is constantly applied to the teat. Early machines operated on this principle, but it was

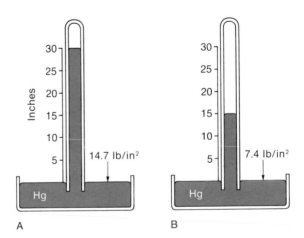

FIGURE 9-2
Measurement of vacuum. A. Barometric pressure at sea level. B. Partial vacuum of 15 inches Hg due to a reduction in the atmospheric pressure.

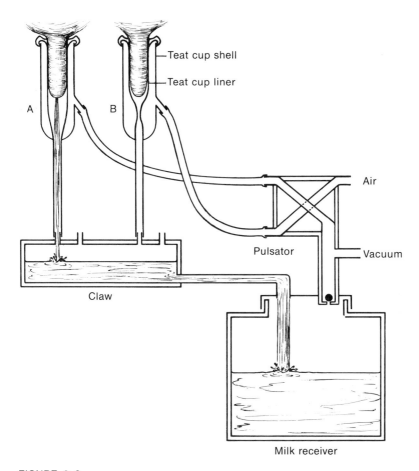

FIGURE 9–3
The milking machine. Milk is removed from the teat by vacuum when the liner is open, as shown in A. The milk moves through the claw to the milk receiver. When the pulsator causes the teat cup liner to close, as in B, milk flow stops.

found that teat irritation and damage soon occurred. This led to the double-action milking machine, which has a teat cup liner within the teat cup shell. The purpose of the liner is to massage the teat and prevent irritation and damage to the teat. A constant vacuum is present on the inside of the liner. The pulsator supplies intermittent atmospheric pressure and a partial vacuum to the space between the teat cup shell and liner. When the pulsator opens the space between the shell and liner to vacuum, equal pressures exist between the outside and the inside of the liner and the liner takes its normal open shape (Part A, Figure 9-3). Milk flows at this phase of the cycle. When air is introduced between the shell and liner, the pressure increases on the outside of the liner and causes it to collapse (Part B, Figure 9-3). The collapse squeezes and massages the teat and at the same time the liner closes below the teat. This prevents the milk from flowing since it closes both the teat meatus and the liner below the teat. This is followed by the introduction of air to A and a partial vacuum to B, causing the liner of A to collapse and the liner of B to open. The opening and closing of the teat cup liner is referred to as one pulsation. Most milking machines operate between 40 and 80 pulsations per minute.

The two basic types of teat cup liners are the moulded and extruded liners. The moulded liner has a mouthpiece, a barrel, and a milk tube moulded into one piece. This is the type shown in Figure 9-3. The extruded liner is made from a straight tube and the mouthpiece is formed by inserting a metal ring somewhat larger than the tube in the upper end. The lower end, the milk tube, is usually made from the bottom part of a moulded liner. Most liners used in the United States are moulded liners.

After the milk is removed from the teat, it travels via the milk tube to the claw, which collects the milk from the four teats. The milk is then transferred to the milk receiver. In the suspended-type milking machine the milk tubes are attached directly to the milk receiver and no claw is present.

Vacuum

The machine factor that causes the greatest change in milk flow rate is the level of vacuum. Increasing the vacuum level increases maximum and average rates of flow (Table 9-1). Increasing the vacuum level has a tendency to cause the teat cups to crawl up on the udder and to increase the machine stripping time and yield (8, 34).

The milking rate is influenced by the vacuum fluctuations in the teat

TABLE 9-1
Effect of vacuum levels on the rate of milking and on machine stripping time.

Vacuum level (inches Hg)	Stripping time (min)	Total milking time (min)	Maximum rate of flow (lb/min)
12	0.6	4.6	8.1
18	0.8	3.8	10.8
24	1.6	4.4	10.6

Source: Schmidt et al. 1963. *Cornell Agr. Expt. Sta. Bull.* 983.

cup liner. A reduction in the rate of milk flow occurs when vacuum fluctuations increase. Vacuum fluctuations occur when large volumes of air
enter the vacuum system. Flooding of the teat cup liners, milk tubes, and
teat cup claws with milk, in addition to elevating milk above the level of
the udder, tends to increase the vacuum fluctuations and decrease the
rate of milk flow. Milking machine design factors that diminish vacuum
fluctuations in the liner are increased bore size of the short milk tube
leading to the claw, pulsation of the teat cups in pairs instead of all four
together, and increasing the volume of the claw. Air admission holes in
the claw help to prevent milk lock and to move the milk from the claw to
the milk receptacle at a faster rate. This greatly decreases the vacuum
fluctuation and increases the average level of vacuum in the liner during
the part of the cycle when milk is flowing. Pressures below the teat in a
narrow-bore liner vary from a few inches to 25 inches Hg vacuum during
a single pulsation cycle in the absence of an air bleed (39). The introduction of air into the barrel of the liner or into the mouthpiece reduces the
vacuum fluctuations and prevents the vacuum from increasing much
above the normal milking vacuum of 15 inches Hg. Teat-end vacuum
fluctuations appear to be one of the more important machine factors associated with new infections and clinical mastitis (8, 10, 25, 35, 42).

The question of whether vacuum enters the test cistern after milking
has not been completely resolved. Vacuum does not enter the teat sinus
during milk flow. Several workers, however, (7, 26) have found vacuum
in the gland sinus of excised bovine udders after the cessation of milk flow.
Caruolo and Marx (7) found similar results in one live cow. Witzel and
McDonald (45) measured the pressure changes in the intact bovine udder
during mechanical milking. They concluded that a pulsating vacuum
developed in the teat sinus at the end of milk flow and that teat sinus
vacuum persisted after inflation collapse (residual vacuum). The vacuum
within the teat during overmilking ranged from two-thirds to full value
of the milking machine vacuum.

Thiel et al. (40) did not agree with the interpretation that the milking
vacuum extends through the streak canal into the teat sinus. They found
that both the gland and the teat sinuses collapse completely under external
air pressure as the last available milk is extracted. The teat sinus is completely free from fluid and is completely collapsed. It appeared that the
gland sinus is in the same condition. They state that the local forces that
tend to separate the opposed walls of the teat sinus give rise to local pressure changes, similar to those occurring when a local force tends to separate the walls of a length of empty layflat plastic tubing. They state that
the stress that tends to separate these opposed walls of the teat sinus
could be expected to account for the vacuum observed by Witzel and

McDonald toward the end of milking. Recent work from Ireland (quoted by Thiel, 38), indicates that the high residual vacuum is a measuring artifact. The Irish investigators used a simple manometric technique and found low values of 4–12 mm Hg vacuum in the teat cisterns, which disappeared as soon as the teat cups were removed. Even though the evidence is not clear-cut, it does appear that a pressure less than atmospheric exists in the teat cistern at least for a short period after milking; however, it does not appear to be as great as first reported. Whether or not this residual vacuum has an effect on aiding the entrance of mastitis organisms or injuring the teat ends has yet to be resolved.

Pulsation Rate and Ratio

The pulsations of a milking machine can be altered in two ways. The number of pulsations per minute and the pulsation ratio can be changed. In machines that operate at a 1:1 pulsation ratio, the teat cup liner is collapsed for the same length of time that it is expanded. Widening the pulsation ratio increases the amount of time that the liner is expanded during each cycle in comparison to the time that it is closed. In a machine operating at a 2:1 ratio, the liners are open twice as long as they are closed.

Changes in pulsation rates and ratios affect the rate of milk flow. Widening the pulsation ratio from a 1:1 ratio increases the rate of milking (Table 9-2). Since the teat cup liner is open for a longer period of time than it is collapsed, it causes the milk to flow for a longer period of time during each cycle. Widening the pulsation ratio has a greater effect on milk flow rate than increasing the pulsation rate; however, the effect is not of the same magnitude as that of increasing the vacuum level. Widening the pulsation ratio increased the machine stripping time and yield in some but not all studies (27, 34).

The milking rate can be increased slightly by increasing the number of pulsations per minute (Table 9-2). The increase in milking rate is best explained by the work of Ardran et al. (2), who showed that increasing the pulsation rate caused the milk to flow for a higher percentage of time during each cycle. Milk flowed 55% of the time in a 1:1 pulsation ratio machine operating at 40 cycles per minute and 74% of the time at 160 cycles per minute. Increasing the pulsation rate of a milking machine also increases the vacuum and pump size requirements of the milking installations because more air must be evacuated with the higher pulsation machines.

The opening of the teat cup liner closely follows the pressure changes in cavity between the liner and teat cup. The half open position of the liner occurs when the pressure differences across the wall of the liner is 3–5

TABLE 9-2
Effect of pulsation rates and ratios on the rate of milking
and on machine stripping time.

Variable	Stripping time (min)	Total milking time (min)	Maximum rate of flow (lb/min)
Pulsation rate			
40	1.1	4.5	9.7
80	1.0	4.3	9.9
120	1.1	4.1	9.7
Pulsation ratio			
1:1	0.9	4.4	9.5
3:1	1.2	4.2	10.8

Source: Schmidt et al. 1963. *Cornell Agr. Expt. Sta. Bull.* 983.

inches Hg. Milk flow starts as soon as the liner begins to open and attains a maximum flow rate for the period of 0.05 seconds to 0.5 seconds from the time that the liner starts to open. At approximately 0.5 seconds, the milk flow rate declines. This also explains why an increase in pulsation rate increases the rate of milk flow—the higher pulsation rate gives more peak flows during each minute. It is suggested that after the teat sphincter muscles have been opened, a considerable time elapses before the full force of the sphincter is exerted to close the streak canal. At pulsation rates above 50 cycles per minute, the streak canal is closed by pressure exerted on the teat by the closing liner. Therefore, at pulsation rates above 50 cycles per minute, the sphincter muscle plays no active part in closing the streak canal, because its response is too slow in comparison to the pulsation rate. Milk flow stops when the collapsing liner is about one-half the normal width below the teat (2, 39, 41).

Other Factors

Adding weights to the teat cup claw and increasing the weight of the teat cups usually result in no change in the milk flow rates, but cause a decrease in machine stripping time and yield. Adding extra weights to the claw causes the units to fall off more often (34).

The effects of floor-type and suspended machines on the milk flow rates and machine stripping time and yield were compared (34). There was no difference in rate of milking between machines, but the suspended machine required less machine stripping time. This effect is similar to that of adding weights to the claw to reduce the machine stripping time.

Within recent years considerable interest has developed on the effect of different types of liners on milking rate and mastitis. Dodd and Clough (13) state that only the mouthpiece and the barrel of the liner have a direct effect on milking rate and machine stripping. The mouthpiece affects the proportion of milk yield obtained as strippings and the barrel affects the rate of milk removal. In a controlled experiment by Schmidt et al. (33), teat cup liners with 2 types of mouthpieces and 3 bore diameters were used for 28-day periods. It was found that there was no significant difference in the rate of milking or in the machine stripping time of the various types of liners (Table 9-3). It was more difficult to keep the narrow-bore liners attached to the cows than the wide-bore liners.

TABLE 9-3
Effect of teat cup liners on milk flow measurements.

Liner		Time before stripping (min)	Stripping time (min)	Maximum rate of flow (lb/min)
Internal diameter	Mouth-piece			
Narrow (⅞")	Solid	4.6	1.9	7.5
Narrow (⅞")	Cushion	4.3	1.9	7.5
Medium (1¹⁄₁₆")	Solid	4.7	1.6	7.7
Medium (1¹⁄₁₆")	Cushion	4.2	1.8	7.9
Wide (1½")	Solid	4.1	1.6	9.4
Wide (1½")	Cushion	4.0	2.3	8.8

Source: Schmidt et al. 1963. *J. Dairy Sci.* 46: 1064.

Cows require a certain amount of time to become accustomed to a new milking machine or treatment. Schmidt et al. (34) found that it took about 7 days for this conditioning process. In addition, it was found that first-calf heifers gave a greater response to a change in vacuum level than the older cows. Their studies also indicated that the selection for fast milking in cows would result in a decrease in machine stripping since there was a significant negative correlation between the stripping yield and the average and maximum rates of milk flow.

9-5 SUMMARY

The rate of milk flow of the dairy cow is determined by the physiological factors of the cow and the physical factors of the milking machine. The best measure of differences in inherited milking rates is the maximum rate of flow, which is defined as the highest milk yield obtained during a specific time interval of milking. The teat orifice is the main physiological factor that affects the rate of milk flow. The size of the orifice governs the rate of flow through the opening and the tonus of the sphincter muscle affects the size of the orifice. The milk flow rate increases with advancing age, but most of this is due to the high milk yield of older cows. In one study, it was found that the Holsteins have a faster rate of milk flow than Ayrshires and Brown Swiss, independent of milk yields. Cows with a fast rate of milk flow are generally the high-producing cows, but the fast rate of milk flow is a result rather than a cause of the increased lactation yield.

Several milking machine factors affect the rate of milk flow. The most important is vacuum level. The teat orifice is opened by a pressure differential across the teat meatus, thus an increase in the vacuum level causes an increase in the rate of milk flow. The effective vacuum level to open the teat meatus is affected by the vacuum fluctuations in the liner. High vacuum fluctuations reduce the rate of milk flow. Vacuum fluctuations can be reduced by providing an air inlet in the claw, by having a wide diameter bore of the short milk tube, and by milking into a weigh jar or a milk line below the level of the udder. Other physical factors of the machine that affect the rate of milk flow are pulsation rate and pulsation ratio. Widening the pulsation ratio has a greater effect on increasing the rate of milk flow than increasing the pulsation rate, but both of these effects are small in comparison to the effect of increasing the vacuum level.

REFERENCES

1. Andreae, U. 1964. *Züchtungskunde* 36:340 (*Dairy Sci. Abstr.* 27:1372, 1965).
2. Ardran, G. M., F. H. Kemp, P. A. Clough, and F. H. Dodd. 1958. *J. Dairy Res.* 25:154.
3. Baxter, E. S., P. M. Clarke, F. H. Dodd, and A. S. Foot. 1950. *J. Dairy Res.* 17:117.
4. Beck, G. H., H. C. Fryer, and D. B. Roark. 1951. *J. Dairy Sci.* 34:58.
5. Brumby, P. J. 1956. *Proc. N. Z. Soc. Animal Prod.* 16:89.
6. Buhr, W. 1958. *Diss. Tierarztliche Hochschule, Hannover* (*Dairy Sci. Abstr.* 22:2543, 1960).
7. Caruolo, E. V., and G. D. Marx. 1962. *J. Dairy Sci.* 45:696.

8. Clarke, D. J., and A. K. Lascelles. 1965. *Aust. J. Exptl. Agric. Anim. Husb.* 5:115.
9. Clough, P. A., and F. H. Dodd. 1957. *J. Dairy Res.* 24:152.
10. Cowhig, M. J. 1969. *Proceedings of the Symposium on Machine Milking.* National Institute for Research in Dairying, Reading, England. p. 15.
11. Desvignes, A., and M. Poutous. 1963. *Ann. Zootech.* 12:17 (*Dairy Sci. Abstr.* 25:2729, 1963).
12. Dodd, F. H. 1953. *J. Dairy Res.* 20:301.
13. Dodd, F. H., and P. A. Clough. 1959. In *Machine Milking,* Ministry of Agriculture Fisheries and Food, London, Bull. 177. Ch. 3.
14. Dodd, F. H., and A. S. Foot. 1953. *J. Dairy Res.* 20:138.
15. Donald, H. P. 1960. *J. Dairy Res.* 27:361.
16. Griffin, T. K., and F. H. Dodd. 1962. *J Dairy Res.* 29:207.
17. Guest, R. W., and S. B. Spencer. 1965. *The Milking Machine System.* Cornell Misc. Bull. 64.
18. Hall, H. S. 1959. In *Machine Milking,* Ministry of Agriculture Fisheries and Food, London, Bull. 177. Ch. 2.
19. Johansson, I., and P. Malven. 1960. *Z. Tierzüch. Zucht.-Biol.* 74:1.
20. Maffey, J. 1961. *Vet. Record* 73:589.
21. Markos, H. G., and R. W. Touchberry. 1966. *J. Dairy Sci.* 49:722.
22. Naito, M., Y. Shoda, H. Kobayashi, Y. Fukushima, and S. Nomura. 1965. *Jap. J. Zootech. Sci.* 36:496.
23. Naito, M., Y. Shoda, J. Nagai, H. Nagasawa, H. Shinohara, and T. Terada. 1964. *Jap. J. Zootech. Sci.* 35:52.
24. Naude, R. T., and A. Smith. 1964. *Proc. S. Afr. Soc. Animal Prod.* 3:101.
25. Nyhan, J. F. 1969. *Proceedings of the Symposium on Machine Milking.* National Institute for Research in Dairying, Reading, England. p. 71.
26. Petersen, W. E. 1944. *J. Dairy Sci.* 27:433.
27. Phillips, D. S. M. 1963. *Proc. Ruakura Fmrs. Conf.*, pp. 219-234.
28. Politiek, R. D. 1962. *Veet.-en Zuivelber.* 5:411 (*Dairy Sci. Abstr.* 25:347, 1963).
29. Politiek, R. D. 1964. *Veet.-en Zuivelber.* 7:313 (*Dairy Sci. Abstr.* 27:2699, 1965).
30. Politiek, R. D. 1965. *Veet.-en Zuivelber.* 8:395 (*Dairy Sci. Abstr.* 28:1089, 1966).
31. Rajamannan, A. H. J., A. C. Linnerud, and E. F. Graham. 1966. *J. Dairy Sci.* 49:32.
32. Rakes, J. M., and G. L. Ford. 1963. *J. Dairy Sci.* 36:369.
33. Schmidt, G. H., R. S. Guthrie, and R. W. Guest. 1963. *J. Dairy Sci.* 46:1064.
34. Schmidt, G. H., R. S. Guthrie, R. W. Guest, E. B. Hundtoft, A. Kumar, and C. R. Henderson. 1963. *Cornell Agr. Expt. Sta. Bull.* 983.
35. Schmidt, G. H., K. O. Switzer, R. W. Guest, and R. S. Guthrie. 1964. *J. Dairy Sci.* 47:761.
36. Schmidt, G. H., and L. D. Van Vleck. 1969. *J. Dairy Sci.* 52:639.
37. Sims, J. A. 1963. *Diss. Abstr.* 23:2279.
38. Thiel, C. C. 1969. *Proceedings of the Symposium on Machine Milking.* National Institute for Research in Dairying, Reading, England. p. 3.
39. Thiel, C. C., P. A. Clough, and D. N. Akam. 1964. *J. Dairy Res.* 31:303.
40. Thiel, C. C., P. A. Clough, F. H. Dodd. 1965. *J. Dairy Sci.* 48:617.

41. Thiel, C. C., P. A. Clough, D. R. Westgarth, and D. N. Akam. 1966. *J. Dairy Res.* 33:177.
42. Thiel, C. C., P. A. Clough, D. R. Westgarth, and D. N. Akam. 1968. *J. Dairy Res.* 35:303.
43. Touchberry, R. W. 1966. *J. Dairy Sci.* 49:722.
44. Venge, O. 1963. *Lantbr. Hogsk. Ann.* 29:187.
45. Witzel, D. A., and J. S. McDonald. 1964. *J. Dairy Sci.* 47:1378.

FACTORS AFFECTING THE YIELD
AND COMPOSITION OF MILK

10-1 MILK SECRETION PROCESS

The constituents of milk are produced by the epithelial cells in two ways. One group of compounds, which includes milk fat, most of the protein components, and lactose, is synthesized in the epithelial cells from blood precursors and then released into the lumen of the alevolus. The remaining milk constituents pass from the blood and move across the epithelial cells or between them into the alveolar lumina without alteration by the cells. In some cases, they are bound to other compounds, but synthesis does not take place within the cells. Details of the secretion of milk fat, lactose, protein, and vitamins and minerals will be covered in later chapters. The secretion of water will be discussed briefly.

The milk of individual first-calf heifers with noninfected mammary glands has a constant amount of sodium, potassium, and lactose. Within a breed, a close inverse relationship exists between the lactose content and the molar sums of potassium and sodium concentrations. This has led to the hypothesis that the water of milk secreted by the alveolar cells arises in two ways: part arises in the secretory cell as water of the potassium-rich intracellular fluid; and part arises as a result of the synthesis of lactose, proteins, and fat, since water moves into the cell to maintain osmotic equilibrium. These two portions are constant within an individual but vary between animals. The constituents primarily responsible for the osmotic pressure of milk are lactose and sodium and potassium and their associated anions. Lactose alone is responsible for more than one-third of the osmotic pressure of normal milk. In addition to the primary secretion of water in milk, a blood plasma transudate, which is rich in sodium and chlorine, contributes to the fluid of milk. This type of secretion appears to be important in the secretion of milk that is associated with advancing lactation, advancing age, and bacterial infection of the udder. Milk secreted during these times has increased percentages of sodium and chlorine and decreased percentages of lactose and potassium (32, 57, 58, 59, 75, 79).

Milk is in osmotic equilibrium with the blood flowing through the udder throughout the period that milk remains in the udder and not just during its formation. Changes in milk composition occur as water moves in and out of the udder in response to changes in the osmotic pressure of blood. The volume of water secreted in the milk is thus changed to maintain osmotic equilibrium between the blood and milk. Since lactose accounts for a large part of the osmotic pressure of milk, an increase in its secretion rate causes an increase in water movement into milk, and, consequently, lactose plays a major role in governing the rate of milk secretion (79, 80).

The potassium:lactose ratio and the potential for lactose content in the milk of individual animals is largely independent of environmental and physiological factors associated with age or stage of lactation. The variation in the lactose content of milk is relatively small and can only be markedly changed by factors that upset the metabolic balance of the udder, such as mastitis (75).

10-2 BLOOD PRECURSORS OF MILK CONSTITUENTS

The rate of milk secretion is partially dependent upon the availability of blood precursors that flow through the mammary gland. This in turn depends upon the rate of blood flow through the udder and the composition and uptake of the blood constituents by the mammary gland. Earlier measurements indicated that the ratio of blood flow to milk yield was about 500:1 for the cow and goat. More recent studies in the conscious lactating goat indicate that the ratio of blood flow to milk yield is 460:1 in high-producing goats and as high as 1,000:1 in low-producing goats. The blood flow:milk yield ratio also increases with advancing lactation and with a drop in yield due to illness (4, 36).

The blood precursors of ruminant milk constituents are shown in Table 10-1. Water, vitamins, and minerals are transferred from the blood plasma to the milk without synthesis. Lactose is synthesized primarily

TABLE 10-1
Blood precursors of the milk constituents in the ruminant.

Milk constituent	Blood Precursor
Water	Water
Lactose	Glucose
Protein	
Casein	Amino acids
β-Lactoglobulin	Amino acids
α-Lactalbumin	Amino acids
Milk serum albumin	Blood serum albumin
Immune globulins	Immune globulins
Fat	
Fatty acids	Acetate, β-hydroxybutyrate, blood lipids
Glycerol	Glucose, glycerol from triglycerides
Minerals	Minerals
Vitamins	Vitamins

from glucose, and casein, β-lactoglobulin and α-lactalbumin are synthesized from amino acids. Milk serum albumin and immune globulins are not synthesized in the mammary gland but transferred as such from the bloodstream. In the ruminant, acetate and β-hydroxybutyrate are precursors of fatty acids up to 16 carbon atoms (C_{16}) in length. A small portion of the C_{12} and C_{14} fatty acids arise from blood C_{16} fatty acids. Milk palmitic acid (C_{16}) comes from the build up of acetate molecules and from palmitic acid of the blood triglycerides. Most of the stearic acid (C_{18}) comes from the blood as such and is not built up from C_2 or C_4 units. Most of the unsaturated fatty acids in the milk are derived from a dehydrogenation of the fatty acids, particularly stearic acid. The mammary gland cannot convert an unsaturated fatty acid, such as oleic, into a saturated fatty acid, such as stearic. Glycerol is mainly synthesized from glucose in the mammary gland, and a small part comes from the triglycerides absorbed from the blood. In the nonruminant, glucose is the primary precursor of the fatty acids (4).

The comparative composition of blood plasma and milk of the cow is shown in Table 10-2. The concentration of carbohydrates and fats is

TABLE 10-2
Comparative composition of blood plasma and milk of the cow.

Blood Plasma		Milk	
Constituent	Percentage	Constituent	Percentage
Water	91.0	Water	87.0
Glucose	0.05	Lactose	4.90
		Casein	2.90
Serum albumin	3.20	α-Lactalbumin	0.52
Serum globulin	4.40	β-Lactoglobulin	0.20
Neutral fat	0.06	Neutral fat	3.70
Phospholipids	0.24	Phospholipids	0.10
Calcium	0.009	Calcium	0.12
Phosphorous	0.011	Phosphorous	0.10
Sodium	0.34	Sodium	0.05
Potassium	0.03	Potassium	0.15
Chlorine	0.35	Chlorine	0.11
Citric acid	Trace	Citric acid	0.20

Source: Maynard and Loosli. 1969. *Animal Nutrition*, 6th ed. New York: McGraw-Hill.

much higher in milk than in the blood. This is also true of the calcium and phosphorous contents. Milk has a lower protein content, especially albumin and globulin, but has a much higher concentration of casein. Blood plasma is also considerably higher in sodium and chlorine than milk. The mammary gland epithelial cells must regulate the mineral composition of milk in some way since the variation in composition is very small.

All of the calcium and 80% of the nitrogen and calories removed from the blood by the udder appear in the milk of the goat. In addition, 80% of the neutral fat and volatile fatty acids taken up by the mammary gland also appear in milk fat. Only 50% of the glucose appears as lactose. The remaining glucose is used for energy. Acetate is also used as a source of energy for the ruminant mammary gland (36).

10-3 HERITABILITY OF MILK COMPONENTS

Because the pricing system of milk in most countries is based upon the fat or solids-not-fat contents, considerable attention has been directed towards determining the heritability of the milk components as well as the phenotypic and genotypic relationships between the various components. In order to make progress in the selection of a trait, it must have a relatively high heritability and, at the same time, enough variation must be present within the species to enable selection to take place. In addition, the trait should be positively correlated with the other desirable and economic traits.

Differences in the milk composition within a species also exist (Table 1-1). Guernsey and Jersey cows have much higher milk fat percentages and somewhat higher protein percentages than the other breeds. However, there is a wide variation in the milk composition among animals within a breed. This variation can be greater than the variation among breeds. An increase in the solids-not-fat (SNF) percentage of milk usually accompanies an increase in milk fat percentage. The phenotypic and genetic correlation between the two is about 0.40. The phenotypic and genetic correlations between the protein and SNF content are 0.81 and 0.94, respectively. Most of the variation in the SNF content of milk is due to the variation in the protein content, since the lactose and mineral contents do not vary much. The fat and lactose contents are positively correlated with a phenotypic correlation of 0.11 and a genetic correlation of 0.37 (33, 35, 54).

The phenotypic correlation between lactation milk yield and fat percentage is approximately -0.20. There is also a negative correlation between lactation milk yield and the SNF and protein percentages. This indicates that selection for milk production results in a slight decrease in the milk fat and SNF percentages. Most of the SNF percentage decrease is due to a decrease in protein percentage. Selection has little effect on the lactose and mineral composition of milk (35).

A large number of studies have been conducted on the heritabilities of milk constituents. The heritabilities for milk fat, protein, SNF, and lactose percentages are in the order of 0.50. The heritability estimates for milk and fat yields are between 0.20 and 0.30 (33).

10-4 FACTORS AFFECTING THE YIELD AND COMPOSITION OF MILK

Colostrum

The first-drawn milk from the mammary gland after parturition is colostrum, which is composed of milk constituents that were secreted by the mammary gland prior to parturition. The composition of colostrum of the Holstein cow, the sow, and the mare is given in Table 10-3. In many states it is illegal to sell milk from the cow for the first 5 days after calving;

TABLE 10-3

Comparison of the composition of colostrum with the composition of normal milk obtained 2–3 weeks after parturition for three species.

Measurement	Holstein Cow (47)[a]		Sow (10)[a]		Mare (71)[a]	
	Colostrum	Milk[b]	Colostrum	Milk[b]	Colostrum	Milk[c]
Total solids (%)	23.9	12.9	20.5	16.9	25.2	11.3
Fat (%)	6.7	4.0	5.8	5.4	0.7	2.0
Protein (%)	14.0	3.1	10.6	5.1	19.1	2.7
Lactose (%)	2.7	5.0	3.4	5.7	4.6	6.1
Ash (%)	1.11	0.74	0.73	0.71	7.72	0.50
Specific gravity	1.056	1.032	—	—	1.076	1.035

[a] Reference number.
[b] 2 weeks after parturition.
[c] 3 weeks after parturition.

however, the gross composition of the milk is normal in approximately 4 to 5 milkings after parturition (47).

The total solids, protein, and ash compositions are higher in colostrum than in the milk obtained 2 or 3 weeks after calving (Table 10-3). The most striking difference is the high protein percentage in colostrum. A large part of this is due to the globulin content, especially the gamma globulins, which contain the antibodies. The antibody titer of blood of the newborn calf is extremely low. The gamma globulin can be absorbed by the calf during its first day of life. The absorption of the intact antibodies from the colostrum allows the newborn to build up an antibody titer, which produces passive immunity against many of the common calfhood diseases. After the first day, the enzymes in the intestines break down the globulin into amino acids, and thus it loses its ability to protect the animal. The loss of ability to absorb intact globulins after the first day may also be due to changes in the absorptive ability of the intestine. The milk fat percentage in colostrum is variable, but colostrum contains a lower lactose content than milk obtained 2-3 weeks later. The importance of colostrum in other species is similar to that in the newborn calf (37).

High levels of lactose can cause scours in calves, therefore the low level of lactose in colostrum may be a built-in protective mechanism to reduce the incidence of scours in the newborn while it consumes colostrum. Colostrum is higher in calcium, magnesium, phosphorus, and chlorine, and lower in potassium than normal milk, but they reach normal levels after a few milkings. The vitamin A content of colostrum milk is about 10 times higher than that of normal milk. This may be related to the protection of the young animals, since the vitamin A content of the body at birth is low. Vitamin A is involved in the protection of animals against diseases (22, 24, 28).

Changes Occurring in a Normal Lactation

The milk production of the dairy cow at calving starts out at a relatively high level and continues to increase to a peak approximately 3–6 weeks after parturition. This is shown in Figure 10-1. This peak may be held for a few weeks, after which the milk production declines until the end of lactation. The rate of decline is defined as the persistency of the animal. Cows with a flatter slope in the lactation curve have a higher persistency. Pregnancy plays a role in the latter part of lactation, causing a marked decrease in the milk production at about the 5th or 6th month of gestation.

The fat, solids-not-fat, and protein contents of the milk are high in early lactation, fall rapidly and reach a minimum during the 2nd to 3rd months of lactation, and then increase towards the end of lactation. This causes an inverse relationship between the yield of milk and percentage composition of these components. The lactose content is low in colostrum, increases to a high value at the beginning of lactation, and declines slightly during the remainder of the lactation. An increase in the SNF and protein contents of milk occurs during the 6th month of lactation; the increase is usually the result of pregnancy. Most reports in the literature indicate that there is no increase in the solids-not-fat and protein percentages of milk during the latter part of lactation when the cows are not pregnant (35, 55, 56, 66).

The composition of mare's milk follows a trend somewhat similar to that of the dairy cow. The total solids, crude protein, and ash percentages drop abruptly from the values of colostrum and then tend to decline slowly thereafter. The values for the 5-day-postpartum and the 4-month-postpartum samples for the following compounds are respectively: total solids, 12.0 and 10.0; crude protein, 3.3 and 2.0; fat, 2.5 and 1.3; and ash, 0.54 and 0.27. The lactose content tends to rise slowly throughout lactation, increasing from a value of 5.9% at 5 days postpartum to 6.5% at 4 months postpartum (71).

The peak lactation in the sow occurs between the 3rd and 5th weeks postpartum. The average fat content of sow's milk declines throughout the first 6 weeks of lactation, the protein content does not change significantly, and the ash content drops slightly at 1–2 weeks postpartum and then increases towards the end of the 6-week sampling period (49). Colenbrander et al. (10) found similar results for protein and ash percentages; the fat percentage remained relatively constant, however, throughout the 6-week lactation period. The lactose content showed a marked rise from

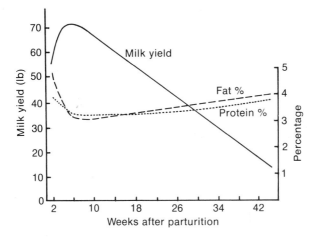

FIGURE 10–1
Lactation curves of milk yield and milk fat and protein
percentages of Holstein cows.

the colostrum content to 1 week postpartum and remained relatively
constant thereafter.

Age and Body Weight at Calving

The amount of milk produced by cows increases with advancing age.
Part of this increase is due to an increase in body weight, which results in
a larger digestive system and a larger mammary gland for the secretion of
milk. A number of studies have separated the body weight and age effects,
particularly as they apply to first-calf heifers.

Advancing age or increased number of lactations results in a gradual
decrease in the percentage composition of milk fat and solids-not-fat.
The drop in fat content is about 0.2% from the first to fifth lactations and
that for solids-not-fat is about 0.4%. Beyond the fifth lactation there
appears to be little further change in either constituent. Much of the
drop in the solids-not-fat contents is due to a drop in lactose content,
whereas the change in the total protein content is relatively small. The
percentage composition of casein decreases, which must result in a com-
pensatory increase in the noncasein protein content. Whether the changes
in milk composition are specifically due to age is hard to determine. The
changes must be considered in light of the selection that has taken place
within the populations. The changes might be brought about by udder
deterioration through normal usage or the increasing incidence of mastitis
with advanced age (33, 35, 55, 56, 66).

Separation of the body weight and age effects on milk production has been reported by a number of workers (5, 8, 17, 18, 39, 41). Milk production increases between 100 to 870 lb for each 100-lb increase in body weight when age is held constant. These figures apply to first-calf heifers as well as to older cows. Erb (17) showed that the increase in milk production per 100 lb body weight is somewhat less than the increase for 100 lb metabolic size (body weight$^{0.70}$). The Holstein population with which he was working had increased milk yields of 430 lb for each 100 lb increase in body weight and 662 lb for each 100 lb increase in metabolic size. When body weight is held constant, there is an increase in milk production with increasing age in months at calving until the animal reaches maturity.

Johansson and Hansson (30) concluded that the effect of age on milk production could be divided into two parts. During the first and second lactations, the yield was directly related to the age at calving. During the third lactation, the yield was independent of the age of calving. During subsequent lactations there was an inverse relationship between milk yield and age at calving. Neither the body weight nor the age at calving plays a significant role in the lactation milk fat percentage.

Gestation

Some of the changes in the milk yield and composition attributed to stage of lactation are due to the effect of gestation. Pregnancy has an inhibitory effect on the milk yield of dairy cows, particularly during the latter part of the lactation. The importance of pregnancy on milk production was demonstrated by McDaniel and Legates (40) who showed that the number of days that a cow was not pregnant during lactation could account for 13.0% of the environmental variation among records of dairy cows.

The effect of pregnancy on milk production does not appear to occur until the 5th month of gestation. Its earliest effect in the normal lactation curve occurs during the 7th month. During the 8th month of pregnancy, there is a marked drying-off effect due to the pregnancy (11).

The way in which pregnancy inhibits lactation has not been determined. It was originally thought that fetal development required a larger amount of nutrients; however, calculations indicate that the energy required for the growth, maintenance, and activity of the full-term calf is equal to that required for the production of 400–600 lb of milk (11). Another possible way in which pregnancy inhibits milk secretion is change in levels of hormones in the body. For instance, a combination of estrogen and progesterone has an inhibitory effect on milk secretion in most animals. It may be that the estrogen and progesterone levels increase up to a level that inhibits secretion. Recent work in mouse mammary gland tissue organ culture indicates that progesterone prevents the rise in activity of α-lactalbumin, one of the two proteins making up the lactose synthetase enzyme (70). It may be that the level of progesterone in the blood during pregnancy increases to a level that interferes with lactose synthesis, which in turn causes a reduction in milk secretion.

During the 4th–5th month of gestation, there is a marked increase in the solids-not-fat content of the milk, accounting for most of the solids-not-fat increase in the latter stages of lactation (78). Parkhie et al. (46) found that cows pregnant for 7 months during their lactations had a significantly higher milk protein content than cows that were not pregnant or pregnant for shorter periods of time. Cows pregnant for less than 7 months did not have higher protein percentages than the nonpregnant cows. There is also an increase in the milk fat percentage as the amount of time that cows are pregnant during the lactation increases (19). It is not possible to determine whether the changes in milk composition are due to pregnancy or whether they are the result of a drop in milk production. In most cases there is an inverse relationship between the milk yield and the milk fat and SNF percentages.

Length of the Dry Period

Most studies indicate that dry periods of less than 6 weeks cause a decrease in milk yield during the next lactation in comparison with a dry period of 6 to 8 weeks. Cows with no or very short dry periods produce between 60–75% of the milk of the control cows that receive a 6- to 8-week dry period. Dry periods over 60 days in length produce no significant increase in the milk yield during the next lactation. Long dry periods decrease the average annual production of the cows by extending the calving interval beyond the normal 13- to 14-month interval and causing a decrease in the lifetime production of the dairy cow (1, 68).

Statistical analyses of the effect of dry-period lengths have shown that they have little effect on the lactation milk production. Part of the non-significant influence of dry-period length in these studies is the fact that a very small number of cows had dry periods less than 6 weeks. If most cows have dry periods longer than 6 weeks, one would not expect to find a relationship between length of dry period and level of milk production. Part of the dry-period length effect is related to the body condition of the cow at calving. Cows in good body condition at calving produce higher milk yields during the following lactation as well as an increased milk fat percentage during the first 3 months of the next lactation than cows in thin body condition at calving (34, 65).

Several attempts have been made to determine the physiological reason that cows need a dry period. Altman (2) found that the frequency of mitosis was greater in nonlactating mammary gland tissue in comparison to lactating tissue of cows in late pregnancy. He indicated that a dry period was necessary to allow for a rapid regeneration of the secretory epithelium before the next lactation. Smith et al. (64) dried off two quarters of two cows 10 weeks before the expected date of parturition and continued to milk the other two quarters throughout gestation. The quarters that were continually milked gave 56% and 62% as much milk during the first 3 months of the next lactations as those quarters that were dried off.

The results obtained so far indicate that a dry period of 6 weeks is essential for maximum milk production during the following lactation. The physiological mechanism responsible for the increase in milk production has not been determined.

Seasonal Effects

The effect of season of calving on the lactation milk production and composition is confounded by breed, the stage of lactation, the climatic condition under which the records are made, and variations in the feeding practices. In the northern part of the United States, the tendency has been towards fall-freshening herds, which confounds the season with stage of lactation effects.

Cows freshening in the fall usually produce more milk than those calving in other seasons. In a mid-western study, Holstein cows freshening during December through March produced approximately 1,300 lb more milk than those calving during July and August. Fall-freshening Holstein cows in New York State at one time produced approximately 1,500 lb more milk than those calving in spring and summer. These differences are becoming less, presumably because of better feeding and management of the cows. Results from North Carolina and Georgia also indicate that cows calving in the winter and spring produce more milk than those calving during the summer (6, 34, 62).

The composition of milk during the different seasons is also affected by lactation trend effects. The percentages of fat and solids-not-fat are usually highest during the winter months, decline in March and April, continue to decline to a low point in July and August, and then start to increase. Fall- and winter-freshening cows have higher lactation percentages of total solids, SNF, and fat than those freshening at other times of the year, because the percentage composition of these three components is high during the fall and winter months, when the milk yield is also high.

In contrast to this, cows calving in North Carolina from May through October had higher average percentage values of milk fat and solids-not-fat than those calving during different seasons of the year (6, 33, 46, 62, 66).

Environmental Temperature Effects

A considerable number of reviews have been published on the effect of temperature and humidity on milk yield and composition (7, 9, 43, 50, 51, 52, 61). The effect of environmental temperature on milk yield and composition is dependent upon the breed of animal. Holsteins and the larger breeds are somewhat more tolerant of the lower temperatures, whereas the smaller breeds, especially the Jersey, and to some extent the Brown Swiss, are much more tolerant of the higher temperatures. Low temperatures have an insignificant effect on the milk yield if extra feed is given to cover the extra energy required to maintain body temperatures. Within the relative humidity range of 60% to 80%, the milk yield is unaffected by temperature changes between 40° and 70° F. Within this range, cows can regulate their body temperatures by physical means without materially altering their heat production. This range of thermal neutrality varies with the breeds, being somewhat higher in the Jersey and Brown Swiss than in the Holsteins. Above the range of thermal neutrality, a marked decrease in milk production occurs with an increase in environmental temperature. At high temperatures, the food consumption decreases and the water consumption increases. At about 105° F, the food consumption and milk production approach zero.

The milk fat content increases with decreasing temperatures below 75° F. The solids-not-fat and total solids contents follow the same pattern as the milk fat percentage. The chloride content of milk increases and the lactose decreases with high environmental temperatures.

Cobble and Herman (9) found that a marked decrease in milk production occurred with environmental temperatures above 80° F for the Holstein, 85° F for the Jersey and Brown Swiss, and 90° F for the Brahmans. A marked increase in milk fat percentage occurred above 90° F. The solids-not-fat percentage continued to decrease with increasing temperatures above 90° F.

Disease

Mastitis affects both the yield and composition of milk. It alters the permeability of the udder tissue and impairs the ability of secretory tissue to synthesize milk constituents. It also destroys the secretory tissue in the udder, consequently lowering the milk production. A decrease in production persists after the abeyance of the clinical signs of mastitis due to a destruction of the secretory tissue (55).

The California Mastitis Test (CMT) is an index of udder inflammation and is directly related to the leucocyte count of the milk. In one experiment (21), individual quarters with abnormal milk were compared with opposite quarters of the same cow that were negative to the California Mastitis Test. Quarters showing test reactions of trace, 1, 2, and 3, produced 9.0%, 19.5%, 31.8%, and 34.4%, respectively, less milk than the quarters that were negative. The presence of pathogenic bacteria in the udder that shows no clinical mastitis causes a decrease in milk yield. Cows infected with mainly *Staphylococcus pyogenes* organisms produced 10% less milk, 11% less solids-not-fat, and 12% less fat during the lactation in comparison with cows free from infection (44).

Milk of cows with clinical mastitis is lower in lactose and potassium and higher in sodium and chloride contents than normal milk. During mastitis, the globulin content increases, serum albumin and proteose contents have smaller increases, and there is a decrease in the casein content. These changes in protein fractions do not change the overall percentage of protein. The changes in the milk fat content are not consistent. In most cases, there is a decrease in the solids-not-fat content of cows with clinical mastitis due to the decrease in the lactose content (55, 60, 73).

Waite and Blackburn (74) categorized the changes in milk composition according to the total cell count of the milk. Milk with a cell count less than 100,000 cells/ml had no subclinical mastitis and no change in the chemical composition of the milk. As the cell count increased from 100,000 to 500,000 cells/ml, there was a decrease in the SNF and lactose contents of the milk. When the cell count was over 1,000,000/ml, the casein content began to decrease.

These studies indicate that the major effect of infection and mastitis on milk composition is on the lactose and mineral contents of the milk brought about by a change in the permeability of the mammary gland epithelium. The changes in the protein content appear after rather severe signs of clinical mastitis.

Body Condition at Calving

The body condition of the cow at calving has an effect on the level of milk production and possibly milk composition. This is in part due to the length of the dry period, since one of the main reasons for advocating a dry period is to allow the animal to rebuild her body stores before the next lactation. Some reports indicate that liberal grain feeding during the dry period increases the milk and fat production during the following lactation. This work was summarized by Schmidt and Schultz (63).

The milk output during early lactation is correlated with the input of energy during the dry period. Catabolism of 100 lb body fat produces as much as 880 lb of milk during early lactation. Most cows lose 100 to 200 lb of body weight after calving, with some cows losing as much as 400 lb. Not all of this loss is body fat, but cows in good body condition at the time of calving have more energy available for the synthesis of milk in early lactation, a time when the animal has a difficult time consuming enough energy to meet her maintenance and milk production requirements (53).

Several studies (23, 25, 81) have shown no beneficial effect of grain feeding during the dry period. In one study (63) three levels of grain were fed during the dry period and it was found that feeding high levels of grain during the dry period did not affect the lactation milk and fat production. All of the cows were in good body condition at the time of drying off and this may be the reason that no differences in production were noted. In another study (16) cows and heifers receiving grain to appetite starting 21 days precalving produced 79 and 119 lb more milk, respectively, during the first 45 days postpartum than cows receiving no grain until after calving. The feeding of grain prepartum turned out to be uneconomical; however, the cows used in the trial were in good condition when they were placed on the trial.

The information on the effect of body condition on milk composition is relatively limited; however, Eckles (12) showed that cows in fat condition at the time of calving produced milk containing higher milk fat percentage than either moderately fleshed or thin cows. Most of the increase in milk fat percentage occurred during the first 2 or 3 months of lactation. In another study (55), the feeding of liberal amounts of grain prior to calving resulted in an increase in fat and SNF percentages for the first few months of lactation.

Plane of Nutrition

Reid (53) states that many low-producing cows would yield more milk if they were provided with more energy. It is a common farm observation that energy is one of the most limiting factors to high milk production. Increasing the energy intake increases the level of milk production toward the cow's inherited potential. The available energy during early lactation plays an important role in the lactation milk production. The milk yield during the early segments of lactation reflects the total lactation yield. Cows with a high level of milk production during early lactation produce considerably more milk than cows starting out at a relatively low level. The relationship of energy intake to milk production is illustrated in a study of two herds by Warner (76). Both herds averaged approximately 50 lb of milk per day during the first month of lactation. One herd had a high persistency with an average daily yield of 44 lb during the 6th month of lactation; whereas the second herd had dropped to 26 lb at this time. Part of the difference between the herds was related to the distribution of the grain fed during the 6-month period. In the first herd, the cows were provided with energy that exceeded the recommended feeding standards during early lactation. The cows in the second herd were underfed during early lactation and overfed during 4th to 6th months of lactation. The cows with the low persistency received about the same amount of grain as the cows in the other herd. This emphasizes the necessity of supplying adequate energy and demonstrates the importance of the distribution of energy during the lactation.

The effect of nutrition on milk composition has been summarized by Laben (33) and Rook (55). Increasing the plane of nutrition by 25–35% above the normal feeding standards causes the SNF percentage to increase by 0.2%. Reductions to 25% below the feeding standards cause a decrease in the SNF percentage of 0.4–0.5%. The changes in the SNF percentages are due largely to the changes in the milk protein content, which in turn are due mostly to changes in the casein content. Underfeeding causes a slight decrease in the lactose content. The effect of the diet on milk fat composition is also related to the change in milk yield. When the diet increases the milk yield, the milk fat percentage tends to decrease.

Dietary Levels of Protein and Fat

Severe underfeeding of protein to dairy animals causes a reduction in the SNF percentage of the milk in addition to a drop in the milk yield. Slight underfeeding of protein to dairy cattle causes a slight decrease in the milk yield and small decreases in the milk content of proteoses, globulin, and nonprotein nitrogen. Increasing the protein content of the diet above the normal recommended standards has no effect on yield and causes only a slight increase in the nonprotein nitrogen content of the milk (55).

About 3–4% fat is needed in the concentrate portion of the ration for maximum milk and fat yields; however, the amount of fat in diet has no consistent effect on milk fat content. The addition of 2 pounds of edible fat to the diet of the cow causes digestive disturbances and leads to a loss of appetite and a fall in milk yield. The effect of specific fats has been reported to modify the milk fat content without affecting milk yield; however, the results are variable and often transient. The exception is the feeding of cod liver oil and certain other highly unsaturated oils, which markedly depress milk fat content without affecting milk yield. Linoleic acid has a similar effect to cod liver oil (13, 55).

Attempts to increase the unsaturated fatty acid composition of milk through feeding have met with limited success. This is partly due to the fact that the rumen microorganisms hydrogenate most of the unsaturated fatty acids in the rumen. The feeding of cottonseed oil as 6% of the concentrate mixture or replacing 15% of the grain allowance with safflower oil reduced the percentage of saturated fatty acids and markedly increased the percentage of unsaturated fatty acids, especially oleic acid; both oils however, caused significant depressions in milk fat percentages. A change in the fatty acid composition of milk occurs during starvation, which results in the short-chain fatty acids being replaced by oleic acid. As much as 80% of the short-chain fatty acids may be replaced by oleic acid (13, 29, 48).

Changes in the Diet

A number of changes in the diet of the dairy cow lead to a depression in milk fat percentage. These have been reviewed by Elliot (13) and Warner (77). One of the earliest rations that was found to depress the milk fat percentage was a high concentrate, restricted roughage ration. Even though the reports differ in the minimum amount of roughage required to produce a decrease in milk fat percentage, Warner (77) concluded that at least 15 pounds of hay or 1½ pounds of hay equivalent should be fed daily to prevent a depression. The physical form of the forage also plays a role in the depression of the milk fat percentage in that fine grinding of the roughage causes a depression. There is much variation in the reports on the fineness of grind, but it appears that definite milk fat depressions occur when the roughage is ground to less than ⅛ inch in length.

The restricted roughage, high concentrate diets are accompanied by a decrease in the level of dietary fiber. The entire ration of the cow should contain at least 17% crude fiber to prevent a depression in milk fat. The level of crude fiber probably plays a role in the milk fat depression when cows are turned out on lush early spring pastures. Concentrates containing flaked corn or other heated starches, such as potato meal, bread or cooked rice, also cause a small decrease in the fat test. In addition, the use of a high corn diet, particularly in pelleted form, causes a decrease in milk fat percentage. Pelleted corn at the level of 35% of the ration will cause a problem by lowering the milk fat test. Expanded grains and pearl millet pastures also cause a depression in milk fat percentage (10, 26, 77).

Rations that depress the milk fat percentage also bring about some characteristic changes in rumen fermentation. There is a decreased molar percentage of acetic acid and an increased molar percentage of propionic acid in the rumen fluid. This reduces the ratio of acetic acid to propionic acid. Van Soest (72) summarized the factors that cause a depression in milk fat test and the theories that have been used to explain the depression. The first theory states that there is a deficiency in the rumen acetic acid production for milk fat synthesis due to the shift in rumen fermentation. The second theory involves a reduction in the amount of β-hydroxybutyric acid in the blood. This acid is taken up by the mammary gland and is used for milk fat synthesis. The third theory is that the glucogenic response during high propionate production suppresses the mobilization of fat from the tissues, and thereby causes a decline in the blood lipids available for milk fat synthesis. Recent work by Baldwin and coworkers (3, 45) supports this latter concept. During milk fat depression, the proportion of stearic acid in milk fat, presumably arising from adipose tissue, is depressed. In addition, the fatty acid esterification in adipose tissue is elevated, which causes the depression in availability of milk precursors to the mammary gland. All of these theories have some experimental observations to support them, but none completely explain all of the ramifications of the causes of the depression in milk fat.

Other changes accompany the depression in the milk fat percentage. They are: a decrease in blood lipids and ketone bodies, an increase in blood glucose, a decrease in rumen pH, increased body weight gains, reduced milk production, decreased short-chain, palmitic, and stearic acid components of the milk fat, and increases in unsaturated fatty acid components of milk fat. The reduction in milk production during a milk-fat-depressing diet has not been obtained in all studies (27, 31).

Some research workers have reported that the feeding of one pound of sodium acetate daily to cows on a fat-depressing diet restored the milk fat percentage to normal; other workers have, however, shown that this is not always effective (13). Sodium butyrate appears to be as effective as acetate, but propionate administration appears to have a further milk-fat-depressing effect. The infusion of propionic acid into the rumen causes a drop in the milk fat percentage and increases the solids-not-fat and protein percentages. Acetic acid infusion causes an increase in milk yield as well as an increase in fat test with no effect on solids-not-fat. The infusion of acetic and butyric acids increases the proportion of C_4-C_{16} acids of milk fat and decreases the proportion of C_{18} acids. Propionic acid infusion decreases the yield of all major component fatty acids of milk except palmitic acid. The infusion of propionic acid and glucose into the blood also decreases the milk fat percentage and increases the percentage of lactose in the milk (13, 20, 67).

The feeding of sodium or potassium bicarbonate, magnesium carbonate, partially delactosed whey, magnesium oxide, and calcium hydroxide prevents part of the depression in the milk fat test caused by a restricted roughage ration. The rumen pH is increased by the minerals, but not by the delactosed whey. The minerals and the whey decrease rumen propionate and increase acetate production. The exact mechanism by which these compounds tend to restore the milk fat percentage has not been clarified (14, 15, 27, 42, 69).

10-5 SUMMARY

Milk is produced by the epithelial cells in one of two ways. Milk fat, lactose, and proteins are synthesized in the cells from the precursors absorbed from the blood. These components are then released into the lumina of the alveoli. The water, mineral, and vitamin components of milk enter the lumen of the alveolus primarily through a diffusion process; however, some of them may be bound to other compounds. Approximately 500 volumes of blood flow through the udder of the cow and goat for each volume of milk produced. The ratio of blood flow to milk yield is higher in lower-producing goats and in animals in late lactation.

Many physiological and environmental factors influence the yield and composition of milk. One of the greatest normal differences in milk composition is that of colostrum. It is the first milk obtained after the initiation of lactation. It has higher percentages of total solids, protein, ash, and lower concentrations of lactose than milk obtained 5 days or later after parturition. The fat composition of colostrum and normal milk varies among species. During a normal lactation curve of the dairy cow the milk yield starts out at a high level, reaches a peak 3–6 weeks after calving, and then gradually declines towards the end of lactation. The milk fat and protein percentages are inversely related to the milk yield. The percentage composition starts out at a moderate level, decreases to a low level during the peak of lactation, and then gradually increases towards the end of lactation.

Among the factors that are related to increases in milk yield of animals, especially the cow, are increased body weight, advancing age, increased plane of nutrition, fall and winter calving, moderate or cool environmental temperatures, and good body condition at calving. Factors that tend to decrease the yield of milk are advancing lactation, advanced stage of gestation, short dry period, spring and summer calving, high environmental temperatures and humidity, diseases that affect the udder or feed intake of the cow, and a decreased plane of nutrition. In most cases, factors that tend to increase the milk yield of the cow tend to decrease milk fat percentage.

Certain changes in the diet of the cow adversely affect the milk fat percentage. Most of these are related to a high concentrate, low roughage diet, which contains a low amount of fiber. The exact reason for the milk fat depression is not known except that the depressed fat percentage is accompanied by a change in rumen fermentation. There is a decrease in rumen acetate production, an increase in the rumen propionate production, and a decrease in the rumen pH. The feeding of sodium or potassium bicarbonate, magnesium bicarbonate, magnesium oxide, and calcium hydroxide, in part, prevent the depression in the milk fat composition caused by a restricted roughage ration.

REFERENCES

1. Ackerman, R. A., R. O. Thomas, and D. F. Butcher. 1967. *J. Dairy Sci.* 50:976.
2. Altman, A. D. 1945. *Vest Zhivot.* 1:85 (*Dairy Sci. Abstr.* 9:287, 1947-48).
3. Baldwin, R. L., H. J. Lin, W. Cheng, R. Cabrera, and M. Ronning. 1969. *J. Dairy Sci.* 52:183.
4. Barry, J. M. 1964. *Biol. Rev.* 39:194.
5. Bereskin, B., and R. W. Touchberry. 1966. *J. Dairy Sci.* 49:869.
6. Blanchard, R. P., A. E. Freeman, and P. W. Spike. 1966. *J. Dairy Sci.* 49:953.
7. Brody, S., A. C. Ragsdale, R. G. Yeck, and D. M. Warstell. 1955. *Mo. Agr. Expt. Sta. Res. Bull.* 578.
8. Clark, R. D., and R. W. Touchberry. 1962. *J. Dairy Sci.* 45:1500.
9. Cobble, J. W., and H. A. Herman. 1951. *Mo. Agr. Expt. Sta. Res. Bull.* 485.
10. Colenbrander, V. F., E. E. Bartley, J. L. Morrill, C. W. Deyoe, and H. B. Pfost. 1967. *J. Dairy Sci.* 50:1966.
11. Dodd, F. H. 1957. In J. Hammond, ed., *Progress in the Physiology of Farm Animals*, Vol. 3. London: Butterworth Scientific Publ. Ch. 20.
12. Eckles, C. H. 1912. *Mo. Agr. Expt. Sta. Bull.* 100.
13. Elliot, J. M. 1962. *Proc. Cornell Nutr. Conf.*, p. 58.
14. Emery, R. S., and L. D. Brown. 1961. *J. Dairy Sci.* 44:1899.
15. Emery, R. S., L. D. Brown, and J. W. Bell. 1965. *J. Dairy Sci.* 48:1647.
16. Emery, R. S., H. D. Hafs, D. Armstrong, and W. W. Snyder. 1969. *J. Dairy Sci.* 52:345.
17. Erb, R. E. 1960. *J. Dairy Sci.* 43:872.
18. Erb, R. E., and U. S. Ashworth. 1961. *J. Dairy Sci.* 44:515.
19. Erb, R. E., M. M. Goodwin, W. N. McCaw, R. A. Morrison, and A. O. Shaw. 1953. *Wash. Agr. Expt. Sta. Circ.* 229.
20. Fisher, L. J., and J. M. Elliot. 1966. *J. Dairy Sci.* 49:826.

21. Forster, T. L., U. S. Ashworth, and L. O. Luedecke. 1967. *J. Dairy Sci.* 50:675.
22. Garrett, O. F., and O. R. Overman. 1940. *J. Dairy Sci.* 23:13.
23. Greenhalgh, J. F. D., and K. E. Gardner. 1958. *J. Dairy Sci.* 41:822.
24. Hansen, R. G., P. H. Phillips, and V. R. Smith. 1946. *J. Dairy Sci.* 29:809.
25. Hathaway, H. D., W. J. Brakel, W. J. Tyznik, and H. E. Kaeser. 1957. *J. Dairy Sci.* 40:616.
26. Hemken, R. W., J. H. Vandersall, and N. A. Clark. 1962. *J. Dairy Sci.* 45:685.
27. Huber, J. T., R. S. Emery, J. W. Thomas, and I. M. Yousef. 1969. *J. Dairy Sci.* 52:54.
28. Huber, J. T., N. L. Jacobson, A. D. McGilliard, and R. S. Allen. 1961. *J. Dairy Sci.* 44:321.
29. Johansson, I., and O. Claesson. 1957. In J. Hammond, ed., *Progress in the Physiology of Farm Animals,* Vol. 3. London: Butterworths Scientific Publ. Ch. 21.
30. Johansson, I., and A. Hanson. 1940. *Kgl. Landtbr. Akad. Handl. Tidskr.* 79:127.
31. Jorgensen, N. A., L. H. Schultz, and G. R. Barr. 1965. *J. Dairy Sci.* 48:1031.
32. Knutsson, P.-G. 1966. *17th Internat. Dairy Congr.* A:129.
33. Laben, R. C. 1963. *J. Dairy Sci.* 46:1293.
34. Lee, J. E., O. T. Fosgate, and J. L. Carmon. 1961. *J. Dairy Sci.* 44:296.
35. Legates, J. E. 1960. *J. Dairy Sci.* 43:1527.
36. Linzell, J. L. 1960. *J. Physiol.* (London) 153:492.
37. Lovell, R., and T. A. Rees. 1961. In S. K. Kon and A. T. Cowie, eds., *Milk: The Mammary Gland and Its Secretion,* Vol. II. New York: Academic Press. Ch. 20.
38. Maynard, L. A., and J. K. Loosli. 1969. *Animal Nutrition,* 6th ed. New York: McGraw-Hill.
39. McDaniel, B. T., and J. E. Legates. 1963. *J. Dairy Sci.* 46:620.
40. McDaniel, B. T., and J. E. Legates. 1965. *J. Dairy Sci.* 48:947.
41. Miller, R. H., and L. D. McGilliard. 1959. *J. Dairy Sci.* 42:1932.
42. Miller, R. W., R. W. Hemken, D. R. Waldo, M. Okamoto, and L. A. Moore. 1965. *J. Dairy Sci.* 48:1455.
43. Moody, E. G., P. J. Van Soest, R. E. McDowell, and G. L. Ford. 1967. *J. Dairy Sci.* 50:1909.
44. O'Donovan, J., F. H. Dodd, and F. K. Neave. 1960. *J. Dairy Res.* 27:115.
45. Opstvedt, J., R. L. Baldwin, and M. Ronning. 1967. *J. Dairy Sci.* 50:108.
46. Parkhie, M. R., L. O. Gilmore, and N. S. Fechheimer. 1966. *J. Dairy Sci.* 49:1410.
47. Parrish, D. B., G. H. Wise, J. S. Hughes, and F. W. Atkeson. 1950. *J. Dairy Sci.* 33:457.
48. Parry, R. M. Jr., J. Sampugna, and R. G. Jensen. 1964. *J. Dairy Sci.* 47:37.
49. Pond, W. G., L. D. Van Vleck, and D. A. Hartman. 1962. *J. Animal Sci.* 21:293.
50. Ragsdale, A. C., S. Brody, H. J. Thompson, and D. M. Worstell. 1948. *Mo. Agr. Expt. Sta. Res. Bull.* 425.

51. Ragsdale, A. C., H. J. Thompson, D. M. Worstell, and S. Brody. 1950. *Mo. Agr. Expt. Sta. Res. Bull.* 460.
52. Ragsdale, A. C., H. J. Thompson, D. M. Worstell, and S. Brody. 1951. *Mo. Agr. Expt. Sta. Res. Bull.* 471.
53. Reid, J. T. 1961. *J. Dairy Sci.* 44:2122.
54. Robertson, A., R. Waite, and J. C. D. White. 1956. *J. Dairy Res.* 23:82.
55. Rook, J. A. F. 1961. *Dairy Sci. Abstr.* 23:251 and 303.
56. Rook, J. A. F., and R. C. Campling. 1965. *J. Dairy Res.* 32:45.
57. Rook, J. A. F., and J. V. Wheelock. 1967. *J. Dairy Res.* 34:273.
58. Rook, J. A. F., and M. Wood. 1958. *Nature* 181:1284.
59. Rook, J. A. F., and M. Wood. 1959. *Nature* 184:647.
60. Rowland, S. J., F. K. Neave, F. H. Dodd, and J. Oliver. 1959. *15th Internat. Dairy Congr.* 1:121.
61. Salman, A. R. 1960. The effect of climate on dairy cattle. M. S. Thesis, Cornell University.
62. Sargent, F. D., K. R. Butcher, and J. E. Legates. 1967. *J. Dairy Sci.* 50:177.
63. Schmidt, G. H., and L. H. Schultz. 1959. *J. Dairy Sci.* 42:170.
64. Smith, A., J. V. Wheelock, and F. H. Dodd. 1966. *J. Dairy Sci.* 49:895.
65. Smith, J. W., and J. E. Legates. 1962. *J. Dairy Sci.* 45:1192.
66. Spike, P. W., and A. E. Freeman. 1967. *J. Dairy Sci.* 50:1897.
67. Storry, J. E., and J. A. F. Rook. 1965. *Biochem. J.* 96:210.
68. Swanson, E. W. 1965. *J. Dairy Sci.* 48:1205.
69. Thomas, J. W., and R. S. Emery. 1969. *J. Dairy Sci.* 52:60.
70. Turkington, R. W., and R. L. Hill. 1969. *Science* 163:1458.
71. Ullrey, D. E., R. D. Struthers, D. G. Hendricks, and B. E. Brent. 1966. *J. Animal Sci.* 25:217.
72. Van Soest, P. J. 1963. *J. Dairy Sci.* 46:204.
73. Waite, R., J. Abbott, and P. S. Blackburn. 1963. *J. Dairy Res.* 30:209.
74. Waite, R., and P. S. Blackburn. 1957. *J. Dairy Res.* 24:328.
75. Walsh, J. P., and J. A. F. Rook. 1964. *Nature* 204:353.
76. Warner, R. G. 1960. Unpublished observations, cited by J. T. Reid, 1961, *J. Dairy Sci.* 44:2122.
77. Warner, R. G. 1965. *Proc. Cornell Nutr. Conf.*, p. 119.
78. Wilcox, C. J., K. O. Pfau, R. E. Mather, and J. W. Bartlett. 1959. *J. Dairy Sci.* 42:1132.
79. Wheelock, J. V., and J. A. F. Rook. 1966. *J. Dairy Res.* 33:309.
80. Wheelock, J. V., J. A. F. Rook, and F. H. Dodd. 1965. *J. Dairy Res.* 32:79.
81. Woodward, W. E., J. B. Shepherd, and R. R. Graves. 1932. *USDA Misc. Publ.* 130.

BIOCHEMISTRY OF MAMMARY GLAND TISSUE

Each mammary gland epithelial cell must perform at least three major functions in the synthesis of milk. First, it breaks down substrates by oxidation to provide energy for the synthetic reactions in the mammary gland. The mitochondria play the predominant role in this process. A second function is to synthesize the components of milk that are not found in the blood, such as lipids, most of the protein, and lactose; this requires the necessary substrates, enzymes, and environment. The percentage composition of the synthesized constituents of milk is quite uniform; consequently, the epithelial cells must in some way control the number of molecules of each component that is secreted. A third function of the cells is to regulate the percentage composition of those milk constituents that are not synthesized in the mammary gland, such as the water, vitamins, and minerals. Again, some regulatory mechanism must exist since the content of these components in milk is quite uniform in healthy lactating mammary glands. The amount of water secreted into the milk is in part dependent upon maintaining a normal osmotic pressure of milk. Water flows through the epithelial cells or spaces between the epithelial cells by diffusion. A fourth possible function of the epithelial cells is to selectively absorb blood precursors of milk constituents from the bloodstream. It is not known whether active transport is involved in the uptake of some of these metabolites. The amount of precursors taken up is in part dependent upon the concentration in the bloodstream. Information in these areas is very limited.

11-1 METHODS OF STUDY

A number of methods have been employed to study the biochemistry of the mammary gland. Four general areas have been investigated. One area has been devoted to determining the relationship of the level of blood precursors absorbed by the mammary gland to milk composition and yield. The second area is devoted to determining the biochemical pathways in the degradation of subtrates and synthesis of milk constituents. A third area is the study of the enzymes involved in the pathways; their levels in the mammary gland prior to, during, and following lactation; and their relationship to limitations in milk yield and composition. A fourth area that has received limited attention is that of measuring the processes of movement of compounds in and out of the epithelial cells.

Arterio-Venous Measurements

A common method to determine the relationship between blood precursors and milk yield and composition is to measure arterio-venous differences across the mammary gland. The ideal setup involves the determination of the chemical composition of the arterial blood flowing into the mammary gland and that of the venous blood leaving the gland. At the same time, the rate of blood flow through the udder must be accurately measured. In this way the amount of blood precursors taken up by the mammary gland can be determined, provided that there are no other blood vessels between the udder and the rest of the body or between the udder halves if the half-udder technique is used. Provisions must also be made either to cut off the lymph flow from the udder or to measure its flow rate and chemical composition.

Measurements of the chemical composition of the arterial and venous blood of the udder have been available for a number of years and have led to information on the relationship between blood precursors and milk constituents. Accurate measurements of the blood flow through the udder of the conscious lactating animal have been made in recent years. The rate of blood flow in the conscious animal is different from that of the animal under anesthesia. In some cases, the arterio-venous measurements have been made on vessels other than those entering the mammary gland. For instance, the carotid artery has been sampled and its blood used for arterial blood samples. In most cases, the venous blood has been obtained from the subcutaneous abdominal vein. The arterio-venous measurements are leading to interesting and valuable information on milk secretion.

Udder Perfusion

A method comparable to measuring arterio-venous differences is the use of udder perfusion. Mammary glands of cows or goats are removed and perfused with whole blood. The blood system of the udder can be isolated so that the other organs of the body do not interfere with the composition of blood flowing through the udder. The rate of blood flow through the udder can be accurately measured. Another advantage of this type of preparation is that specific compounds can be added to the arterial blood flowing through the udder and its effect on the milk secretion can be measured without having it changed by the liver or other organs. The milk from the gland can be obtained at intervals with the aid of oxytocin. One major limitation of this technique is that the mammary gland ceases to function after a period of 12 hours. The rate of milk secretion declines after a few hours.

Tissue Studies

Mammary gland tissue slices have been used to study the biochemistry of the gland. These are usually incubated with appropriate substrates and enzymes to study the synthesis of various compounds. In many cases, tissue slices from various stages of lactation as well as prepartum and involuted mammary gland tissue have been used to determine changes in measurements, such as respiratory quotient, oxygen uptake, and lactic acid production.

A modification of the tissue slice technique is the organ culture technique. Small pieces of mammary gland tissue are grown in media for varying periods of time. In most cases, the hormones required for the growth and secretion have been studied in these tissues. This method can be used to determine the relation between blood precursors and milk composition if sufficient tissue is present to synthesize enough milk for chemical analysis.

A further modification of the tissue slice technique is one of cellular fractionation. The cells are disrupted by mechanical or other means and specific components of the cell separated by differential centrifugation. In most cases, components, such as the mitochondria, microsomes, and the supernatant fraction, are incubated with specific substrates and enzymes to determine their relationship to the specific metabolism of a substance in the mammary gland.

Measurement of Enzyme Levels

Considerable attention has been directed towards the measurement of specific intermediates in metabolism as well as the presence of specific enzymes in the mammary gland tissue. These measurements are made during the various stages of development, secretion, and involution of the mammary gland tissue. The measurement of the enzyme levels can determine whether particular biochemical pathways exist in the cell and whether the enzyme level is a rate-limiting step in the metabolism of the gland. The presence or absence of particular intermediates gives additional information on the pathways of metabolism that are present in the tissue.

Radioactive Labeling

Many of the previous methods include the use of radioactive isotopes. In most cases, the isotopes do not delineate pathways of metabolism but often serve as a basis for deciding between various possible pathways in the mammary gland. The use of isotopes has also been used to measure the rate of secretion of various components within the mammary gland. A particular radioactive label is attached to the compound to be measured and the radioactivity is measured instead of the chemical composition of that compound.

11-2 AVAILABLE BLOOD PRECURSORS FOR MILK CONSTITUENTS

The mammary gland is dependent upon the blood flowing through the gland for its source of energy substrates and precursors for milk constituents. The amount of metabolite available is dependent upon the rate of blood flow through the udder and its uptake by the mammary gland. In some cases, a large concentration of metabolite flows through the udder, but the uptake by the mammary gland is negligible.

Many of the metabolites absorbed from the gastro-intestinal tract are changed by organs, such as the liver, before they reach the mammary gland. For instance, propionic acid is absorbed in large quantities from the rumen mucosa. It is converted to glucose by the liver before it reaches the mammary gland; consequently, the amount of propionic acid available to the mammary gland is extremely small. It has been shown that propionic acid can be utilized by the guinea pig mammary gland in the citric acid cycle; however, since most of the propionate is converted to glucose before it reaches the mammary gland, it has very little quantitative significance (15).

The approximate arterio-venous (A-V) differences of various metabolites across the ruminant mammary gland have been summarized by Barry (6, 7). He has calculated the average amount of each metabolite available per 100 g of milk. This was calculated by multiplying the arterio-venous difference of the metabolite by 500 or 375. It was assumed that approximately 500 volumes of whole blood, or 375 volumes of plasma, flow through the mammary gland for each volume of milk that is produced, a value obtained in the goat at the height of lactation (12). The results are given in Table 11-1. It will be noted that glucose, acetate, β-hydroxybutyrate, and triglyceride fatty acids are the major precursors of milk constitutents. The value for each amino acid is relatively low, but combining all the amino acids gives a relatively high figure. Barry

TABLE 11-1
Approximate arterio-venous (A-V) differences across the lactating mammary gland.

| Compound | Animal | Arterial conc. (mg/100 ml) | | A-V difference (mg/100 ml) | Amount of compound (g available/ 100 g milk) |
		Whole blood	Plasma		
Glucose	Goat	50.0	—	16.0	8.0
Acetate	Goat	9.0	—	5.7	2.9
Formate	Goat	0.7	—	0.2	0.08
β-Hydroxybutyrate	Goat	—	6.0	3.7	1.4
Acetoacetate	Goat	—	0.25	0.1	0.04
Lactate	Cow	4.0	—	0.2	0.1
Pyruvate	Cow	0.4	—	0.05	0.02
Triglyceride fatty acids	Goat	—	22.0	13.2	4.9
Free long-chain fatty acids	Goat	—	16.0	0.6	0.2
Glycerol	Goat	—	0.5	0.1	0.04
Each free amino acid	Cow	—	1.0	0.6	0.2
CO_2	Goat	25.0	—	-3.3	1.6

Source: Barry. 1966. *Outlook on Agriculture* 5:129.

(6, 7) concluded that all of the essential amino acids and a large proportion of the nonessential acids in casein and β-lactoglobulin come from the free amino acids absorbed from the blood. Glycerol and fatty acids are the important components of milk fat; however, free glycerol and free fatty acid absorption from the bloodstream is low and contributes little to the precursors for milk fat synthesis. Hartman (9) found somewhat higher blood and arterio-venous values of lactate than those reported by Barry (7); however, if the assumptions made by Barry are applied, only 0.4 g of lactate would be available for 100 g of milk. This would contribute only a small portion of the precursors for lactose.

The two major components used for energy by the mammary gland are glucose and acetate. It was originally thought that acetate provided the bulk of the carbon dioxide produced by the ruminant mammary gland (6, 7). Barry (6, 7) calculated that if 30% of the fatty acids of milk were synthesized from blood acetate, an A-V difference of 2.5 mg acetate/100 ml of whole blood would be required for these acids. The mean A-V difference of acetate was 5.7 mg/100 ml. The negative A-V difference for carbon dioxide in Table 11-1 indicates that more CO_2 leaves the udder than enters it. In order to account for the negative A-V difference of 3.3 mg carbon dioxide, an A-V difference of 8.2 mg of acetate or glucose would be required; however, only 3.2 mg of acetate/100 ml of blood are available for oxidation to carbon dioxide (5.7 minus 2.5 mg). It is thus apparent that acetate provides less than one-half of the energy and CO_2 in the ruminant mammary gland.

In an experiment by Annison and Linzell (3), it was found that acetate accounted for 21-33% and glucose accounted for 29-49% of the mammary gland CO_2 that was expired. Sufficient acetate was left to provide 17-45% of the milk fat. Of the glucose that was taken up and oxidized by the mammary gland a more than adequate amount was left over to form all the milk lactose and glycerol. About 30% of the mammary CO_2 that was expired was unaccounted for from either acetate or glucose metabolism. Neither stearic acid nor free long-chain fatty acids of blood are responsible for the remaining 30% of the mammary CO_2 that is expired, since stearic acid is not oxidized by the mammary gland (7, 11).

11-3 ENERGY PRODUCTION AND UTILIZATION

Each epithelial cell generates its own energy for the synthetic processes by the oxidation of compounds that are absorbed by the cell. Glucose and acetate are the primary sources of energy in the ruminant mammary gland, whereas glucose is the primary source of energy in the nonruminant mammary gland. The mitochondria are cell organelles in which the oxidation of substrates takes place and the energy is released for utilization within the cell. During the oxidation of compounds, two types of energy are released: free or useful energy and entropy, which is useless or degraded energy. Since the living cell must maintain a constant temperature, it cannot use energy in the form of heat for synthetic reactions and must therefore use the free energy. The cells extract the free energy from the chemical bonds of the glucose and the acetate and convert it into sources of energy that can be utilized by the cell for its synthetic processes. The common method of utilizing the released energy is in the form of a high energy bond of adenosine triphosphate (ATP). The universal function of all mitochondria is to couple the oxidation of substrates to the synthesis of ATP, which in turn is used for the synthetic processes within the cell.

The ATP Molecule

The ATP molecule (Figure 11-1) carries the free energy resulting from the oxidation of compounds. During the oxidation process, ATP is regenerated from adenosine diphosphate (ADP) and inorganic phosphate (P_i) by the formation of a high energy bond between the terminal phosphate group of ADP and the inorganic phosphate. In some instances, two terminal phosphate groups are attached to adenosine monophosphate (AMP) to generate the high energy bond. The bond between the terminal carbon atom and the first phosphate group is not a high energy bond.

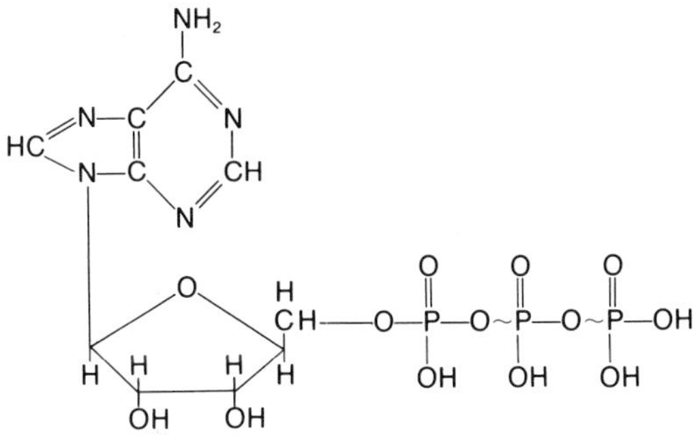

FIGURE 11-1
The ATP molecule is composed of adenine, ribose, and three phosphate molecules. The ATP molecule captures free energy in the high energy bonds ($\sim$) between the phosphate groups. The captured energy is then used for the synthetic processes.

Upon hydrolysis of this bond, an energy exchange of -1 to -5 kilo-calories per mole (kcal/mole) occurs. When either of the two terminal phosphates are hydrolyzed, from -5 to -15 kcal/mole are liberated. These are referred to as high energy bonds. There are also other high energy compounds found in nature and a large percentage of these are associated with a terminal phosphate group.

After the generation of the ATP molecule, it can be used in synthetic processes. Instead of the terminal phosphate group being split off and the free energy released as heat, the terminal phosphate group is transferred to a specific acceptor molecule. The acceptor molecule with the phosphate group has had its energy content raised to a level that enables it to participate in an energy-requiring process, such as the biosynthesis of fats, carbohydrates, or proteins. The ADP molecule resulting from the removal of the terminal phosphate group from ATP can be reused for the generation of ATP. This is done by coupling ATP formation to the oxidation of substrates.

Formation of ATP

Plant and animal cells form ATP in two ways: (1) substrate level phosphorylation and (2) oxidative phosphorylation linked to electron transport. These processes capture part of the energy released during the breakdown of substrates within the cell. Both processes are important in the formation of ATP; however, 90% of the ATP is formed from phosphorylation that is linked to the electron transport system.

During the breakdown of carbohydrates, some of the intermediates become phosphorylated. Some of these phosphorylations result in the development of high energy bonds. In the further breakdown of the phosphorylated compounds, the phosphate groups are released to ADP to form ATP. There are two ADP phosphorylations in the Embden-Meyrhof glycolytic pathway (Figure 11-3). The enzymes that catalyze these phosphorylation steps are soluble in the cytoplasm, whereas the enzymes involved in electron transport linked to oxidative phosphorylation are found in mitochondria.

The oxidative phosphorylation linked to the electron transport system is shown in Figure 11-2. The cell utilizes the energy available in the substrates by a gradual oxidation instead of an abrupt one. An abrupt oxidation would result in a marked liberation of heat. The substrate is oxidized by a compound that has a slightly higher oxidation potential than the initial substrate. This compound is again oxidized by another compound that has a slightly higher oxidation potential. This is continued until a high oxidation potential is reached equivalent to that of oxygen. In this way, a small amount of energy is released at each oxidation instead

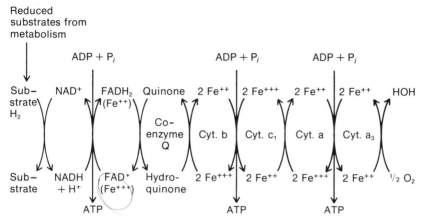

FIGURE 11-2
Oxidative phosphorylation linked to the electron transport system (see text).

of a sudden release. These oxidation-reduction reactions involve the transfer of hydrogen ions and electrons. A dehydrogenase activates the hydrogen atoms in the substrate; the atoms are accepted by the carrier nicotinamide adenine dinucleotide (NAD^+) and then by flavin adenine dinucleotide (FAD^+).

An electron is removed from each hydrogen ion by cytochrome b or c leaving protons (H^+). Coenzyme Q has recently been discovered to be part of the electron transport system; however, its exact function is not known at this time. The exact number of cytochromes involved in electron transport is not known. The electrons are passed from one cytochrome to another in order of b, c_1, a, and, finally, to a_3. At this stage the protons react with oxygen ($\frac{1}{2} O_2$) and 2 electrons to form water. In this process 2 hydrogen atoms have been removed and they and their electrons have been passed down the cytochrome chain to combine with $\frac{1}{2} O_2$ to form water. As the electrons pass down the chain, utilizable energy becomes available to form an ATP molecule from ADP and phosphate. Three ADP molecules are phosphorylated for each 2 hydrogen atoms and electrons that pass down the cytochrome chain, forming 3 moles of ATP. If the first NAD^+ step is bypassed in the electron transport system and the hydrogen ions and electrons picked up by FAD^+, only 2 moles of ATP are formed. This occurs in the citric acid cycle when succinate is oxidized to fumarate (Figure 11-4). The exact reason for bypassing the first step is not known.

In addition to being carriers of hydrogen ions and electrons to the cytochrome system, reduced NAD^+ (NADH) and reduced nicotinamide adenine dinucleotide phosphate (NADPH) also play an important role in supplying hydrogen ions in synthetic process. This is especially true of NADPH, which supplies hydrogen ions in the reductive processes of fatty acid synthesis.

The NADH, NADPH, and ATP molecules are generated in the mammary gland epithelial cells by three pathways. These will be discussed in detail.

Embden-Meyerhof Glycolytic Pathway

This pathway was elucidated by G. Embden and O. Meyerhof in the period between 1920 and 1940. These reactions occur in the absence of oxygen. The steps involved in glycolysis are shown in Figure 11-3. Several monosaccharides can be utilized in this pathway, but the major monosaccharide available to the mammary epithelial cell is glucose, and, consequently, its oxidation will be discussed. Glucose is absorbed from the bloodstream and it must be phosphorylated before it can undergo oxidation. Glucose is phosphorylated in the 6th carbon position by a phosphate group from ATP. The enzymes required for the different steps are given in Table 11-2. Glucose 6-phosphate is converted into fructose 6-phosphate. A second ATP molecule is required to phosphorylate fructose 6-phosphate in the 1 carbon (C-1) position to produce fructose 1, 6-diphosphate. Fructose 1, 6-diphosphate is cleaved between the C-3 and C-4 atoms to form dihydroxyacetone phosphate and glyceraldehyde 3-phosphate. These two compounds are interchangeable.

TABLE 11-2
Enzymes and cofactors involved in the steps of the Embden-Meyerhof pathway of glycolysis, as shown in Figure 11-3.

Step	Enzyme	Cofactors
1	Glucokinase	Mg^{++}, ATP
2	Phosphoglucose isomerase	
3	Phosphofructokinase	Mg^{++}, ATP
4	Aldolase	
5	Phosphoglyceraldehyde dehydrogenase	NAD^+
6	3-Phosphoglyceric acid kinase	Mg^{++}, ADP
7	Phosphoglyceromutase	
8	Enolase	Mg^{++}
9	Pyruvic acid kinase	Mg^{++}, K^+, ADP
10	Lactic acid dehydrogenase	$NADH_2$

Source: White et al. 1968. *Principles of Biochemistry*, 4th ed. New York: McGraw-Hill.

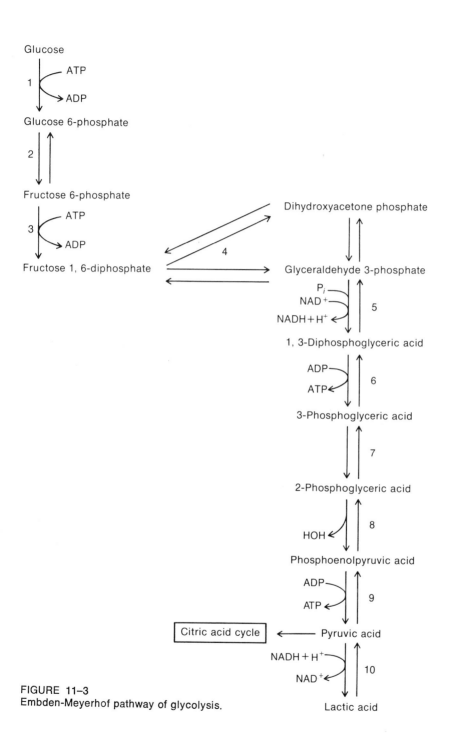

FIGURE 11–3
Embden-Meyerhof pathway of glycolysis.

Unless dihydroxyacetone phosphate is utilized for other purposes, it is converted into glyceraldehyde 3-phosphate, thus producing two 3-carbon units from each glucose molecule. Phosphate is added at reaction 5 and at the same time NAD^+ is reduced to NADH. The process creates a high energy bond on the phosphate group on the C-1 atom. The hydrogen ions and electrons transferred to the NAD^+ molecule can be transferred to the cytochrome system (electron transport system) to produce three ATP molecules. One ATP molecule is produced at reaction 6, in which the high energy phosphate group on the C-1 atom of 1, 3-phosphoglyceric acid is transferred to ADP. This ATP is formed by substrate level phosphorylation. The 3-phosphoglyceric acid is converted into 2-phosphoglyceric acid. Water is removed from 2-phosphoglyceric acid to form phosphoenolpyruvic acid and in the process a second high energy phosphate bond is formed. This high energy phosphate is transferred to ADP at reaction 9 to produce a second ATP molecule by substrate level phosphorylation. The removal of the phosphate group produces pyruvic acid, which can enter the citric acid cycle or be reduced to lactic acid. If it is reduced to lactic acid, $NADH + H^+$ provides the hydrogen ions.

The net synthesis of this process is as follows:

$$1 \text{ glucose} + 2\,ATP + 2\,ADP \longrightarrow 2 \text{ lactic acids} + 4\,ATP$$

or

$$1 \text{ glucose} + 2\,ADP + 2\,ATP + 2\,NAD^+ \longrightarrow$$

$$2 \text{ pyruvic acids} + 4\,ATP + 2\,NADH + H^+ (6\,ATP)$$

The 6 molecules of ATP are formed when 2 molecules of $NADH + H^+$ are passed to the electron transport system. Three molecules of ATP are formed for each $NADH + H^+$ passed through the system.

Citric Acid Cycle

The citric acid cycle is the final common pathway of metabolism. (Other names for this cycle are the tricarboxylic acid cycle and the Krebs cycle in honor of the man who elucidated a large portion of the cycle.) The citric acid cycle causes the final degradation of 2, 3, and possibly 4 carbon units from carbohydrate, fat, and protein metabolism by a combination of decarboxylations and dehydrogenations. In the process of decarboxylation and dehydrogenation, oxygen is consumed and CO_2 and water are given off. Energy is released in the form of ATP.

In carbohydrate metabolism the citric acid cycle picks up the pyruvic acid from glycolysis. The pyruvic acid is converted to an active form of acetic acid, acetyl coenzyme A (acetyl CoA). In the process of forming acetyl CoA, pyruvic acid is decarboxylated and two hydrogen ions are released and are picked up by NAD⁺ (Figure 11-4). The NADH + H⁺ then transfers the hydrogen ions and the electrons to the cytochrome system. Acetyl CoA then combines with oxaloacetic acid to form citric acid and in the process the CoA is split off. Citric acid is converted to isocitric acid through an intermediate, cis-aconitic acid. Isocitric acid is decarboxylated and two hydrogen ions are removed to form α-ketoglutaric acid. The hydrogen ions are picked up by NADP⁺ and transferred to the cytochrome system. The α-ketoglutaric acid is decarboxylated, two hydrogen ions are removed from it and transferred to NAD⁺, and CoA is added to form succinyl CoA. Succinyl CoA is converted to succinic acid by the removal of CoA. During this process a phosphate group is attached to the CoA. The CoA transfers its high energy phosphate group to either ADP or guanosine diphosphate (GDP). The GTP (GDP + P_i) transfers its terminal phosphate group to ADP to form an ATP molecule. One high energy ATP molecule is thus formed at the substrate level.

Succinic acid is dehydrogenated to form fumaric acid. In the process the hydrogen ions and electrons are picked up by FAD⁺ and transferred to the cytochrome system. In this case, only 2 ATP molecules are formed because the H⁺ and electrons enter the cytochrome system at FAD⁺ instead of NAD⁺ or NADP⁺. Fumaric acid is converted to malic acid by the addition of water. Malic acid is dehydrogenated with the hydrogen ions and electrons being picked up by NAD⁺. Again three ATP molecules are formed after the hydrogen ions and electrons pass through the cytochrome system. The dehydrogenation of the malic acid forms oxaloacetic acid, which can pick up another acetyl CoA molecule. This results in the complete degradation of acetyl CoA molecule with the regeneration of oxaloacetic acid for continuing the cycle. The enzymes that catalyze these reactions are given in Table 11-3.

The net energy production of the breakdown of a glucose molecule via the Embden-Meyerhof pathway and citric acid cycle is as follows:

1 glucose + 2 ATP + 2 ADP + 2 NAD⁺ ⟶

2 pyruvates + 4 ATP + 2 NADH + H⁺ (6 ATP)

2 pyruvates + 2 ADP + 6 NAD⁺ + 2 NADP⁺ + 2 FAD⁺ ⟶

6 CO₂ + 4 H₂O + 2 ATP + 6 NADH + H⁺ (18 ATP)

+ 2 NADPH + H⁺ (6 ATP) + FADH₂ (4 ATP)

NET: 1 glucose + 2 ATP ⟶ 40 ATP

SUM: 1 glucose ⟶ 38 ATP

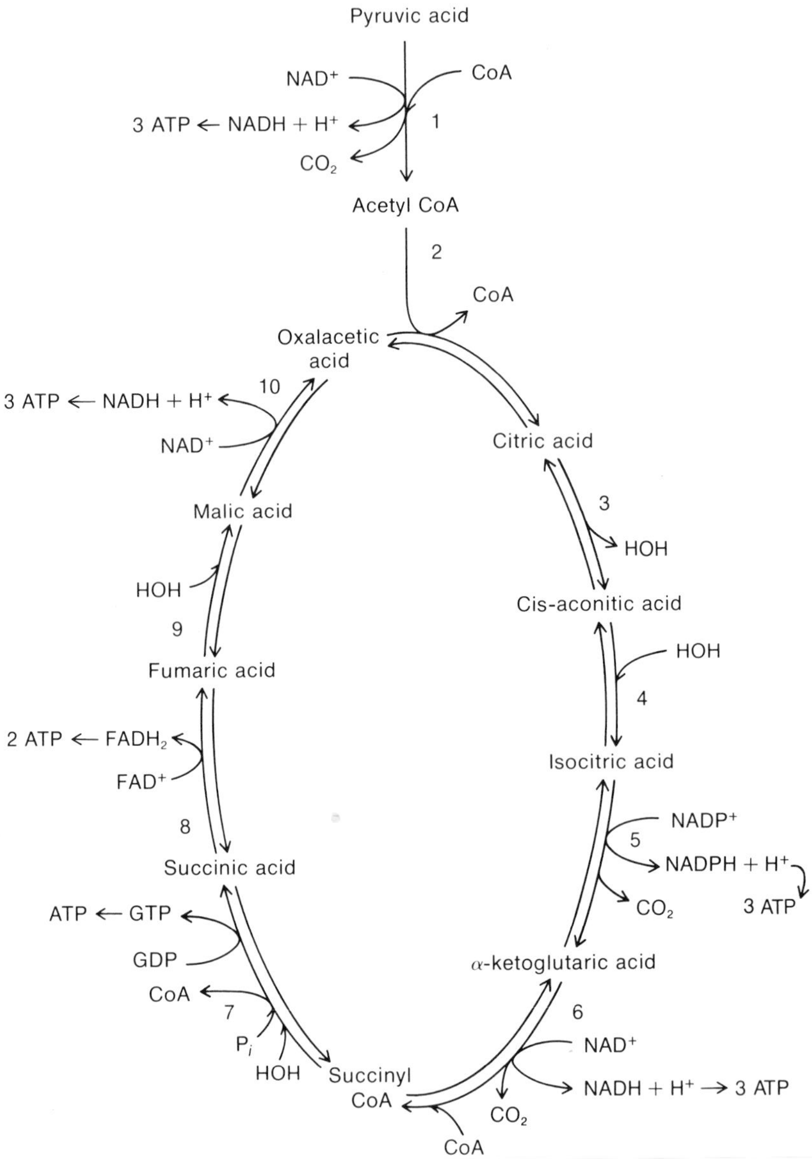

FIGURE 11-4
Citric acid cycle.

TABLE 11-3
Enzymes and cofactors involved in steps of the citric acid cycle,
as shown in Figure 11-4.

Step	Enzyme	Cofactors
1	Pyruvate oxidase	Thiamine-pyrophosphate NAD^+, CoA, Mg^{++}, lipoic acid
2	Citrate condensing enzyme (citrate synthetase)	—
3	Aconitase	—
4	Aconitase	—
5	Isocitrate dehydrogenase	Mn^{++}, $NADP^+$
6	α-Ketoglutarate dehydrogenase	Thiamine-pyrophosphate, lipoic acid, CoA, NAD^+
7	Succinyl thiokinase	—
8	Succinate dehydogenase	Fe^{++} flavin
9	Fumarase	—
10	Malate dehydrogenase	NAD^+

Source: White et al. 1968. *Principles of Biochemistry*, 4th ed. New York: McGraw-Hill.

If the energy content of the terminal pyrophosphate bond of ATP is 8 kcal/mole, the oxidation of 1 mole of glucose yields 304 kcal of energy (8×38) trapped in the form of ATP. The heat of combustion of glucose is 686 kcal/mole; therefore, the oxidation of glucose to form ATP has an efficiency of 44% (304/686). Fifty-six percent of the energy is lost as heat during ATP formation.

Pentose Phosphate Pathway

Another important pathway in the mammary gland for the breakdown of glucose is the pentose phosphate pathway or shunt. Other names for this pathway are: hexose monophosphate pathway or shunt, phosphogluconate oxidative pathway, and the Warburg-Dickens-Horecker pathway. The steps in this pathway are outlined in Figure 11-5 and the summation of the carbon units involved is given in Figure 11-6. The pathway proceeds by the decarboxylation of the C-1 carbon of the glucose molecule. In the process, glucose is shortened to a 5-carbon unit and the hydrogen ions are picked up by $NAPD^+$ to form $NADPH + H^+$. The oxidations occur at steps 1 and 3 in Figure 11-5. Thus 2 $NADPH + H^+$ are formed for each glucose molecule that enters the pentose phosphate pathway and these can lead to 6 ATP molecules. The pentose phosphate pathway is important in the mammary gland in the formation of fatty acids from

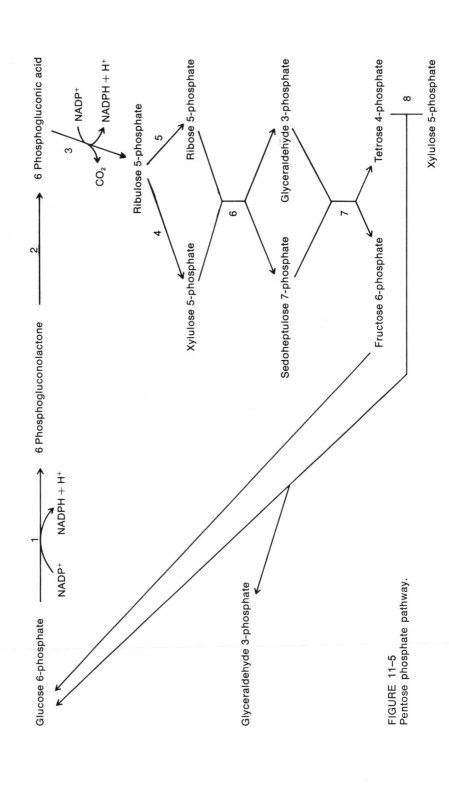

FIGURE 11-5
Pentose phosphate pathway.

acetic acid and β-hydroxybutyric acid. NADPH + H$^+$ serves as a hydrogen ion donor in the reductive reactions in fatty acid synthesis.

Ribulose 5-phosphate is changed to ribose 5-phosphate by an isomerase enzyme and to xylulose 5-phosphate by an epimerase enzyme (Table 11-4). These two 5-carbon units are converted to a 7- and a 3-carbon unit by a transketolase reaction in which the first two carbon atoms of xylulose 5-phosphate are attached to the C-1 carbon of ribose 5-phosphate to give a 7-carbon unit. This leaves the 3-carbon unit, glyceraldehyde 3-phosphate. The 3- and 7-carbon units are in turn converted to fructose 6-phosphate and a 4-carbon unit by a transaldolase reaction. Fructose 6-phosphate can be converted to glucose 6-phosphate and re-enter the cycle. Tetrose 4-phosphate can combine with another xylulose 5-phosphate to produce fructose 6-phosphate and glyceraldehyde 3-phosphate. Two glyceraldehyde 3-phosphate molecules can be converted into fructose 1, 6-diphosphate by a reversal of glycolysis. Glyceraldehyde 3-phosphate can also be used for glycerol synthesis. Ribose 5-phosphate can be used in the synthesis of nucleic acids.

TABLE 11-4
Enzymes involved in steps of the pentose phosphate pathway, as shown in Figure 11-5.

Step	Enzyme
1	Glucose 6-phosphate dehydrogenase
2	Lactonase
3	Phosphogluconate dehydrogenase
4	Phosphopentose epimerase
5	Phosphopentose isomerase
6	Transketolase
7	Transaldolase
8	Transketolase

Source: White et al. 1968. *Principles of Biochemistry*, 4th ed. New York: McGraw-Hill.

The carbon units involved in the pentose phosphate shunt are summarized in Figure 11-6. In order to balance the equations, 6 glucose units are converted into 6 pentoses. The net result of the degradation of 6 glucoses is the regeneration of five 6-carbon units and the complete degradation of one glucose. Two NADPH + H$^+$ molecules are generated for each glucose molecule that was reduced to a 5-carbon unit. For the 6 glucose units entering the cycle, 12 NADPH + H$^+$ units have been generated, which are equivalent to 36 ATP. One ATP molecule was

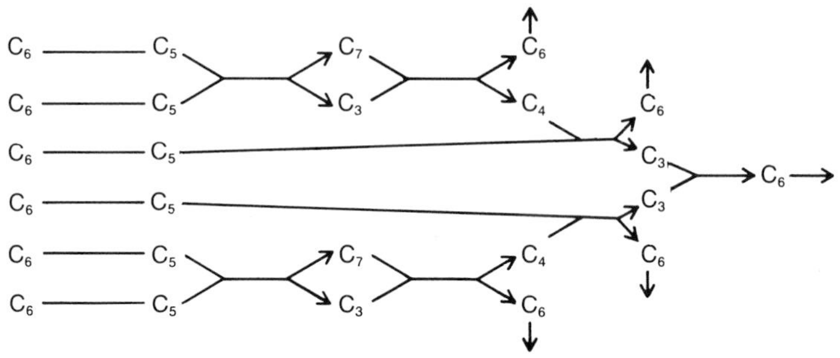

Sum: 6 glucose + 6 O_2 + 12 $NADP^+$ → five 6-carbon units + 6 CO_2 + 6 H_2O
+ 12 NADPH + H^+ (36 ATP)

FIGURE 11–6
Summary of the carbon units involved in the pentose phosphate pathway.

required to phosphorylate the glucose that was degraded; therefore, a net synthesis of 35 ATP molecules occurred. If 8 kcal/mole are captured in each high energy ATP bond, a total of 280 kcal/mole of free energy is captured. This results in an efficiency of 41% (280/686), which is quite comparable to that of the Embden-Meyerhof pathway.

The pentose phosphate pathway is present in mammary gland tissue. The evidence for this comes from several sources. Wood et al. (16) injected glucose labeled in the 1- and 6-carbon positions into the dairy cow. It was found that the specific activity of the CO_2 was much greater after glucose 1-[14] C was injected than after glucose 6-[14] C injection. This indicated that the pentose cycle occurred in the udder, since the pentose phosphate pathway involves the decarboxylation of C-1 of glucose. Other evidence includes: (1) the levels of glucose 6-phosphate dehydrogenase and 6 phosphogluconate dehydrogenase increase markedly at parturition, (2) mammary gland tissue *in vitro* preferentially oxidized the C-1 atom of glucose rather than the C-6, (3) the detection of intermediates of the cycle in mammary gland tissue, and (4) the randomization of the radioactive label in galactose after the injection of specifically labeled hexoses is consistent with the operation of the pentose phosphate cycle in the lactating udder (8).

It is impossible to determine the exact amount of glucose oxidized by the pentose phosphate pathway; however, Abraham et al. (2) estimated that 60% of the total glucose is metabolized through this cycle in the rat mammary gland at the peak of lactation. It has also been shown that the pentose phosphate pathway accounts for about half of the glucose atoms incorporated into acetyl CoA in rat mammary tissue (1, 13). In the perfused cow udder, 60-70% of the glucose utilized was used for lactose synthesis, 20-30% was oxidized via the pentose phosphate shunt and less than 10% was metabolized via the Embden-Meyerhof pathway (17). These results indicate that this pathway plays a major role in the metabolism of glucose in the mammary gland.

Mammary Gland Enzyme Levels

A number of studies have been conducted on the presence and level of enzymes in ruminant and nonruminant mammary gland tissue. In several recent studies (4, 5) a number of enzymes involved in glycolysis, the pentose phosphate pathway, fat synthesis, lactose synthesis, protein synthesis, mitochondrial activity, and enzymes related to the general metabolic status have been studied. The onset of lactation in the rat is characterized by a rapid increase in the activity of all enzymes studied. Comparable results were obtained in the guinea pig during late pregnancy and lactation. In contrast to this, there was no marked increase in activity of the enzymes studied in the cow. Baldwin (4) concluded that the initiation of lactation in the cow does not involve the sudden acquisition of enzymatic potential for milk synthesis, but that the enzymes are already present during pregnancy and that other factors determine the rate of activity after the initiation of secretion. He also concluded that the differences in enzyme levels were not related to differences in milk composition among the species.

Jones (10) studied seven enzymes related to milk secretion and found that hypophysectomy of the rat resulted in a marked decline in activity of all enzymes within a 12- to 16-hour period. Removal of the litter caused a similar change in pattern of enzyme activity within 24 hours after weaning.

Attempts have been made to determine the rate of control of particular pathways. It has been shown that the pentose phosphate pathway is not limited by the enzymes of the pathway but is limited by the reoxidation of NADPH, which in turn is largely dependent upon the rate of fatty acid synthesis (10).

There is no question that enzymes are required for the various biochemical pathways. Measurements of these enzymes and their levels in mammary gland tissues have given little information on how their rate of activity affects the rate of a particular pathway. Additional evidence must be gathered to determine if the rate of activity of an enzyme is a rate-limiting factor in the milk secretion process.

11-4 SUMMARY

Each epithelial cell in the mammary gland must perform several functions. It must break down substrates to provide energy for the synthetic processes within the mammary gland. It must then synthesize the components of the milk that are not found in the blood, such as fat, lactose, and protein. The cells also regulate the composition of milk by controlling the amounts of the constituents that are not synthesized in the mammary gland, such as water, vitamins and minerals.

The major blood precursors for the formation of milk are glucose, acetate, β-hydroxybutyrate, triglyceride fatty acids, and amino acids. The two major sources of energy are glucose and acetate. Other compounds are absorbed and utilized by the mammary gland; however, they do not make significant contributions to the quantitative aspects of the milk composition, even though their qualitative aspects are extremely important.

The energy used for the synthetic processes within the mammary gland is formed by the oxidation of compounds absorbed by the cell. These compounds are broken down mainly in the mitochondria. During the oxidation of the compounds, the useful energy is transferred to high energy bonds of adenosine triphosphate (ATP). ATP is generated from adenosine diphosphate (ADP) and inorganic phosphate either by substrate level prosphorylation or by oxidative phosphorlylation linked to electron transport. Approximately 90% of the ATP is formed via the electron transport system.

The ATP molecule is utilized in energy-requiring synthetic processes. The terminal phosphate group of ATP is transferred to a specific acceptor molecule. The acceptor molecule thus has its energy content raised to a level at which it can participate in the energy-requiring processes within the cell, such as the synthesis of triglycerides, lactose, and proteins. The liberated ADP molecule can be reused for the generation of ATP.

Energy is generated in the epithelial cell by one of three pathways. The Embden-Meyerhof glycolytic pathway degrades glucose and other hexose molecules into two lactic acids with the generation of ATP at the substrate level phosphorylation. The last compound formed before lactic acid in the cycle is pyruvic acid, which can enter the citric acid cycle. The citric acid cycle is the final common pathway of metabolism. In addition to the pyruvic acid from carbohydrate metabolism, the citric acid cycle can also utilize acetyl CoA from fatty acid metabolism and the carbon skeletons from amino acid metabolism. Before it enters the citric acid cycle, the pyruvate is converted to acetyl CoA. The acetyl CoA is picked up by oxaloacetic acid to form citric acid. In transversing the cycle the acetyl CoA is broken down to CO_2 and HOH and the oxalo-acetic acid is regenerated. The oxaloacetic acid then picks up another acetyl CoA molecule to continue another cycle. During the breakdown of acetyl CoA, ATP molecules are formed by substrate level oxidation and oxidative phosphorylation linked to electron transport system.

A third pathway operating in the mammary gland is the pentose phosphate pathway, or shunt. In this pathway, hexose units, namely glucose, are broken down with the liberation of $NADPH + H^+$. The $NADPH + H^+$ can transfer its hydrogen ions and electrons to the electron transport system to form ATP or it can supply the hydrogen ions for the reductive stages of fatty acid synthesis. The latter appears to be its primary function in the mammary gland epithelial cell. Breakdown products of the pentose phosphate shunt are also involved in nucleic acid synthesis. The pentose phosphate shunt is the major pathway for the oxidation of glucose in the epithelial cell.

Studies of the enzyme activities in the mammary gland have shown that the rat mammary gland is characterized by a rapid increase in activity of all enzymes at the onset of lactation. In the cow, however, there is no sudden acquisition of enzymatic potential for milk synthesis. Hypophysectomy causes a marked decline in the activity of all of the enzymes that have been studied. These changes appear similar to those occurring during the involution process. Differences in enzyme levels occur among species, but they are not related to the differences in the composition of the milk.

REFERENCES

1. Abraham, S., and I. L. Chaikoff. 1959. *J. Biol. Chem.* 234:2246.
2. Abraham, S., P. F. Hirsch, and I. Chaikoff. 1954. *J. Biol. Chem.* 211:31.
3. Annison, E. F., and J. L. Linzell. 1964. *J. Physiol.* 175:372.
4. Baldwin, R. L. 1966. *J. Dairy Sci.* 49:1533.
5. Baldwin, R. L., and L. P. Milligran. 1966. *J. Biol. Chem.* 241:2058.
6. Barry, J. M. 1964. *Biol. Rev.* 39:194.
7. Barry, J. M. 1966. *Outlook on Agriculture* 5:129.
8. Folley, S. J. 1961. *Dairy Sci. Abstr.* 23:511.
9. Hartmann, P. E. 1966. *Aust. J. Biol. Sci.* 19:495.
10. Jones, E. A. 1967. *Biochem. J.* 103:420.
11. Lauryssens, M., R. Verbeke, and G. Peeters. 1961. *J. Lipid Res.* 2:383.
12. Linzell, J. L. 1960. *J. Physiol.* 153:492.

13. McLean, P. 1964. *Biochem. J.* 90:271.
14. White, A., P. Handler, and E. L. Smith. 1968. *Principles of Biochemistry,* 4th ed. New York: McGraw-Hill.
15. Willmer, J. S., and H. Gutfreund. 1963. *Biochem. J.* 89:29p.
16. Wood, H. G., R. Gillespie, R. G. Hansen, W. A. Wood, and H. J. Hardenbrook. 1959. *Biochem. J.* 73:694.
17. Wood, H. G., G. J. Peeters, R. Verbeke, M. Lauryssens, and B. Jacobson. 1965. *Biochem. J.* 96:607.

MILK PROTEIN SYNTHESIS

12-1 MILK PROTEIN COMPONENTS

Milk protein is made up of a number of specific proteins, with casein being the most important component. The protein fractions of cow's milk are given in Table 12-1. This nomenclature is taken from the third revision by the American Dairy Science Association Committee on Milk Protein Nomenclature. Table 12-1 gives only the general classifications of the various protein components; however, many variants of a_s-casein, K-casein, β-casein, γ-casein, α-lactalbumin and β-lactoglobulin are present. The variants of the protein fractions have different chemical compositions and they are identified by their electrophoretic mobility. The variants reflect the action of autosomal genes that are transmitted from parent to offspring by simple Mendelian inheritance. It is now possible to relate some of the variants of casein and the other proteins to the blood type of the animal. As additional genetic variants are discovered, the nomenclature will be revised.

The protein α-lactalbumin is found in the skim milk of many species. Recently, it has been shown to be one of the two protein components of

TABLE 12-1
Fractions and some properties of proteins in cows' milk.

Protein (contemporary nomenclature)	Approx. % of skim milk protein	Isoelectric point	Molecular weight	Number of variants identified
a$_s$-Casein	45-55	4.1	23,000	6
K-Casein	8-15	4.1	19,000	2
β-Casein	25-35	4.5	24,100	7
γ-Casein	3-7	5.8-6.0	30,650	4
α-Lactalbumin	2-5	5.1	14,437	2
β-Lactoglobulin	7-12	5.3	36,000	6
Blood serum albumin	0.7-1.3	4.7	69,000	
IgG immunoglobulin				
IgG1	1-2		150,000 to	
IgG2	0.2-0.5		170,000	
IgM immunoglobulin	0.1-0.2		900,000 to	
			1,000,000	
IgA immunoglobulin	0.05-0.10		300,000 to	
			500,000	
Proteose-peptone	2-6	3.3-3.7	4,100 to	
fraction			200,000	

Source: Rose et al. 1970. *J. Dairy Sci.* 53:1.

lactose synthetase (6). In order to be active, lactose synthetase requires an A protein, galactosyltransferase, and a B protein, α-lactalbumin. The α-lactalbumin by itself does not have any catalytic activity.

12-2   PRECURSORS OF MILK PROTEIN

Casein, β-lactoglobulin, and α-lactalbumin make up about 90–95% of the protein of milk. These three proteins are synthesized in the udder, therefore their precursors will be considered in detail. Blood serum albumin, the immune globulins, and γ-casein are not synthesized in the mammary gland and are apparently absorbed as such from the blood. The three possible sources of blood precursors of the milk proteins synthesized in the udder are: peptides, plasma proteins, and free amino acids. The concentration of peptides in the blood plasma is below the amount needed to provide 10% of the amino acids in the protein formed in the udder (3).

Plasma proteins may provide a small proportion of the essential amino acids for the synthesis of the components formed in the udder. To determine the relationship between plasma proteins and milk protein, Campbell and Work (5) produced plasma proteins labeled with ^{14}C-glycine and infused them into two lactating rabbits. They found that the activities of the glycine and serine of the milk proteins were never more than 10% of those of the plasma proteins. From this they concluded that at least 90% of the free glycine and serine in milk must come from sources other than plasma proteins. This is the basis for the conclusion that less than 10% of the milk proteins synthesized in the udder arise from plasma proteins.

The free amino acids absorbed by the mammary gland provide most of the nitrogen required for the synthesis of milk protein. Almost all of the free amino acids absorbed by the mammary gland are incorporated into milk protein, since the free amino acids make up less than 10% of the milk protein nitrogen (14). The amino acid composition of milk of the cow and sow is shown in Table 12-2. The evidence for the incorporation of amino acids into milk protein comes from two sources, arteriovenous studies and radioactive isotope studies.

TABLE 12-2
Approximate amino acid content of the total milk protein of cow's and sow's milk.

Essential amino acids[a] (g/100 g protein)			Nonessential amino acids[a] (g/100 g protein)		
Acid	*Cow*	*Sow*	*Acid*	*Cow*	*Sow*
Arginine	3.6	5.6	Alanine	3.6	[b]
Histidine	2.7	2.5	Aspartic acid	7.2	5.1
Isoleucine	5.6	5.1	Cystine	0.7	1.6
Leucine	9.7	8.2	Glutamic acid	23.0	11.2
Lysine	7.9	6.0	Glycine	2.0	2.0
Methionine	2.5	1.5	Proline	9.2	[b]
Phenylalanine	5.2	4.2	Serine	5.8	5.8
Threonine	4.6	4.1	Tyrosine	5.1	5.5
Tryptophan	1.3	1.3			
Valine	6.6	5.2			

Source: Block and Weiss. 1956. *Amino Acid Handbook*. Springfield, Ill.: C. C. Thomas.
[a] Based upon essential amino acids for rat (Rose. 1938. *Physiol. Rev.* 18:109).
[b] Value not given.

Essential Amino Acids

Two recent studies have related the arterio-venous differences of free amino acids to the composition of milk protein of the goat and the dairy cow (10, 16). The experiment with the goat (10) included measurements of the arterio-venous difference of the amino acids as well as the rate of blood flow and the percentage composition of the amino acids of the milk protein, whereas the work with the dairy cow (16) included only arterio-venous differences. The rate of blood flow and the composition of the milk were estimated from previous but similar studies. In both studies it was found that the essential amino acids, arginine, histidine, isoleucine, leucine, lysine, threonine, and valine, were absorbed in sufficient quantities to account for all of the amino acids in the protein components formed in the udder. The uptake of phenylalanine by the goat udder was sufficient to account for the concentration of that amino acid in the protein; however, it was less than sufficient in the dairy cow. This insufficiency may be due in part to errors in the assumptions that were made in calculating the blood flow and milk protein composition of the dairy cow. The arterio-venous differences for methionine were less than adequate in both studies. Mephan and Linzell (10) concluded that the uptake values for methionine were probably underestimated and since methionine is an essential amino acid, it was probably absorbed in amounts sufficient to provide all of the methionine residues in milk protein. The results of these studies indicate that the arterio-venous differences of the essential amino acids are sufficient to account for almost, if not all, of these amino acids in the milk protein.

Further evidence for the necessity of absorbing the essential amino acids comes from the work of Schingoethe et al. (13). Bovine and rat mammary organ cultures grown in the absence of any of the essential amino acids showed a significant reduction in milk protein synthesis. Rat cells demonstrated a requirement for tyrosine and bovine cells, a requirement for cystine.

Nonessential Amino Acids

Some of the nonessential amino acids are absorbed as free amino acids from the bloodstream and some are synthesized in the mammary gland. From arterio-venous studies, it has been shown that sufficient glutamic acid and tyrosine are absorbed from the blood by the goat udder to account for these amino acid components in milk protein and that sufficient glutamine is absorbed from the cow's blood to account for the glutamine content of milk protein (10, 16). Verbeke and Peeters (16) found that the uptake of aspartic acid, asparginine, glutamic acid, serine, and proline in the cow was not sufficient to account for these amino acid residues in the protein synthesized in the mammary gland. The arterio-venous differences and the amino acid residue requirements in the goat's milk was somewhat more variable (10). In some cases, there was a definite deficiency of the amino acid absorption from the blood and in other cases the arterio-venous differences were sufficient to account for the protein amino acids. The arterio-venous difference of serine was not sufficient to account for that component of milk protein in the goat, whereas the uptake of arginine was greatly in excess of the requirement of arginine residues in the milk.

Radioactive isotopes have also been used to study the blood precursor-milk composition relationships. Specifically labeled amino acids are injected into the blood, and the milk and blood samples are obtained after various intervals and measured for their specific activities. The specific activity of the precursor can be compared to that of the product, from which the calculation of the amount of precursor responsible for a particular component in the milk can be made. In addition, the specific activities of the various amino acids of the milk protein can be analyzed to determine whether a particular amino acid was converted into another amino acid in the mammary gland. Results of these types of studies have been summarized by Barry (2). He concluded that 70% of the glutamine, glutamic acid, and tyrosine, and 50% of the proline and aspargine in casein came from the free amino acids absorbed from the bloodstream. Less than 20% of the glutamine, glutamic acid, and aspargine residues were synthesized in the mammary gland from blood glucose.

The results of the radioisotope studies generally support the conclusions obtained from the arterio-venous studies. Barry (3) concludes that at least half of the nonessential amino acids in casein and β-lactoglobulin are derived directly from the blood without exchange of atoms with other metabolites.

The extent of synthesis of nonessential amino acids in the mammary gland epithelial cells is not known. Most of the synthesis involves the interconversion of various amino acids to form sufficient amino acids for milk protein synthesis. For example, ornithine is absorbed in considerable quantity by the mammary gland, but it does not appear in the milk. It is mainly converted to proline by the epithelial cell (17).

Some *de novo* synthesis of amino acids can take place in the mammary gland. Verbeke et al. (15) perfused isolated cow udders with blood containing labeled acetate and propionate. They found an appreciable specific activity in the nonessential amino acids, glutamic acid, aspartic acid, serine, and glycine. In the propionic experiments, a marked activity was also detected in alanine. Schingoethe et al. (13) showed that bovine and rat mammary cells grown in organ culture did not have a reduction in milk protein synthesis in the absence of alanine, aspartic acid, asparagine, glutamic acid, glutamine, glycine, proline, or serine. These results support the concept that some of the nonessential amino acids can be synthesized in the mammary gland.

12-3   PROTEIN SYNTHESIS

The bionsynthesis of milk protein has recently been reviewed by Baldwin (1) and Larson (8). For details on the incorporation of the amino acids into protein, the reader is referred to these reviews or a recent textbook in biochemistry. The present knowledge on the synthesis of proteins will be reviewed briefly.

Protein synthesis takes place in the epithelial cell and is controlled by genes, which contain the genetic material, deoxyribonucleic acid (DNA). The sequence of protein synthesis is brought about by the following scheme, which includes replication of DNA, transcription of ribonucleic acid (RNA) from DNA, and translation, which is the formation of protein according to the information on RNA.

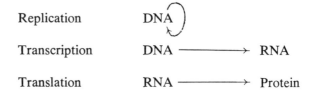

Replication	DNA
Transcription	DNA ⟶ RNA
Translation	RNA ⟶ Protein

Replication involves the separation of the two strands of DNA and the duplication of both strands by a base-pairing procedure. Replication occurs prior to cell division, and thus has no direct role in protein synthesis. Transcription involves the production of RNA on the DNA strands. The RNA molecules move to the cytoplasm and play an active role in the synthesis of protein. Translation involves the processes by which the amino acids are brought together and joined to form the proteins; this is done at the ribosomes.

Transcription

In transcription, three types of RNA molecules are formed. They are: messenger RNA (mRNA), transfer or soluble RNA (tRNA or sRNA), and ribosomal RNA (rRNA). All RNA molecules are formed from the DNA material within the nucleus by a base-pairing procedure, comparable to that occurring during the DNA replication process. The two strands, or a part of the two strands, of the DNA molecule separate and the bases of the RNA molecule to be formed pair with the bases on the DNA molecule. Thus cytosine and guanine, uracil and adenine, and adenine and thymine line up opposite each other on the DNA and RNA chains. RNA differs from DNA in that uracil replaces thymine, and the pentose in RNA is ribose, whereas in DNA it is deoxyribose. Only one strand of the DNA is copied *in vivo* whereas both strands are copied *in vitro*.

Translation

Translation is a complex process which first requires the attachment of an amino acid to a transfer RNA molecule according to the following scheme.

Amino acid $+$ tRNA $+$ ATP $\longrightarrow$

$$\text{Amino acyl} \sim \text{tRNA} + \text{AMP} + P_i\text{-}P_i$$

This step requires an amino-acid-activating enzyme as well as the energy from ATP. Each amino acid has its own specific activating enzyme. ATP is utilized to raise the energy level of the amino acid so that the amino acid can participate in the reaction.

There is at least one tRNA for each amino acid and some amino acids have more than one. The tRNA molecule has about 80 nucleotides with a terminal sequence of cytidylyl-cytidylyl-adenosine. The amino acid is attached to either the 2' or 3' hydroxyl group of the terminal adenosine molecule. The tRNA also has a specific sequence of 3 bases, called an anticodon, which recognizes a triplet of bases on the corresponding mRNA, commonly called the codon. It is not the amino acids but the transfer RNA that recognizes the site on the messenger RNA. This was shown by Lipmann (9) who prepared an amino acyl $\sim$ RNA complex of cysteine with the cysteine-activating enzyme. The amino acid portion of the molecule was reduced to alanine. He used a mRNA in his test system that incorporated cysteine but not alanine. He found that alanine was incorporated into the protein, thus proving that it was the transfer RNA, and not the amino acid, that recognized the site on the messenger RNA.

Protein synthesis occurs on the ribosomes. The majority of the ribosomes are attached to the double-layer membrane of the endoplasmic reticulum, but some appear free in the cytoplasm. The ribosome is made up of two subunits, and these are denoted as 30S and 50S subunits from sedimentation behavior in the ultracentrifuge. Both contain ribosomal RNA. The rRNA brings the amino acyl~ tRNA complex and mRNA together for the synthesis of protein.

The mRNA in some way becomes attached to the rRNA. The amino acids are brought to these sites by tRNAs. The amino acyl~tRNA and the growing protein molecule are attached to the larger subunit and the mRNA binds to the smaller subunit. The triplet of bases on mRNA acts as the codon for the specific amino acid. The anticodon of the tRNA recognizes the codon and places the amino acid in the starting position. Proteins start from the amino end and grow toward the carboxyl end. The second amino acid is then brought into place by a second tRNA and this progress continues until the protein is formed. As each subunit is added, the ribosome moves relative to the mRNA, thus the ribosome moves along the mRNA. As the ribosome moves over the codon, a new amino acyl ~ tRNA moves into position. This process requires two different enzymes as well as the high energy compound, guanosine triphosphate (GTP). The proposed scheme for this is as follows:

Ribosomes

$$(AA \sim tRNA)_n + GTP \longrightarrow$$

$$AA_1\text{-}AA_2\text{-}AA_3\text{-}\ldots\text{-}AA_n + GDP\ (GMP?) + tRNA_n.$$

At the same time the peptide bond between the carboxyl group of one amino acid and the amino group of the second amino acid is formed. After the peptide bond formation, the tRNA is liberated into the cytoplasm so that it can gather another amino acid. It appears that each ribosome at a given time contains only one messenger RNA chain and one growing polypeptide chain.

Most of the evidence on protein synthesis has been obtained from bacteria. Larson (8) summarized the evidence to support the concept that this is probably the mode of synthesis of milk proteins. His evidence is as follows: (1) the major milk proteins are synthesized from free amino acids; (2) amino-acid-activating enzymes and those forming amino acyl ~ tRNA complexes have been found in mammary gland tissue; (3) antibiotics such as actinomycin and puromycin inhibit protein synthesis (actinomycin inhibits DNA-dependent RNA synthesis and puromycin inhibits the incorporation of amino acids at the ribosomal level); (4) studies on variations in individual milk proteins indicate that their synthesis is under genetic control; and (5) the universal nature of the mechanism of protein synthesis appears to hold for a variety of organisms including the mammalian systems.

Control of Protein Synthesis

The amount of protein in milk is rather constant; therefore some control mechanism must be present in the mammary gland. Larson (8) reviewed some of the possible control mechanisms for protein synthesis. Two of these involve feedback inhibition and inhibition by repression. In both cases, the accumulation of the end-products results in an inhibition of enzyme action and a decrease in protein synthesis. Feedback inhibition inhibits enzyme action early in protein formation and repression occurs later in the pathway. It is not known whether repression occurs at the transcription or the translation site.

Larson (8) also reviewed the control of protein synthesis by the operator and regulator genes proposed by Jacob and Monod (7). In this scheme, DNA is made up of a series of sites or cistrons, each one corresponding to a gene. A series of cistrons are closely linked together on the genetic map to form an area called an operon. All of the cistrons within the operon are under the control of a common gene, the operator gene. When the operator gene is open, all of the cistrons within the operon synthesize mRNA and when it is closed no mRNA synthesis occurs. The operator gene can be closed by a specific repressor. The activity of the repressor is controlled by another specific material, the effector. The messenger RNA synthesis can be started by an inactivation of the repressor by an effector. Thus the cistrons within the operator can synthesize mRNA, which in turn leads to the formation of several enzymes or proteins, the special activity of that operon. Another type of effector can activate the repressor, which stops the formation of mRNA. Thus, the starting and stopping of protein synthesis can be under the control of repressors and effectors. Whether this particular mechanism works in the mammary gland is yet to be determined. This may be an area in which the hormones act in the control of protein synthesis and directing new functions of cells.

12-4 SUMMARY

Milk protein is made up of a number of specific proteins. Among the major components are casein, α-lactalbumin, and β-lactoglobulin. Each major component is broken down into subunits based upon their molecular weight, isoelectric point, and other chemical properties. The chemical composition of some of the components of the protein is determined by the genetic make-up of the animals. It is now possible to relate the variants of the milk protein to the blood type of the animal.

The major portion of the protein is synthesized within the mammary gland, including most of the casein, α-lactalbumin, and β-lactoglobulin. Gamma casein, blood serum albumin, and the immune globulins are absorbed as preformed proteins from the blood.

Most of the protein synthesized by the epithelial cells is synthesized from amino acids that are absorbed from the bloodstream. This has been determined by measuring arterio-venous differences across the mammary gland and relating the uptake by the mammary gland to the composition of the amino acids in milk protein. In addition, radioactive isotopes have been used to follow the pathways of incorporation of labeled elements of amino acids into the proteins in the milk. The peptides in the blood plasma provide less than 10% of the amino acids in milk protein. Plasma proteins may provide a small portion of the essential amino acids of milk protein synthesized in the mammary gland; however, less than 10% of these proteins come from plasma proteins. The essential amino acids must come from the bloodstream and most of the nonessential amino acids are also absorbed as amino acids from the blood. In some cases, nonessential amino acids are produced from other amino acids. For instance, there is a considerable uptake of ornithine by the mammary gland, but no ornithine is found in the milk protein. It appears to be converted to proline by the epithelial cell. The nonessential amino acids can also be synthesized in the mammary gland from carbohydrates and volatile fatty acids, such as glucose and acetic acid.

The mechanism of synthesis of protein from amino acids appears to be comparable to that found in most other protein-synthesizing cells. It is controlled by the deoxyribonucleic acid (DNA) in the nucleus of the cell. The DNA is responsible for the production of three types of ribonucleic acid (RNA), i.e., messenger RNA, transfer RNA, and ribosomal RNA. The messenger RNA carries the code or template for the formation of a specific sequence of amino acids into a protein. Messenger RNA is synthesized within the nucleus and then travels to the ribosomes, which line the endoplasmic reticulum in the cytoplasm. Ribosomes are also located as free units in the cytoplasm. The ribosomes contain ribosomal RNA. The third RNA, transfer RNA, picks up a specific amino acid within the cell and transfers it to the ribosome containing the ribosomal and messenger RNAs. The amino acid is activated in the presence of a specific activating enzyme and ATP to form an amino acyl $\sim$ tRNA complex. At the ribosome, the transfer RNA recognizes the code on the messenger RNA and places the amino acid in its proper sequence. The amino acid is then connected to the growing chain of amino acids by a peptide bond and the transfer RNA moves to the cytoplasm to pick up another amino acid. Each amino acid has a specific transfer RNA. The formation of the protein molecule is referred to as a translation process and requires energy in the form of guanosine triphosphate (GTP) as well as specific amino acids.

REFERENCES

1. Baldwin, R. L. 1969. In H. H. Cole and P. C. Cupps, eds. *Reproduction in Farm Animals,* 2nd ed. New York: Academic Press. Ch. 16.
2. Barry, J. M. 1961. In S. K. Kon and A. T. Cowie, eds., *Milk: The Mammary Gland and Its Secretion,* Vol. I. New York: Academic Press. Ch. 10.
3. Barry, J. M. 1964. *Biol. Rev.* 39:194.
4. Block, R. J., and A. B. Weiss. 1956. *Amino Acid Handbook.* Springfield, Ill.: C. C. Thomas.
5. Campbell, P. N., and T. S. Work. 1952. *Biochem. J.* 52:217.
6. Ebner, K. E., and U. Brodbeck. 1968. *J. Dairy Sci.* 51:317.
7. Jacob, F., and J. Monod. 1961. *J. Molecular Biol.* 3:318.
8. Larson, B. L. 1965. *J. Dairy Sci.* 48:133.
9. Lipmann, F. 1963. *Progress in Nucleic Acid Research* 1:247.
10. Mepham, T. B., and J. L. Linzell. 1966. *Biochem. J.* 101:76.
11. Rose, D., J. R. Brunner, E. B. Kalan, B. L. Larson, P. Melnychyn, H. E. Swaisgood, and D. F. Waugh. 1970. *J. Dairy Sci.* 53:1.
12. Rose, W. C. 1938. *Physiol. Rev.* 18:109.
13. Schingoethe, D. J., E. C. Hageman, and B. L. Larson. 1967. *Biochim. Biophys. Acta* 148:469.
14. Shahani, K. M., and H. H. Sommer. 1951. *J. Dairy Sci.* 34:1010.
15. Verbeke, R., S. Aqvist, and G. Peeters. 1957. *Arch. Internat. Physiol. Biochim.* 65:433.
16. Verbeke, R., and G. Peeters. 1965. *Biochem. J.* 94:183.
17. Verbeke, R., G. Peeters, A. M. Massart-Leen, and G. Cocquyt. 1968. *Biochem. J.* 106:719.

MILK FAT SYNTHESIS

13-1 MILK FAT COMPOSITION

Fat is one of the major components of milk and the most variable. It is influenced by nutrition and environment to a greater extent than the other milk components. There is more variation in the percentage of milk fat among animals within a species than in any other major milk constituent. There is also considerable variation in the percentage and composition of the milk fat among species.

Milk fat is composed primarily of triglycerides. Bovine milk fat, for instance, contains only 1% other lipids (21). The general formula for a triglyceride is shown in Figure 13-1, in which three fatty acids, R-1, R-2, and R-3, are esterified to glycerol. The percentage composition of fatty acids attached to the glycerol molecule in human, pig, cow, and goat milks is given in Table 13-1. The most striking difference between the ruminant and the nonruminant milk fat is the relatively high percentage of short-chain fatty acids in ruminant milk fat. Human and pig milk fat also contain higher amounts of unsaturated fatty acids than that of ruminants. Milk fats from other nonruminants have fatty acid compositions comparable to those of the human and pig.

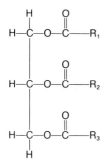

FIGURE 13–1
Formula for a triglyceride. Three fatty acids, R_1, R_2, and R_3, are attached to a glycerol molecule. The fatty acids vary in carbon chain length and degree of unsaturation.

TABLE 13-1
Percentage of fatty acids in triglycerides of milk fat.

Fatty acid	Carbon length	% moles in triglycerides			
		Human	Pig	Goat	Cow
Saturated					
Butyric	4	—	⟍	7	10
Caproic	6	—		5	3
Caprylic	8	—	2	4	1
Capric	10	2		13	2
Lauric	12	8	⟍	7	3
Myristic	14	9	2	12	9
Palmitic	16	23	29	24	21
Stearic	18	9	6	5	11
Unsaturated					
Oleic	18:1	34	35	17	31
Linoleic	18:2	7	14	3	5
Other	—	8	12	3	4

Source: Hilditch and Williams. 1964. *The Chemical Composition of Natural Fats*, 4th ed. New York: John Wiley.

13-2 PRECURSORS OF MILK FAT

Information about the precursors of fatty acids and glycerol of milk fat come from two sources. One source is the measurement of arteriovenous differences of metabolites across the mammary gland. The second is the measurement of the radioactivity of the various milk fat components following the injection of radioactive-labeled precursors into the animal.

The arterio-venous (AV) differences of the milk fat precursors are shown in Table 11-1. Barry (6) calculated the grams of each precursor that are available for 100 grams of milk. The precursors of milk fat that are taken up by the mammary gland in sufficient quantities for milk fat synthesis are glucose, acetate, β-hydroxybutyric acid, and triglycerides.

The 18-carbon unit (C_{18}) fatty acids of milk fat and some of the C_{16} fatty acids come almost entirely from the triglycerides of chylomicra and low-density lipoproteins of the blood. Negligible amounts of free fatty acids (FFA) absorbed from the blood appear in the milk. The arterio-venous differences of FFA are extremely small; however, there is a substantial decrease in the radioactivity of FFA from the bloodstream. This indicates that there is a substantial uptake of the FFAs, but this is compensated by an almost equal release of FFA into the venous blood leaving the udder, giving a small but variable net FFA uptake by the mammary gland. There is no significant arterio-venous difference of phospholipids, sterols, or sterol esters in the goat mammary gland (3, 5, 7).

From one radioactivity study (15), it was estimated that 25% of the total milk fatty acids of the cow were derived from dietary fatty acids. Riis et al. (37) infused labeled fatty acids into a lactating cow and concluded that 50% of the milk fatty acids were derived from plasma lipids. These acids are predominantly long-chain fatty acids, therefore a large proportion of the carbon atoms come from the plasma triglyceride fatty acids. Barry (5) estimated that 30% of the carbon atoms of milk fat were derived from acetate and the remainder came from plasma fatty acids. Groves and Larson (16) concluded that 40-60% of the lipid components were derived from blood serum lipids. From these studies it appears that at least half of the fatty acids in bovine milk come from β-lipoprotein triglycerides in the blood.

The information on the precursors for nonruminant milk fat is somewhat limited. Barry (5) states that it is highly probable that a large proportion of the milk fat comes from plasma triglycerides. He also states that there is a significant synthesis of fatty acids within the rat and rabbit mammary gland epithelial cells from glucose and possibly acetate. Considerable radioactivity in C_{12}, C_{14}, and C_{16} fatty acids of sow's milk was demonstrated after the infusion of labeled glucose, indicating the conversion of glucose into milk fat in this species (32).

In the ruminant mammary gland, there is a negligible amount of fatty acids synthesized from glucose. It was first thought that this was due to the fact that glucose does not form acetyl CoA in ruminant mammary gland tissues, but recent evidence indicates that it is due to a lack of citrate lyase enzyme activity. Acetyl CoA is formed in the mitochondria from pyruvate. The formed acetyl CoA cannot pass directly to the cytoplasmic compartment and is converted into citrate, which apparently passes without difficulty into the cytoplasm because it is in relatively high concentrations in the milk. In the rat mammary gland the citrate is cleaved by the citrate lyase enzyme to form acetyl CoA units, which can be used for fatty acid synthesis. Since the activity of this enzyme is low in most ruminant tissues, the number of acetyl CoA units formed from glucose that are available for fatty acid synthesis is much lower in ruminant mammary gland than in the nonruminant glands. The acetyl CoA used by the ruminant mammary gland for milk fat synthesis is formed primarily from acetate in the cytoplasm (17).

13-3 SYNTHESIS OF MILK FAT

Synthesis of Short-chain Fatty Acids

The demonstration that the short-chain fatty acids with carbon lengths up through C_{16} were formed in the mammary gland was made by Popják et al. (35, 36). Radioactive-labeled acetate was injected into the blood of goats. The specific activity of the milk fat was much higher than that of the plasma fatty acids, indicating that the acetate was incorporated into milk fat. The relative specific activities of the various fatty acids after ^{14}C-acetate injection were as follows: C_4, 34; C_6, 63; C_8, 84; C_{10}, 100; C_{12}, 71; C_{14}, 30; C_{16}, 30; $C_{18:0}$, 1.5; and $C_{18:1}$, 0.9. If the C_{10} fatty acid was derived entirely from acetate, the figures indicate the percentage of the other acids formed from acetate. The involvement of acetate for the synthesis of fatty acids up to C_{14}, and to some extent C_{16}, has been verified by a large number of workers. Annison et al. (2, 3) calculated that the specific activities of the C_4-C_{14} fatty acids of milk fat were 75-90% of that of blood acetate, again indicating that these acids arise primarily from blood acetate. They also calculated that 21-23% of the carbon dioxide produced by the mammary gland came from acetate. Acetate accounted for less than 1% of the long-chain fatty acids. The small amount of propionic acid incorporated into milk fat is used as a 3-carbon unit to which acetate units are added to form odd-numbered carbon fatty acids (13, 22).

Popják et al. (36) injected labeled acetate into the goat and measured the radioactivity in the milk fatty acids. They found that the carboxyl carbon of the C_6 acid had 2.5 times as much radioactivity as the remainder of the labeled carbon atoms. If all of the C_6 fatty acid had arisen from acetate, the labeling should have been the same in the C-2, C-4, and C-6 atoms. They suggested that some of the C_6 fatty acids arose from the condensation of labeled acetate with unlabeled β-hydroxybutyrate. They also suggested that half of the molecules of the C_4 acid came directly from β-hydroxybutyrate. In contrast to this, Kumar et al. (28) infused blood containing ^{14}C-labeled β-hydroxybutyrate and found that the C_6 fatty acid of cow's milk had a higher specific activity than the C_4 fatty acid. This suggests that β-hydroxybutyrate is not a specific precursor of the C_4 acid. It has been suggested that the β-hydroxybutyrate is incorporated into milk fat of cows, goats, and rabbits without cleavage (29, 33). In a more recent study (31) the infusion of β-hydroxybutyrate into the lactating goat indicated that about 40% of this molecule was broken down into C_2 fragments. The exact mechanism of utilization of β-hydroxybutyrate for milk fat synthesis is not clear at the present time. From labeling and arterio-venous studies, it does appear that the β-hydroxybutyrate plays a role in milk fat synthesis. The incorporation probably proceeds by two routes, one in which β-hydroxybutyrate is cleaved into C_2 units and incorporated as acetyl CoA and the second in which it serves as a starting carbon chain for the addition of C_2 units.

Synthesis of Long-chain Fatty Acids

From the early work of Popják et al. (35, 36), it was shown that approximately 30% of palmitic acid was derived from acetate. The arterio-venous differences of palmitic acid are quite high and are comparable to those of stearic acid. Barry (5) concludes that most of the palmitic acid comes from the blood triglycerides. This is supported by the continuous labeled-acetate infusions of Annison et al. (3), who demonstrated that palmitic acid had one-fourth the radioactivity of blood acetate, indicating that palmitic acid was partly derived from acetate but mostly from plasma triglycerides. The injection of labeled palmitic acid into the bloodstream resulted in a substantial amount of the radioactivity being transferred directly into palmitic acid of the milk fat. Barry (5) also suggested that part of the C_{14} fatty acids in milk fat came from a degradation of the palmitic acid, a C_{16} acid, in the mammary gland and that a small number of C_{12} units arose in a similar manner. Gerson et al. (14) infused acetic acid into the lactating dairy cow for 30 hours and indicated that a large proportion of the palmitic acid could be synthesized from acetate, but by a slower pathway than that of the shorter-chain fatty acids.

The stearic and oleic acids are derived from the triglycerides of chylomicra and low density lipoproteins in the blood. More stearic acid than oleic acid is absorbed from plasma blood lipids. In addition, goat's milk fat contains 3 to 4 times as much oleic acid as stearic acid, which suggests that stearic acid is converted into oleic acid by the mammary gland. It has been shown that stearic acid can be converted to oleic acid by the bovine and sow mammary glands and the enzymes responsible for the desaturation process have been isolated. Oleic acid, however, cannot be converted into stearic acid by the mammary gland (5, 7, 9).

The transformation of blood stearic and blood oleic acid into the C_{18} fatty acids of milk fat has been confirmed by a number of workers. Gerson et al. (14) used a continuous infusion of radioactive acetate and found that oleic acid had a higher specific activity than stearic acid. They suggested that precursors other than stearic acid might be involved in the synthesis of oleic acid. They also suggested that the formation of the C_{18} and higher molecular weight acids might involve the chain elongation pathway, instead of a direct absorption from the bloodstream. In contrast to this, Popjak et al. (35, 36) and Barry (5) indicated that negligible amounts of $C_{18:0}$ and $C_{18:1}$ acids came from blood acetate in the goat. It has been suggested that the mammary gland has a large pool of long-chain fatty acids that can serve as an endogenous source of fatty acids for the synthesis of milk glycerides (18, 31).

The preponderence of evidence suggests that the C_{18} fatty acids are absorbed from the blood as either stearic or oleic acid. Stearic acid can be converted into oleic acid. A small amount of C_{18} acids might arise from precursors other than stearic or oleic acid; however, it is insignificant from a quantitative standpoint.

Glycerol Synthesis

The arterio-venous differences of free glycerol indicate that it provides less than 10% of the glycerol portion of the milk triglycerides. A substantial amount of glycerol is absorbed with the blood triglycerides. The presence of the enzyme, glycerolkinase, in the mammary gland shows that glycerol 3-phosphate for triglyceride synthesis can be derived from glycerol. Most of the glycerol is synthesized from blood glucose. The enzyme, glycerol 3-P dehydrogenase is present in the rat mammary gland. This indicates that glycerol 3-phosphate can be derived from glucose via dihydroxyacetone phosphate in the Embden-Meyerhof Pathway. Radioactive isotope studies also support the conclusion that glycerol is derived through the Embden-Meyerhof Pathway. The glycerol 3-phosphate concentration rises nearly threefold at the time of parturition in the guinea pig mammary gland tissue (4, 5, 27, 34).

West et al. (40) conclude that a substantial or complete hydrolysis of the plasma triglycerides occurs at the capillary wall and precedes their uptake by the mammary gland. The hydrolysis in this area would not affect the arterio-venous differences of free glycerol since these measurements are made on blood entering and leaving the mamary gland. No accurate measurements are available to indicate the amount of glycerol that arises from the various sources, but estimates indicate that circulating blood glucose can potentially supply 70% of the milk lipid glycerol, whereas the lipoprotein glycerides can supply about 50% (5, 24).

13-4   BIOCHEMICAL PATHWAYS

The oxidation of fatty acid through β-oxidation occurs through a stepwise degradation of the acid with the liberation of 2-carbon units, acetyl CoA. The acetyl CoA units can enter the citric acid cycle. The fatty acid is first activated to form a fatty acyl CoA, which requires Coenzyme A and ATP (Step 1, Figure 13-2). In Step 2, two hydrogen ions are removed from the C-2 and C-3 atoms and transferred to FAD^+. Water is then added to form a hydroxyl group on the third carbon atom. The two hydrogen ions on the third carbon atom are transferred to NAD^+. The NADH and FADH can release their hydrogen ions and electrons to the cytochrome system with the production of ATP. During Step 5, a split occurs between the C-2 and C-3 atoms to yield acetyl CoA. At the same time a second CoA enzyme is added to the remaining fatty acid to again produce a fatty acyl CoA. This procedure of the stepwise elimination of 2-carbon units is repeated until the entire fatty acid is oxidized. Fatty acid oxidation is relatively unimportant in mammary gland tissue (1).

Fatty acids are synthesized from acetate and other fatty acids in one of two ways. The mitochondrial system forms fatty acids by a reversal of β-oxidation (Figure 13-2). This system is present within the mitochondria and is primarily involved in lengthening short-chain fatty acids. The reversal of β-oxidation requires both NADH and NADPH. Under physiological conditions, the thiolase reaction that catalyzes the condensation of acetyl CoA and acyl CoA (Step 5, Fig. 13-2) to form the β-ketoacyl CoA, does not favor the synthetic process (8). The equilibrium can be shifted towards condensation and synthesis in the presence of NADH and β-hydroxyacyl dehydrogenase (39).

The second system is located primarily in the cytoplasm of the cell and produces palmitic acid from acetyl CoA without the participation of mitochondrial fatty acid oxidative enzymes. This system of fatty acid synthesis requires CO_2 or bicarbonate, Mn^{++}, NADPH, and a biotin-containing enzyme, acetyl carboxylase. The steps in this formation are shown in Figure 13-3. The carbon atom picked up from bicarbonate is

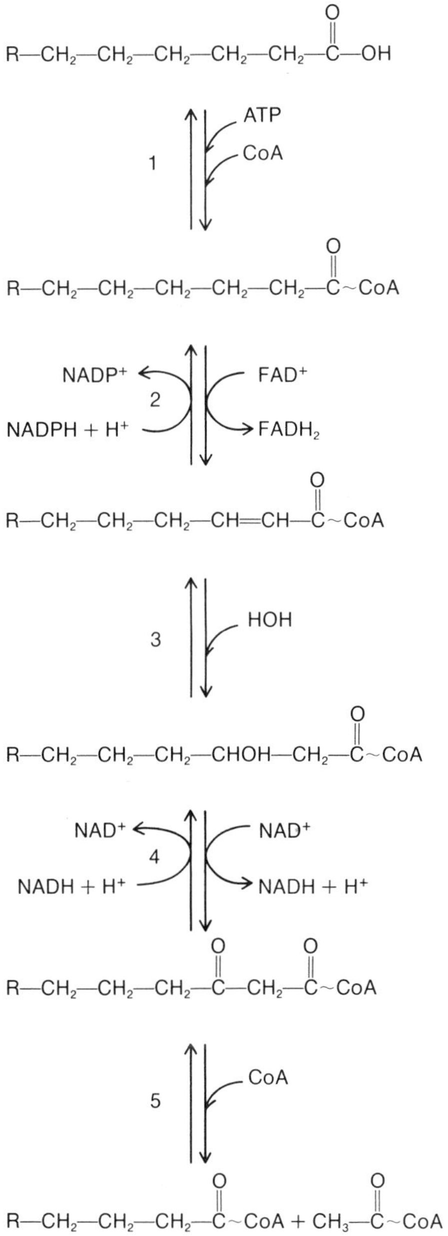

FIGURE 13–2
Fatty acid oxidation (β-oxidation).
Enzymes involved in the steps are:

(1) Thiokinase

(2) Fatty acid-CoA dehydrogenase

(3) enoyl hydrase

(4) β-hydroxyacyl dehydrogenase

(5) β-ketoacyl thiolase

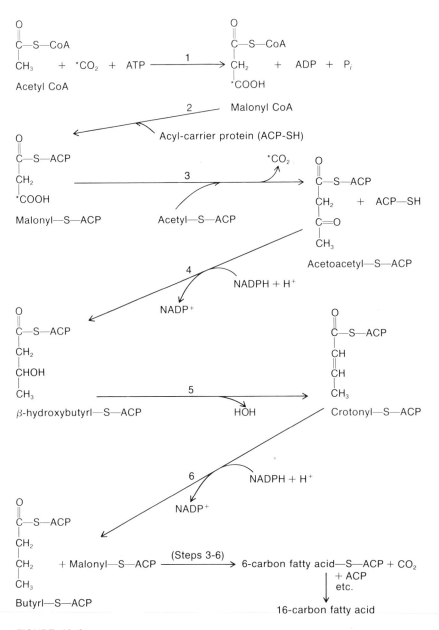

FIGURE 13–3
Fatty acid synthesis through malonyl CoA. ACP and CoA are written as ACP-SH and CoA-SH to indicate their active acyl activation sites. See text for discussion.

labeled with an asterisk so that it can be followed in the pathway. The enzymes in this pathway are given in Table 13-2.

Malonyl CoA, after formation, combines with acyl-carrier protein (ACP). All intermediates in fatty acid synthesis appear to be protein

TABLE 13-2
Enzymes involved in steps of fatty acid synthesis through malonyl CoA, as shown in Figure 13-3.

Step	Enzyme
1	Acetyl carboxylase (biotin)
2	—
3	β-ketoacyl-ACP synthetase
4	β-ketoacyl-ACP reductase
5	Enol-ACP hydrase
6	Crotonyl-ACP reductase

Source: White et al. 1968. *Principles of Biochemistry*, 4th ed. New York: McGraw-Hill.

bound to ACP. The malonyl-S-ACP combines with acetyl-S-ACP to form acetoacetyl-S-ACP with the liberation of ACP-SH. The condensation of the acetyl-S-ACP and malony-S-ACP results in the liberation of CO_2, a process that shifts the overall reaction equilibrium towards synthesis (8). The reduction of acetoacetyl-S-ACP requires NADPH to form a hydroxyl group on the β carbon. When NADH is substituted for NADPH, the rate of fatty acid synthesis decreases by 75% (8). Water is then removed from this molecule (Step 5) to form crotonyl-S-ACP. This introduces a double bond between the C-2 and C-3 atoms, NADPH is again required to reduce this molecule to butyrl-S-ACP. If this is liberated from ACP, butyric acid is formed. In most cases, the butyrl-S-ACP combines with another molecule of malonyl-S-ACP to form a C_6 fatty acid with the liberation of CO_2 and ACP-SH. A stepwise condensation with further malonyl-S-ACP units occurs with the final formation of palmitic acid. The NADPH molecules are supplied primarily by the pentose phosphate pathway.

The malonyl CoA pathway has been demonstrated to be present in mammary gland tissue. The enzymes involved in fatty acid synthesis through malonyl CoA occur in both the microsomes and the soluble-enzyme fraction in a wide variety of tissues (11, 12, 29).

The proportion of the fatty acids synthesized in the mammary gland that arise through the malonyl CoA and acetyl CoA (reversal of β-oxidation) pathways is not known. The evidence for these two pathways in mammary gland tissue is conflicting. Dils and Popják (11) concluded that the malonyl CoA pathway is the major route for the biosynthesis of fatty acid from acetate in the lactating rat mammary gland tissue. They found that virtually no synthesis of fatty acids from acetate takes place when the biotin-mediated carboxylation of acetyl CoA to malonyl CoA is inhibited by avidin. Lachance and Marais (30) concluded that the mammary glands of rabbits synthesized C_4 and C_6 fatty acids via the acetyl CoA pathway and the intermediate- and long-chain fatty acids via malonyl CoA and possibly chain elongation. Bu'Lock and Smith (10) fed labeled fatty acids to rabbits and followed the synthesis of milk fatty acids after the labeled fatty acids were degraded. They concluded that the uniform alternate labeling of the C_2-C_{10} fatty acids indicated that these were synthesized via the malonyl CoA pathway. The C_{12}-C_{18} fatty acids had a higher radioactivity in the carboxyl end, which they concluded to be due to chain elongation.

Gerson et al. (14) used two different methods of administering ^{14}C-acetic acid to the dairy cow. The single injection of ^{14}C-acetic acid resulted in the typical picture of fatty acid synthesis. The C_4-C_{14} fatty acids were derived primarily from acetate. The C_{18} fatty acids were derived primarily from blood triglycerides. When the ^{14}C-acetate was infused for a 30-hour period, three groups of fatty acids were present in the mammary gland. The groups are as follows: C_2-C_{10}, C_{12}-C_{16}, and C_{18} fatty acids. They suggested that the C_2-C_{10} fatty acids arose from acetate through the acetyl CoA pathway. The C_{12}-C_{16} fatty acids arose through the malonyl CoA pathway, and part of the C_{18} fatty acids involved the chain elongation pathway. Further work is needed to clarify the role of these two pathways in milk fat synthesis for the various species; however, most research workers indicate that the malonyl CoA pathway is the major pathway for the synthesis of C_4 to C_{16} fatty acids from acetate.

13-5   ESTERIFICATION OF FATTY ACIDS

The esterification of fatty acids on the glycerol molecule does not occur in a random order. Analysis of the triglycerides of cow's milk fat indicates that the C_{12}-C_{16} fatty acids are primarily concentrated on the C-2 atom of glycerol. The short-chain fatty acids, namely C_4 and C_6, are primarily located on the C-1 and C-3 atoms. The stearic acid is also esterified preferentially on C-1 and C-3 atoms of glycerol. The fatty acids derived from blood triglycerides and those acids synthesized within the mammary gland are not segregated onto different glycerol moleclules (20, 38).

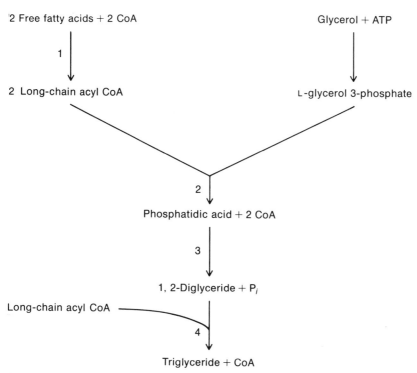

FIGURE 13–4
Proposed pathway for esterification of fatty acids (by Kennedy, 1961,
Fed. Proc. 20:934).

The accepted pathway for the esterification of the fatty acids on glycerol is that proposed by Kennedy (23). This is shown in Figure 13-4 and the enzymes are listed in Table 13-3. This was worked out for liver and intestine and has also been shown to be present in adipose tissue. Evidence for the existence of the Kennedy Pathway in mammary gland tissue

TABLE 13-3
Enzymes and cofactors involved in the steps of triglyceride formation, as shown in Figure 13-4.

Step	Enzyme	Cofactors
1	Acid CoA ligase	ATP, Mg^{++}
2	Acyl CoA L-glycerol 3-phosphate acyltransferase	—
3	L-α-phosphatidate phosphohydrolase	—
4	Acyl CoA 1,2-diglyceride 0-acyltransferase	—

indicates the incorporation of fatty acids by rat mammary gland tissue requires ATP, Mg^{++}, and CoA. Also particulate fractions of goat mammary gland catalyze the esterification of both glycerol 3-phosphate and diglyceride. In addition, it has been demonstrated that the palmitoyl-transferase enzyme (required for Step 2 in Figure 13-4) is present in lactating guinea pig mammary glands. It is suggested that the transferase might be a suitable point at which the pathway of fat synthesis might be regulated since palymitoyl CoA stands as a branch point in the metabolism and since the esterification of glycerol 3-phosphate represents an interaction of two major areas of metabolism (26).

The monoglyceride pathway of fatty acid esterification, which is present in the intestine, may function in the mammary gland. In this pathway, 1, 2-diglyceride is formed from the direct acylation of 2-monoglyceride (25).

13-6 SUMMARY

Milk fat is the most variable component of milk. This is true for the percentage composition of the fat and the fatty acid composition of the triglycerides within and among species. Most of the milk fat is made up of triglycerides. The major precursors for milk lipids are glucose, acetate, β-hydroxybutyrate acid, the triglycerides of the chylomicra, and the low-density lipoproteins from the blood. The short-chain fatty acids from C_4 to C_{14} and some of the palmitic acid are synthesized within the mammary gland from acetate derived as absorbed acetate in the ruminant or from glucose in the nonruminant animal.

The ruminant mammary gland can not utilize acetyl CoA formed from glucose in the mitochondria. The β-hydroxybutyrate is also used for fatty acid synthesis. Part of this is utilized as the starting carbon chain for the addition of C_2 units and part is cleaved into C_2 units and utilized as acetyl CoA units for fatty acid synthesis.

Approximately 30% of the palmitic acid is derived from acetate and the remainder comes from the triglycerides in the blood. Stearic and oleic acids come primarily from the plasma triglycerides. Stearic acid is absorbed in greater quantities from the blood than oleic acid, yet oleic acid is the most prevalent C_{18} fatty acid in milk. Stearic acid can be converted to oleic acid by the bovine, goat, and sow mammary gland; however, oleic acid cannot be saturated to form stearic acid.

Free glycerol from the bloodstream provides less than 10% of the glycerol portion of milk triglycerides. Most of the glycerol comes from the synthesis of glycerol 3-phosphate from glucose by the Embden-Meyerhof Pathway and the remainder comes from the glycerol portion of the lipoprotein glycerides. It has been shown that glucose can potentially supply 70% of the milk lipid glycerol.

Two routes of fatty acid synthesis are probable in the mammary gland; however, the malonyl CoA pathway appears to be the predominant one. The acetyl CoA pathway is a reversal of β-oxidation; however, the evidence for its importance in the mammary gland is conflicting. The malonyl CoA pathway produces palmitic acid from the acetyl CoA in the cytoplasm of the cell and does not require the participation of mitochondrial fatty-acid-oxidative enzymes, which are required for reversal of β-oxidation. The malonyl CoA pathway requires CO_2, Mn^{++}, NADPH, and a biotin-containing enzyme, acetyl carboxylase. In this pathway, acetyl CoA is carboxylated to form malonyl CoA, which is joined to an acyl-carrier protein. This protein complex is then attached to an acetyl CoA molecule to form a β-hydroxybutyrl compound. This is then hydrogenated to form a butyrl protein complex. The addition of a second malonyl CoA molecule increases the chain length to 6 carbons. Additions of malonyl CoA molecules are repeated until palmitic acid is formed. The enzymes necessary for these pathways are present in the mammary gland.

Two pathways for the esterification of fatty acids may be present in the mammary gland; however, it appears that the phosphatidic acid pathway is the most common. In this pathway, two long-chain acyl CoA molecules are attached to L-glycerol 3-phosphate to form phosphatidic acid. The phosphate molecule is then removed to form 1,2-diglyceride. A third long-chain acyl CoA molecule is attached to the 1,2-diglyceride to form the triglyceride. The second pathway that may be involved is the formation of 1,2-diglyceride from the acylation of 2-monoglyceride.

REFERENCES

1. Annison, E. F., S. Fazakerley, J. L. Linzell, and B. W. Nichols. 1965. *Biochem. J.* 94:21p.
2. Annison, E. F., and J. L. Linzell. 1964. *J. Physiol.* 175:372.
3. Annison, E. F., J. L. Linzell, S. Fazakerley, and B. W. Nichols. 1967. *Biochem. J.* 102:637.
4. Baldwin, R. L., and L. P. Milligan. 1966. *J. Biol. Chem.* 241:2058.
5. Barry, J. M. 1964. *Biol. Rev.* 39:194.

6. Barry, J. M. 1966. *Outlook on Agriculture* 5:129.
7. Barry, J. M., W. Bartley, J. L. Linzell, and D. S. Robinson. 1963. *Biochem. J.* 89:6.
8. Bennett, T. P., and E. Frieden. 1966. *Modern Topics in Biochemistry.* New York: Macmillan Co.
9. Bickerstaffe, R., and E. F. Annison. 1968. *Biochem. J.* 108:47p.
10. Bu'Lock, J. D., and G. N. Smith. 1965. *Biochem. J.* 96:495.
11. Dils, R., and G. Popják. 1962. *Biochem. J.* 83:41.
12. Ganguly, J. 1960. *Biochim. Biophys. Acta* 40:110.
13. Garton, G. A. 1963. *J. Lipid Res.* 4:237.
14. Gerson, T., F. B. Shorland, G. F. Wilson, and C. W. S. Reid. 1968. *J. Dairy Sci.* 51:356.
15. Glascock, R. F., W. G. Duncombe, and L. R. Reinius. 1956. *Biochem J.* 62:535.
16. Groves, T. D., and B. L. Larson. 1965. *Biochim. Biophys. Acta* 104:462.
17. Hardwick, D. C. 1966. *Biochem. J.* 99:228.
18. Hardwick, D. C., J. L. Linzell, and T. B. Mepham. 1963. *Biochem J.* 87:4p.
19. Hartmann, P. E., and A. K. Lascelles. 1964. *Aust. J. Biol. Sci.* 17:935.
20. Hilditch, T. P., and P. N. Williams. 1964. *The Chemical Composition of Natural Fats*, 4th ed. New York: John Wiley.
21. Jack, E. L., and L. M. Smith. 1956. *J. Dairy Sci.* 39:1.
22. James, A. T., G. Peeters, and M. Lauryssens. 1956. *Biochem. J.* 64:726.
23. Kennedy, E. P. 1961. *Federation Proc.* 20:934.
24. Kinsella, J. E. 1968. *Biochim. Biophys. Acta* 164:540.
25. Kinsella, J. E., and R. D. McCarthy. 1968. *Biochim. Biophys. Acta* 164:518.
26. Kuhn, N. J. 1967. *Biochem. J.* 105:213.
27. Kuhn, N. J. 1967. *Biochem. J.* 105:225.
28. Kumar, S., L. Lakshmanan, and J. C. Shaw. 1959. *J. Biol. Chem.* 234:754.
29. Kumar, S., V. N. Singh, and R. Keren-Paz. 1965. *Biochim. Biophys. Acta* 98:221.
30. Lachance, J. P., and R. Marais. 1965. *Biochem. Biophys. Res. Comm.* 20:269.
31. Linzell, J. L., E. F. Annison, S. Fazakerley, and R. A. Leng. 1967. *Biochem. J.* 104:34.
32. Linzell, J. L., T. B. Mepham, E. F. Annison and C. E. West. 1967. *Biochem. J.* 103:42p.
33. Luick, J. R., and K. K. Kameoka. 1966. *J. Dairy Sci.* 49:98.
34. McBride, O. W., and E. D. Korn. 1964. *J. Lipid Res.* 5:442.
35. Popják, G., T. H. French, and S. J. Folley. 1951. *Biochem. J.* 48:411.
36. Popják, G., T. H. French, G. D. Hunter, and A. J. P. Martin. 1951. *Biochem. J.* 48:612.
37. Riis, P. M., J. R. Luick, and M. Kleiber. 1960. *Amer. J. Physiol.* 198:45.
38. Smith, L. M., C. P. Freeman, and E. L. Jack. 1965. *J. Dairy Sci.* 48:531.
39. Wakil, S. J. 1961. *J. Lipid Res.* 2:1.
40. West, C. E., E. F. Annison, and J. L. Linzell. 1967. *Biochem. J.* 104:59p.

LACTOSE, MINERALS, VITAMINS

14-1 LACTOSE

Lactose is a disaccharide made up of a glucose and a galactose molecule. The two molecules are joined by a beta linkage between the C-1 atom of galactose and the C-4 atom of glucose (Figure 14-1). Lactose is found almost exclusively in milk and in the mammary glands of animals. Small amounts are occasionally found in some plants; however, it is present in very low concentrations. The mechanism of formation in plants also appears to be different from that in animals (19).

Biochemical Pathway of Lactose Synthesis

The proposed scheme for lactose synthesis is given in Figure 14-2. Glucose is first phosphorylated in the C-6 position. In the presence of a mutase enzyme, the phosphate group is moved to the C-1 position (Table 14-1). Glucose 1-phosphate then unites with uridine triphosphate (UTP) to form uridine diphosphate glucose (UDP-glucose) with the liberation of pyrophosphate (P_i-P_i). UDP-glucose is then converted into UDP-

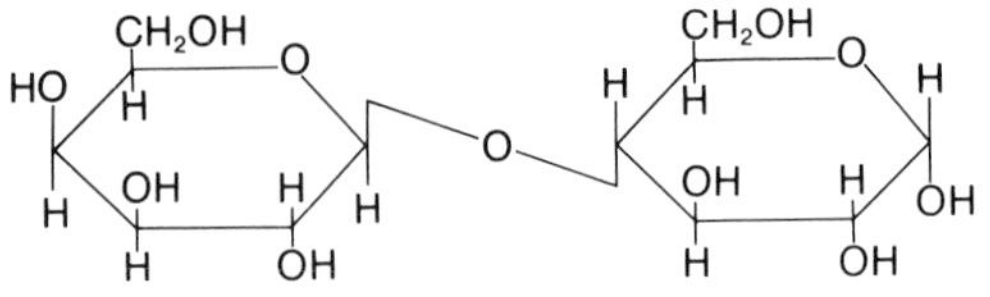

FIGURE 14–1
Lactose composed of a molecule of galactose (A)
joined to a molecule of glucose (B) by a β linkage
between C-1 of galactose and C-4 of glucose.

Glucose + ATP $\xrightarrow{\quad 1 \quad}$ glucose 6-P + ADP

Glucose 6-P $\xrightarrow{\quad 2 \quad}$ glucose 1-P

Glucose 1-P + UTP $\xrightarrow{\quad 3 \quad}$ UDP-glucose + pyrophosphate (P_i—P_i)

UDP-glucose $\xrightarrow{\quad 4 \quad}$ UDP-galactose

UDP-galactose + glucose $\xrightarrow{\quad 5 \quad}$ lactose + UDP

FIGURE 14–2
Proposed pathway of lactose synthesis.

galactose in the presence of an epimerase enzyme. The UDP-galactose combines with glucose to form lactose with the liberation of UDP. It was originally thought that glucose 1-phosphate was the acceptor of the galactosyl molecule with the production of lactose 1-phosphate (9), which was then converted to lactose with the liberation of the phosphate ion in the presence of a phosphatase enzyme. More recent work has demon-

TABLE 14-1
Enzymes required for the steps of lactose synthesis,
as shown in Figure 14-2.

Step	Enzyme
1	Hexokinase
2	Phosphoglucomutase
3	UDP-glucose pyrophosphorylase
4	UDP-galactose 4-epimerase
5	Lactose synthetase

strated that free glucose, rather than glucose 1-phosphate, is the galactosyl acceptor in the formation of lactose. This evidence has been found in the rat mammary glands, the perfused udder, and the intact lactating cow (4, 7, 10, 32).

The activities of the enzymes involved in lactose biosynthesis have been studied in mammary gland tissues of various species. It has been found that the UDP-galactose 4-epimerase and UDP-glucose pyrophosphorylase activities increase markedly after the onset of lactation in the rat, the guinea pig, and the rabbit. The phosphoglucomutase activity also increases at the onset of lactation in the rat and guinea pig. In contrast to these species, there is no marked increase in the activity of these three enzymes in the cow's mammary gland after the onset of lactation. It is concluded that the initiation of lactation in the cow does not involve the sudden acquisition of enzymatic potential for milk synthesis, but that the enzymes are already present during pregnancy and that a factor other than increased enzyme activity causes the onset of lactation. Hypophysectomy causes a marked decrease in the UDP-glucose pyrophosphorylase and phosphoglucomutase activities in the rat (2, 12, 14).

The lactose synthetase activity of the rat mammary gland increases very markedly during lactation from an almost zero value on the last day of pregnancy. This increase in lactose synthetase activity parallels the increase in tissue lactose content. A comparison of the activity of lactose synthetase with the other enzymes in the pathway of lactose biosynthesis indicates that the activity of the lactose synthetase may be a rate-limiting step in milk secretion (17). Lactose synthetase is a complex of two proteins. The A protein of this complex is a nonspecific galactosyltransferase that is normally present in many tissues besides the mammary gland. The A protein can transfer galactose from UDP-galactose to compounds such as N-acetyl glucosamine, but not to glucose. The B protein is α-lactalbumin, which is present in relatively high concentrations in milk. A combination of the A and B proteins can unite UDP-galactose to glucose to form lactose (6, 8, 18). Progesterone appears to repress the formation of α-lactalbumin during pregnancy. When the concentration of plasma progesterone decreases at parturition, the rate of α-lactalbumin synthesis increases (28).

Precursors of Lactose

Most of the glucose and galactose in the synthesis of lactose come from glucose or from substances that are rapidly converted to glucose (19). Barry (3) summarized the arterio-venous differences and concluded that blood glucose is the principal precursor of lactose in the goat and in the cow. He stated that some of the carbon atoms of lactose, especially the galactose residue, originate from other compounds, such as acetate and glycerol.

The arterio-venous differences for glucose are about twice that required for lactose synthesis, consequently the remaining glucose can be utilized for energy and glycerol production. The role of blood glucose in lactose synthesis and milk production has been reviewed by Linzell (22) and Rook et al. (24). Since glucose is the primary precursor of milk lactose and because milk is maintained isotonic with the blood, Rook et al. (24) concluded that a reduction in lactose secretion caused a reduction in water secretion into the milk, and consequently a reduction in milk yield. Linzell (22) also suggested that the availability of glucose to the mammary gland can be a limiting factor for maximum milk secretion. Kleiber et al. (15) injected labeled glucose into the cow and found that it contributed about 85% of the carbon in lactose. They also concluded that acetate and lactate become important sources of lactose carbons in the intact animal, probably only after their conversion in tissues, such as the liver, to compounds that can be utilized for lactose formation by the mammary gland.

Studies with radioactive isotopes indicate that not all of the galactose comes from the plasma glucose and that not all of the galactose is formed from glucose via the scheme proposed in Figure 14-2. There are several lines of evidence for this, which have been summarized by Leloir and Cardini (19). The administration of uniformly labeled glucose (glucose labeled in all carbon atoms) results in equal radioactivity in the glucose and galactose parts of the lactose molecule. When glucose is labeled in the C-1 position, the radioactivity of the galactose molecule is less than that of the glucose molecule. If UDP-glucose were converted to UDP-galactose as shown in Figure 14-2, the labeling should be the same. When ^{14}C-labeled acetate is injected into the artery of the mammary gland, about 90% of the total radioactivity of the lactose molecule appeared in galactose, with little appearing in the glucose molecule. Most of the radioactivity appeared in the C-4 position of the galactose molecule.

When glycerol 1,3-^{14}C is provided to the mammary gland, galactose contains much more ^{14}C than glucose and most of the labeled carbon atoms are in the C-4 and C-6 positions of galactose (30). This distribution does not support the concept that glycerol is converted into glucose or galactose by a reversal of the Embden-Meyerhof Pathway. If it were, there should be equal labeling in the C-1, C-3, C-4 and C-6 atoms. Bartley et al. (4) obtained further information that indicated that little carbon from the 3-carbon units entered the hexose phosphate pool by a reversal of the Embden-Meyerhof Pathway. Hansen et al. (10) suggested that the higher labeling in the C-4 and C-6 atoms might be explained by a transaldolase-like exchange with UDP-galactose. In this mechanism a

3-carbon unit is exchanged with a 3-carbon unit of the galactose molecule. There is no definite evidence that this mechanism takes place in the mammary gland. A similar transaldolase-type of reaction with triose phosphate and fructose phosphate could explain the high labeling of the C-4 atoms (30).

The mammary gland appears to have two hexose pools from which lactose is synthesized. The one pool is a free glucose pool that is used as the galactosyl acceptor and the second is a hexose phosphate pool that contributes some of the galactose molecules. In the rat, galactose 1-phosphate can be converted to UDP-galactose, and thus enter the lactose synthesis pathway directly instead of being first converted to UDP-glucose. The enzyme galactose 1-phosphate uridyl-transferase, which catalyzes the conversion of galactose 1-phosphate to glucose 1-phosphate, is absent or has negligible activity in the mammary gland (4).

An alternative mechanism to explain why the galactose and glucose molecules of lactose are differently labeled is that a particular architecture within the cell permits compartmentalization of certain enzymes. In this way, the substrate pools are not in equilibrium with each other, and thus equal labeling of the two hexose sugars would not occur (30).

Part of the difference in the ^{14}C distribution pattern between galactose and glucose can also be explained by the operation of the pentose phosphate pathway. Wood et al. (29) injected glucose 2,6-^{14}C into the artery of the dairy cow. The glucose in lactose was labeled almost exclusively in the C-2 and C-6 positions, indicating that glucose was a direct precursor of the glucose in lactose. The galactose was labeled in the C-2 and C-6 positions, but also contained considerable activity in the C-1, C-2 and C-5 positions. When glucose 6-^{14}C was injected, both the glucose and the galactose of lactose were almost exclusively labeled in the C-6 position. This indicated that the C-2 atom of glucose was transferred at random to the C-1, C-3, and C-5 atoms of galactose, but C-6 of glucose was not transferred to other carbon positions of glucose or galactose. The authors considered that the pentose phosphate pathway was the mechanism by which C-2 was converted into the C-1 and C-3 atoms. They proposed that the C-5 labeling occurred by way of aldolase and triose phosphate isomerase reactions which formed glyceraldehyde 2,3-^{14}C phosphate, which then exchanged with a 3-carbon unit of fructose 6-phosphate by means of a transaldolase reaction. In this way glucose 2-^{14}C was converted to C-5 of galactose, but C-6 of glucose was not converted into the C-1 of galactose.

Wood et al. (31) also found that the injection of glucose 2-^{14}C into the dairy cow resulted in the glucose molecule being labeled in the C-2 position and the ^{14}C was found extensively in the C-1 and C-3 positions of galactose. They concluded that the galactose was formed from glucose through a hexose phosphate intermediate and the movement of carbon atoms occurred through reactions of the pentose phosphate cycle. They estimated the proportion of glucose metabolized by the pentose cycle for cells making lactose to be 23% in one experiment and 30% in another experiment. They also calculated that less than 10% of the glucose was metabolized by the Embden-Meyerhof Pathway and approximately 60-70% was converted into lactose. For the entire cow, Black et al. (5) ha e concluded that 40% of the total glucose used by the cow is metabolized via the pentose phosphate pathway. They state that the value is higher for specific organs, such as the mammary gland.

The results of these trials indicate that the glucose molecule in lactose is not changed from plasma glucose but acts as the galactosyl acceptor. Most of the galactose comes from glucose, but some of the galactose in lactose arises from a scheme other than that shown in Figure 14-2. The incorporation of glycerol into galactose is brought about by an exchange with 3-carbon units of galactose or fructose through a transaldolase reaction. Some *de novo* synthesis of galactose may occur in the mammary gland. From a quantitative standpoint, however, glucose is still the most important precursor of galactose.

Galactosaemia

Galactosaemia is a human disease in which the galactose molecule cannot be utilized. Feeding milk to human infants with this disease leads to an increase in the size of the liver and spleen, ascites, cataracts, and feeble-mindedness. When the galactose is removed from the diet, a rapid regression of the symptoms occurs. The feeding of galactose to these individuals causes an accumulation of galactose 1-phosphate in the red blood cells and lenses of the eye. The enzyme galactose 1-phosphate uridyl transferase converts galactose 1-phosphate and UDP-glucose into glucose 1-phosphate and UDP-galactose (see Figure 14-3). This enzyme is absent

$$\text{Galactose} + \text{ATP} \xrightarrow{\quad 1 \quad} \text{galactose 1-P} + \text{ADP}$$

$$\text{Galactose 1-P} + \text{UDP-glucose} \underset{\longleftarrow}{\overset{2}{\longrightarrow}} \text{UDP-galactose} + \text{glucose 1-P}$$

$$\text{UDP-galactose} \underset{\longleftarrow}{\overset{3}{\longrightarrow}} \text{UDP-glucose}$$

$$\text{UDP-glucose} + P_i - P_i \xrightarrow{\quad 4 \quad} \text{glucose 1-P} + \text{UTP}$$

FIGURE 14–3
Steps in the conversion of galactose into glucose. The enzymes involved in the steps are: (1) Galactokinase, (2) Galactose 1-phosphate uridyl transferase, (3) epimerase, and (4) UDP-glucose pyrophosphorylase.

in the galactosaemic individual, thus the galactose molecule cannot be converted into glucose. The galactosaemic adult has only about 1% of the normal capacity to oxidize lactose or galactose. A clinical test has been devised to determine whether a newborn individual has the ability to utilize galactose normally (16, 19).

14-2 MINERAL SECRETION

Mineral Composition of Milk

The major mineral constituents of cow's milk are shown in Table 14-2. The two most important minerals from a nutritional standpoint are calcium and phosphorus. Only 25% of the calcium, 20% of the magnesium, and 44% of the phosphorus are in a soluble form; whereas the total amount of other major mineral constituents is in soluble form. The calcium and magnesium in the insoluble form are in chemical or physical combination with caseinate, phosphate, and citrate. This provides a mechanism by which milk can contain a high concentration of calcium, and at the same time, maintain normal osmotic equilibrium with the blood. The buffering capacity of milk is due to its composition of citrates, phosphates, bicarbonates, and protein. The action of these substances keeps the hydrogen concentration of milk close to a pH of 6.6 (13, 21, 26).

TABLE 14-2
Major mineral constituents of cow's milk.

Mineral	Percentage of total composition	Percentage in soluble form
Calcium	0.12	25
Phosphorus	0.10	44
Potassium	0.15	100
Chlorine	0.11	100
Magnesium	0.01	20
Sodium	0.05	100

Calcium and Phosphorus

The casein and inorganic phosphates of milk come from the inorganic phosphate of the plasma. The calcium in the milk comes from the blood calcium, which is derived from the feed and from the skeleton. Blood calcium is in equilibrium with the calcium in the skeleton. Generally speaking, it is difficult to increase the calcium content of milk by increasing the calcium content of the feed because of this equilibrium. During early lactation most high-producing cows are deficient in calcium intake. Increasing the Vitamin D level of the feed increases the calcium absorption from the intestinal tract but will not increase the milk calcium content. Injection of ^{45}Ca into the blood and monitoring of the calcium content of the milk indicates that the calcium appears in the milk a few hours after administration. This lag in calcium appearance in the milk can best be explained by the presence of a calcium reservoir in the udder (13, 26).

Regulation of Mineral Composition of Milk

Information on the regulation of the mineral composition of milk is lacking. Considerable attention has been directed to this, but it is not known whether the epithelial cells absorb minerals from the blood in proportion to the concentration in the blood or whether they selectively absorb them. In addition, it is not known whether some of the absorbed minerals are selectively released from the epithelial cell either into the milk or back into the blood. Because of the consistent concentration of the milk minerals, some sort of regulatory mechanism must be present.

Relationship of Lactose, Sodium, Potassium, and Chlorine Contents

Rook and Wheelock (25) summarized the relationship between lactose, sodium, potassium, and chlorine contents of milk. Animals that are free from infections have constant amounts of lactose, potassium, and sodium in their milk. The constant amounts are characteristic of each individual animal. Within a breed there is a close inverse relationship between the lactose content of milk and the molar sum of sodium and potassium contents. There is also a close inverse relationship between the lactose and potassium contents of milk. Milk is in osmotic equilibrium with blood, and the lactose, potassium, sodium, and chlorine contents of milk are responsible for its osmotic pressure; therefore, water moves into the cell and lumen of the alveolus to maintain osmotic equilibrium. This explains the movement of water into milk and, in part, the control of the volume of milk produced, but does little to indicate the control of the movement of ions into the milk. Lactose is secreted by the epithelial cell, but it is not definitely known whether the ions pass through the epithelial cell or between cells.

Increased sodium and chlorine concentrations appear in the milk under certain circumstances. One concept to explain this favors the view that the milk secreted by the alveolar cell has a constant composition and that, in the lumen of the alveolus, it is mixed with a secretion that is a diluent of blood serum and has approximately the same concentrations of potassium, sodium, and chlorine as that of blood serum. It is suggested that the diluent filters into the alveolar lumina without passing through the epithelial cells. When the volume of the milk secreted by the epithelial cells is decreased, the proportion of the diluent from the blood rises and could explain the changes in ionic composition of milk during late lactation, after infections, or with other treatments (25).

An alternate explanation for the variations in the sodium and chlorine contents of milk is that milk secreted by the cell is richer in sodium and chlorine than that obtained from the gland at milking. As the fluid moves from the alveoli through the ducts into the cisterns of the gland, a resorption of sodium and chlorine takes place. Such a resorption would be against a concentration gradient and probably linked to ATP. A reduction in blood supplied to the ducts or an interference with the resorption process would increase the sodium and chlorine contents of milk (25).

It is generally accepted that sodium and potassium diffuse into the cell from the extracellular fluid. Because the concentration of potassium is high and that of sodium is low within the cell, it appears that these concentrations are maintained by the action of a sodium "pump," which is ATP-dependent. This "pump" transfers sodium out of the cell and potassium into it. These are only sketchy indications of the control of the ionic composition of milk (25).

Trace Mineral Composition

The trace mineral composition of cow's milk is shown in Table 14-3. In addition to the minerals listed, others appear in minute quantities. These are aluminum, barium, bromine, chromium, lead, lithium, nickel, radium, rubidum, selenium, silicon, silver, strontium, tin, titanium, and vanadium. Zinc is found in relatively large amounts in milk in comparison to the other components. About 12% of the total zinc is present in the dissolved form and the remainder is associated with the caseinate particles (1, 23).

Most of the trace minerals are in organic complexes and the concentration of some of them is higher in the fatty portion than in the solids-not-fat portion of the milk. Iron and copper appear to be in protein-bound complexes that are adsorbed on the surface of the fat globules. Except for copper and iron, the feeding of supplements with high amounts of the trace elements increases the amount of these elements in cow's and ewe's milk. The increase varies from relatively slight with zinc to considerable with cobalt, manganese, and molybdenum, to a very marked extent with

TABLE 14-3
Trace mineral constituents of cow's milk.

Mineral	Parts per million
Arsenic	0.05
Boron	0.2
Cobalt	0.001
Copper	0.13
Fluorine	0.15
Iodine	0.04
Iron	0.45
Manganese	0.03
Molybdenum	0.05
Zinc	3.7

Source: Archibald, 1958. *Dairy Sci. Abst.* 20:711;
Smith. 1959. *Physiology of Lactation,* 5th ed. Ames,
Iowa: Iowa St. Univ. Press.

iodine. The content of iron and copper in milk cannot be increased, even if the content of these elements in the diet is markedly increased. Diets low in copper, however, reduce the amount of element normally present in the milk (1). Colostrum contains several times the amount of trace elements found in normal milk.

The method by which the trace mineral content of milk is controlled is not known. To a large extent, it appears dependent upon the concentration of minerals in the blood reaching the mammary gland. It has been shown that the mammary gland has the ability to concentrate iodine similar to the iodine concentration mechanism of the thyroid. It also appears that the transfer of iodine into milk is in part an active process and that iodine does not readily diffuse across the mammary gland membranes during passive transfer (20).

14-3 VITAMIN SECRETION

The mammary gland cannot synthesize vitamins; consequently, it is dependent upon the blood supply for the vitamins it secretes into the milk. The vitamins may be synthesized by bacteria in the rumen, converted from provitamin and precursors in the liver, small intestine, and the skin, or come directly from the feed sources. The vitamin content of milk is shown in Table 14-4. The vitamins are usually classified as fat- and water-soluble vitamins. The fat-soluble vitamins are A, D, E and K. Vitamins

A and E are not synthesized by rumen bacteria or the body, consequently animals are dependent upon the feed for these vitamins.

TABLE 14-4
Vitamin content of whole milk of four species of mammals.

	Cow	Goat	Pig	Human
	(In International Units per liter)			
Vitamin A	1511	2074	1036	1898
Vitamin D	13.7-33.0	23.7	79	22
	(In milligrams per liter)			
Thiamine	.45	.40	.70	.16
Riboflavin	1.81	1.84	2.21	.36
Nicotinic acid	.97	1.87	8.35	1.47
Pantothenic acid	3.57	3.44	5.28	1.84
Vitamin B_6	.66	.07	0.40	.10
Biotin	.032	.039	.014	.008
Folic acid	.0029	.0024	.0039	.002
Vitamin B_{12}	.0044	.0006	.0016	.0003
Choline	125	150	206	90
Ascorbic acid	21.8	15	140	43
Vitamin E	1.01	—	—	6.64
Inositol	110	210	—	330

Source: Hartman and Dryden. 1965. *Vitamins in Milk and Milk Products.* American Dairy Science Assoc., Champaign, Ill.

Fat-soluble Vitamins

Vitamin A   Vitamin A and its precursors, the carotenoids, are usually grouped together as the vitamin A content, or activity, of milk. Plants contain primarily carotenoids and animal tissues contain primarily vitamin A. The carotenoids, especially β-carotene, can be converted into vitamin A by the wall of the small intestine. The efficiency of this conversion is relatively small in dairy cattle. A difference in efficiency exists among the dairy breeds. Jerseys and Guernseys convert a smaller percentage of carotene into vitamin A. For instance, Guernsey milk fat contains approximately three times as much carotene as Holstein milk fat. This accounts for the very yellow color of the Guernsey and Jersey milk. The Holstein breed converts more of the carotene into vitamin A and Holstein milk fat contains approximately 60% more true vitamin A than Guernsey milk fat. In addition to cow's milk, human milk and mare's milk contain both vitamin A and carotenoids, whereas goat's, ewe's, buffalo's and sow's milk contains only vitamin A. The carotenoids in the milk appear as part of the fat phase as well as part of a protein complex. In the fat phase they are present in the fat globule membrane (11, 21, 26, 27).

The carotene and vitamin A contents of the milk are greatly influenced by the dietary intake of carotenoids. The vitamin A activity of cow's milk during grazing is 1.5 to 15 times higher than it is during the winter months. On the average, market milk during winter has about one-half the vitamin A content of that during the summer months when cows are on pasture. The feeding of vitamin A and carotene can increase the vitamin A activity in milk fat by 3 to 5 times. The feeds that are particularly high in β-carotene are those containing thin green leaves. Silages usually provide more carotene than hays. Corn silage, on the other hand, is only a fair source of carotene because the corn plant is not ensiled until it is relatively mature. When high levels of vitamin A and carotene are fed, from 0.1–6% of them appear in the milk, indicating a relatively inefficient conversion. With low intakes, the efficiency of conversion is higher. The liver can store relatively large amounts of vitamin A, consequently a decrease in the carotene content of the feed will not show up immediately as a change in the vitamin A activity of the milk. Colostrum is a very rich source of vitamin A activity. It has 4 to 25 times the vitamin A activity of normal milk. Except for this high level of activity in colostrum, there is no change in vitamin A activity with stage of lactation (11, 21, 26, 27).

Vitamin D   Vitamin D in milk is present as vitamin D_2, which results from the irradiation of ergosterol in the feed, and vitamin D_3, a derivative of 7-dehydrocholesterol, which is produced by the direct action of ultraviolet rays of the sun on the animal. The amount of vitamin D in the milk is directly related to the ergosterol in the feed and the exposure of the animal to sunlight. During the summer months, the average vitamin D content of milk is 33 IU per liter and it decreases to an average value of 13.7 during the winter months. Vitamin D contents are higher in plants that are exposed to the sun during curing. Green plants, silages, and artificially-dried grasses are low in vitamin D content. The efficiency of converting activated sterols in the feed into vitamin D is relatively low in that only 0.5–2.4% of these appear in the milk. There is a relationship between the amount of vitamin D in the milk and the fat content of the milk. Milk from Jersey and Guernsey cows has a higher vitamin D content than that of Holsteins. Colostrum contains 3 to 10 times more vitamin D than normal milk (11, 21, 26).

Vitamins E and K   The form of vitamin E in cow's milk is α-tocopherol. The amount of α-tocopherol in the milk is related to that in the diet, the concentration being twice as high during the summer when cows are grazing on green plants than during the winter. Increasing the tocopherol content of the diet increases the vitamin E content of milk. Colostrum contains 2.5 to 7 times the vitamin E content of normal milk. The vitamin E may act as an antioxidant in milk fat; however, its exact function in milk has not been elicited.

Milk is a relatively poor source of vitamin K. Unlike the other fat-soluble vitamins, the concentration of vitamin K in the milk cannot be affected by its supply in the diet, because large quantities can be synthesized in the rumen (11, 21).

Water-soluble Vitamins

B Vitamins The B vitamins are synthesized by the microflora in the rumen. The bacteria are broken down in the intestinal tract and the ruminant animal can utilize the liberated B vitamins for its body functions. For this reason, the concentration of the B vitamins in the milk cannot be affected greatly by the diet of the ruminant animal. Ruminant milk contains only appreciable quantities of riboflavin, inositol, and pantothenic acid; however, a quart of milk will supply 33–50% of the thiamine, 85–140% of the riboflavin, 25–60% of the vitamin B_6, 33% of the pantothenic acid, at least 20% of the choline, and 20% of the biotin requirements of the average adult daily. The B vitamin concentration of the milk of the simple-stomached animal can be influenced by the B vitamin concentration in the diet. Unlike most B vitamins, the riboflavin content can be changed in the milk of the cow. Changing from a winter ration to fresh pasture feeding increases the riboflavin content by 20–50%. Jersey and Guernsey milk is much higher in riboflavin content than Ayrshire or Holstein milk. Colostrum also contains much higher contents of thiamine, riboflavin, vitamin B_6, choline, folic acid, and vitamin B_{12} than normal milk (11, 21, 26).

Vitamin C Vitamin C in milk is in two active forms: ascorbic acid, a stable reduced form, and dehydroascorbic acid, a reversibly oxidized form. The vitamin C content of milk is little affected by a cow's ration, her age, breed, stage of lactation or season of year except that colostrum is 10–60% higher in vitamin C than normal milk. Ruminant animals can synthesize the vitamin in the body, but humans cannot, and therefore the ascorbic acid content of human milk can be increased by increasing the levels in the diet. If the vitamin C content of the ruminant diet is increased, the excess vitamin C is quickly destroyed by the bacteria or excreted. Milk is not an important source of vitamin C for the human since a large part of that in fresh milk is destroyed before it reaches him (11, 21, 26).

14-4   SUMMARY

Lactose

The major component of most milks is lactose, which is a disaccharide made up of a glucose and a galactose molecule. The principal precursor of lactose is blood glucose. In the mammary gland, the glucose molecule is phosphorylated to form glucose 6-phosphate, which is then converted into glucose 1-phosphate. The glucose 1-phosphate is united with uridine triphosphate (UTP) to form uridine diphosphate glucose (UDP-glucose). The UDP-glucose is then converted to UDP-galactose. The UDP-galactose is united with free glucose to form lactose with the liberation of UDP. The last step in the synthesis of lactose is catalyzed by the enzyme lactose synthetase, which is composed of two protein molecules. These molecules, the A and B proteins, must be united in order to produce an active enzyme. The B protein of this enzyme is α-lactalbumin, a common component of milk. It appears that progesterone represses the formation of α-lactalbumin during pregnancy. After the fall of plasma progesterone at parturition, the α-lactalbumin concentration can build up to an extent to form lactose synthetase to allow the initiation of lactose synthesis. This may be the rate-limiting enzyme in the initiation of lactation process in some animals.

Galactosaemia

Galactosaemia is a human disease in which the galactose molecule cannot be utilized, because of a deficiency of the enzyme galactose 1-phosphate uridyltransferase. This enzyme converts galactose 1-phosphate and UDP-glucose into glucose 1-phosphate and UDP-galactose. If galactose feeding is continued to humans with this deficiency, it accumulates in their bodies, and they develop such symptoms as increased size of liver and spleen, ascites, cataracts, and feeble-mindedness. Galactosaemic individuals must consume a diet devoid of galactose.

Minerals

The major mineral constituents of milk are calcium, phosphorus, potassium, chlorine, sodium, and magnesium. Potassium, chlorine, and sodium are wholly in soluble form; some of the other three major ions are in soluble form and some are linked with the colloidal portion of casein, phosphates, and citrates. The buffering capacity of the milk is due to the citrates, phosphates, and bicarbonates along with the proteins in the milk. The action of these substances keeps the pH of milk close to 6.6. The calcium in milk comes from the diet as well as the skeleton. The blood serum calcium is in equilibrium with that of the skeleton. For this reason, it is difficult to increase the calcium content of milk by increasing the calcium content of the feed. The inorganic phosphate of the blood serum is the precursor of the phosphates in milk.

There is considerable evidence to indicate that dairy animals free from infections have constant amounts of lactose, potassium, sodium, and chlorine in their milk. The constant amount is characteristic of each individual animal. There is a close inverse relationship between the lactose content of milk and the molar sum of the sodium and potassium contents. In addition, there is a close inverse relationship between the lactose and potassium contents of the milk. It appears that the water moves into the milk to maintain osmotic equilibrium with that of blood; consequently, the secretion of lactose, potassium, sodium, and chlorine determines the volume of milk produced. The mechanisms that control the amount of these ions and the lactose that go into the milk have not been described.

Milk also contains trace amounts of other minerals. On a quantitive basis, however, these are relatively small amounts, with the exception of zinc. Except for copper and iron, feeding high amounts of trace minerals increases the amount in cow's and ewe's milk. Only slight increases occur with zinc, but marked increases can occur in the iodine content of milk with feeding large amounts of iodine.

Vitamins

Vitamins cannot be synthesized by the mammary gland; therefore, it is dependent upon the blood supply for the vitamins secreted into the milk. Generally, the vitamin content of milk can be increased by increasing the vitamin content of the blood supplying the mammary gland. The ruminant animal is dependent upon the feed supply and exposure to sunlight for its fat-soluble vitamins, A, D, and E. Vitamin A is supplied by feeds in the form of β-carotene, which is converted to Vitamin A by the intestinal wall. Increasing the carotene or vitamin A content in the diet, as occurs during pasture grazing, increases the vitamin A activity of the milk by as much as 15 times. Colostrum is a very rich source of vitamin A. The vitamin D in cow's milk comes from the activation of ergosterol in the feed or from the animal's exposure to sunlight, which activates 7-dehydrocholesterol in the skin of the animal. Increasing either the feed sources of ergosterol or the exposure to sunlight increases the vitamin D of milk. Milk produced in the summer has a much higher vitamin D content than winter milk. Colostrum has 3 to 10 times more vitamin D than normal milk. The vitamin E content of milk can also be increased by increasing the vitamin E content in the diet; however, the significance of the vitamin E content of milk has not been determined. Vitamin K is in low concentration in milk and cannot be affected by dietary supplies.

The B vitamins are synthesized by the microflora in the rumen, consequently changes in the B vitamin contents of the diet do not change the contents in milk, except for riboflavin. The riboflavin content of milk can be increased by switching cows from a winter feeding regime to pasture feeding. Colostrum is higher in most of the B vitamins. The ascorbic acid (vitamin C) content of cow's milk cannot be changed by dietary contents, because it is synthesized by the ruminant's body. Colostrum has somewhat higher amounts of vitamin C than normal milk. Humans cannot synthesize vitamin C, therefore, the content of this vitamin in human milk is influenced by the amount in the diet.

REFERENCES

1. Archibald, J. G. 1958. *Dairy Sci. Abstr.* 20:711.
2. Baldwin, R. L. 1966. *J. Dairy Sci.* 49:1533.
3. Barry, J. M. 1964. *Biol. Rev.* 39:194.
4. Bartley, J. C., S. Abraham, and I. L. Chaikoff. 1966. *J. Biol. Chem.* 241:1132.
5. Black, A. L., M. Kleiber, E. M. Butterworth, G. B. Brubacher, and J. J. Kaneko. 1957. *J. Biol. Chem.* 227:537.
6. Brew, K. 1969. *Nature* 223:671.
7. Carubelli, R., B. Taha, R. E. Trucco, and R. Caputto. 1964. *Biochim. Biophys. Acta* 83:224.
8. Ebner, K. E., and U. Brodbeck. 1968. *J. Dairy Sci.* 51:317.
9. Folley, S. J. 1961. *Dairy Sci. Abstr.* 23:511.
10. Hansen, R. G., H. G. Wood, G. J. Peeters, B. Jacobson, and J. Wilken. 1962. *J. Biol. Chem.* 237:1034.
11. Hartman, A. M., and L. P. Dryden. 1965. *Vitamins in Milk and Milk Products.* American Dairy Science Association, Champaign, Ill.
12. Heitzman, R. J. 1968. *J. Endocrinol.* 40:81.
13. Johansson, I., and O. Claesson. 1957. In J. Hammond, ed., *Progress in the Physiology of Farm Animals.* London: Butterworths Scientific Publ. Ch. 21.
14. Jones, E. A. 1967. *Biochem. J.* 103:420.
15. Kleiber, M., A. L. Black, M. A. Brown, C. F. Baxter, J. R. Luick, and F. H. Stadtman. 1955. *Biochim. Biophys. Acta* 17:252.

16. Komrower, G. M. 1967. *Proc. Royal. Soc. Med.* 60:1155.

17. Kuhn, N. J. 1968. *Biochem. J.* 106:743.

18. Larson, B. L. 1969. *J. Dairy Sci.* 52:737.

19. Leloir, L. F., and C. E. Cardini. 1961. In S. K. Kon and A. T. Cowie, eds., *Milk: The Mammary Gland and Its Secretion,* Vol. I. New York: Academic Press. Ch. 11.

20. Lengemann, F. W. 1965. *J. Dairy Sci.* 48:197.

21. Ling, E. R., S. K. Kon, and J. W. G. Porter. 1961. In S. K. Kon and A. T. Cowie, eds., *Milk: The Mammary Gland and Its Secretion,* Vol. II. New York: Academic Press. Ch. 17.

22. Linzell, J. L. 1967. *J. Physiol.* 190:347.

23. Parkash, S., and R. Jenness. 1967. *J. Dairy Sci.* 50:127.

24. Rook, J. A. F., J. E. Storry, and J. V. Wheelock. 1965. *J. Dairy Sci.* 48:745.

25. Rook, J. A. F., and J. V. Wheelock. 1967. *J. Dairy Res.* 34:273.

26. Smith, V. R. 1959. *Physiology of Lactation,* 5th ed. Ames, Iowa: Iowa St. Univ. Press.

27. Thompson, S. Y. 1968. *J. Dairy Res.* 35:149.

28. Turkington, R. W., and R. L. Hill. 1969. *Science* 163:1458.

29. Wood, H. G., R. Gillespie, S. Joffe, R. G. Hansen, and H. Hardenbrook. 1958. *J. Biol. Chem.* 233:1271.

30. Wood, H. G., S. Joffe, R. Gillespie, R. G. Hansen, and H. Hardenbrook. 1958. *J. Biol. Chem.* 233:1264.

31. Wood, H. G., G. J. Peeters, R. Verbeke, M. Lauryssens, and B. Jacobson. 1965. *Biochem. J.* 96:607.

32. Wood, H. G., P. Schambye, and G. J. Peeters. 1957. *J. Biol. Chem.* 226:1023.

UDDER ABNORMALITIES

15-1 MASTITIS

Mastitis is the most costly disease of dairy cows. Annual losses due to this disease have been estimated to range from $225,000,000 to $1,000,000,000. This is the cost of losses in milk production due to sub-clinical and clinical mastitis, and of the treatment, culling, and replacement of infected cows.

A blind quarter resulting from the destruction of secretory tissue due to mastitis is shown in Figure 15-1. Figure 15-2 contrasts normal secretory tissue to that undergoing atrophy as a result of mastitis. Survey figures indicate that at least 50% of the cows in the United States are infected with pathogenic organisms in an average of two quarters per cow. Similar survey figures published 30 to 40 years ago are little different from those of today, indicating that relatively little progress has been made in the control of the disease (3, 57).

The greatest loss due to mastitis is the loss of milk production. Approximately 20% of the lactation yield is lost after moderate to severe cases of clinical mastitis (40). Milk production of quarters of the same cows

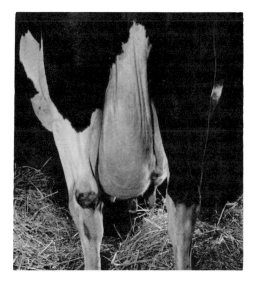

FIGURE 15-1
A blind quarter resulting from a severe
clinical case of mastitis.

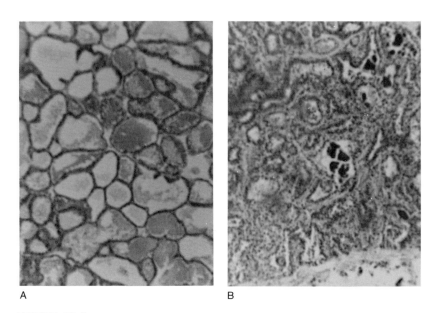

A   B

FIGURE 15-2
Contrast between normal secretory tissue, A, and secretory tissue undergoing
severe atrophy, B, as a result of clinical mastitis.

showing differences in the California Mastitis Test (CMT) reactions were compared (12). The CMT is a measure of the leucocyte numbers in milk, which is in turn a measure of the inflammation of the mammary gland; the higher the test reaction, the more severe the inflammation. Test reactions of trace, 1, 2, and 3 were associated with average decreases in milk production of 9.0%, 19.5%, 31.8%, and 43.4%, respectively, in comparison to the opposite quarters that were negative to the CMT reaction. In one study (46), the lactation yields of milk, solids-not-fat, and fat of infected cows were depressed by 10%, 11%, and 12%, respectively, in comparison to noninfected cows. In another study (66), quarters infected throughout the dry period or becoming infected in the dry period produced 35% less milk after calving than the noninfected quarters of the same udder. Milk from quarters showing high CMT reactions also have decreased percentages of total solids, fat, solids-not-fat, and lactose (1, 53).

Definitions

Mastitis is the reaction of the mammary gland to injury (3). This response is called inflammation and it is an attempt by the udder to destroy or neutralize the irritant and prepare the way for repair so that the mammary gland can return to normal function. Many definitions have been used to define different classes of mastitis. A distinction must be made between the evidence of the inflammation, clinical mastitis, and the cause of the mastitis, which in most cases is bacteria. The presence of the bacteria within the mammary gland is referred to as an infection. The noninfectious type of mastitis is that observed after an injury or trauma to the mammary gland. Newbould and Neave (42), however, never found inflammation of a mammary gland in the absence of infection in their study.

Infectious mastitis can be divided into several categories. Subclinical mastitis usually refers to the presence of infectious organisms within the mammary gand, but no visible abnormalities are present. Clinical mastitis refers to the presence of abnormal milk or an abnormal mammary gland. Clinical mastitis is usually described as subacute, acute, and septic. Subacute or mild clinical mastitis is one in which the milk shows abnormal consistency or color. Acute or severe clinical is one in which the mammary gland shows the symptoms of inflammation, such as heat, pain, redness, and swelling. Septic mastitis is characterized by generalized symptoms, such as fever, stiffness, evidence of pain and lack of appetite. Chronic mastitis refers to the condition in which the cow's milk periodically shows abnormalities and then returns to normal.

The Infection Process

Mastitis Pathogens   At least 20 different kinds of organisms are capable of causing infection of the mammary gland; however, 99% of mastitis is caused by *Streptococcus agalactiae (Strep. ag.), Streptococcus dysgalactiae, Streptococcus uberis* and *Staphylococcus aureus (S. aureus)* and bacillary organisms, which include coliform and Pseudomonas organisms (23). Well over 90% of the mammary gland infections are caused by streptococci and staphylococci organisms (36, 57). Survey figures on the percentage of infected cows are shown in Table 15-1. It is commonly stated that approximately 50% of the cows are infected in an average of two quarters per cow (3); however, the data in Table 15-1 indicate that approximately 30–40% of the quarters are infected. The percentages of quarters and cows infected with *Strep. ag.* on initial surveys in the New York State Mastitis Control Program are considerably higher than those infected on all surveys. Many of the dairymen entering the New York program and having initial surveys have probably experienced the problem of their cows having abnormal milk. A relationship appears to exist between the amount of abnormal milk and the incidence of *Strep. ag.* infection (64).

Streptococcus agalactiae is considered to be an obligate parasite of the mammary gland (23); however, it has recently been shown that it is a fairly common organism in the genito-urinary tract and pharynx of humans, especially women (57). For the most part, the elimination of *Strep. ag.* from the mammary glands prevents it from being a major threat to the dairy cows in the herd. Most of the other organisms involved in mastitis are found in the environment; however, the main reservoir of these organisms in a dairy herd is infected udders (39).

Relationship between Infection and Clinical Mastitis   There is considerable confusion about the relationship between infection and clinical mastitis. A simple diagram (Figure 15-3) helps to explain the situation. The milk from a noninfected mammary gland is sterile; however, the exterior of the teat is routinely exposed to pathogens. An infection occurs if the pathogens are present, if the mammary gland is susceptible to the invasion of the bacteria through the streak canal, and if the organisms are allowed to multiply within the mammary gland. The streak canal is the major path of entry for bacteria into the mammary gland. An infection is diagnosed when pathogenic bacteria can be cultured from fresh milk of a quarter and when the milk has a raised leucocyte count.

The method by which bacteria penetrate the teat canal is not known. It may occur as a single step, in stages, or by continuous growth of the

TABLE 15-1
Percentage of quarters and cows infected with mastitis pathogens.

Pathogen	Percentage of quarters infected		Percentage of cows infected		
	N.Y. Research Project (57)[a]	England (34)[a]	N.Y. State Mastitis Control Program- Initial Surveys	Conn. (54)[a]	N.Y. Farm Survey (64)[a]
Strep. agalactiae	12.4	} 11.0	27.0	23.0	18.7
Strep. dysgalactiae	1.1		} 18.0	} 8.0	} 25.8
Strep. uberis	6.9				
Staph. aureus	16.7	17.0	13.0	18.0	22.9
Other	2.9	0.7	1.0	1.0	3.5

[a] Reference number.

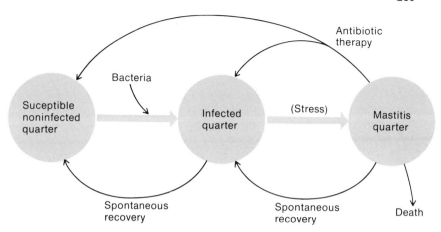

FIGURE 15–3
Possible sequence of events in the development of infection and mastitis.
(From Dodd et al. 1964. *J. Dairy Sci.* 47:1109.)

organisms through the canal (36). Evidence for the direct passage of organisms through the canal during milking was provided by McEwen and Samuel (18); however, the experiment was conducted under somewhat abnormal conditions.

After the gland becomes infected, a number of possible events may occur at any time, some within a few hours, but some may occur up to several years after the infection is established. Some infections disappear by spontaneous recovery and others are eliminated by therapy. The infected mammary gland can become mastitic as shown by gross changes in the composition of milk or the typical signs of inflammation of the mammary gland. From 2–16% of the cows with infected quarters show signs of clinical mastitis at any one time depending upon the method of detection. Abnormal milk or inflammation of the gland is usually diagnosed by the milker and, in most cases, the gland is treated with antibiotics. This usually causes the inflammation to subside and the mammary gland returns to an infected state. If the antibiotic therapy is completely effective, the infection as well as the clinical signs are eliminated. Some glands showing abnormal milk return to the infected state without therapy. A small percentage of the clinical quarters become so acute as to cause systemic infections and cause septic mastitis. In severe cases the cow may die (7).

Factors Influencing the Establishment of Infection   The level of infection in a dairy herd remains relatively constant. Thus the proportion of cows that become infected during a period of time must equal the proportion of cows whose udders go from an infected to a noninfected state. First-calf heifers at calving are relatively free from mastitis infections. In one study (30), however, it was found that of 950 heifers calving in 16 herds, 11.8% of the heifers and 4.1% of the quarters were infected on the day of calving. *Streptococcus uberis, Streptococcus dysgalactiae, Staphylococcus aureus* were the most common organisms found in these heifers. Only 2 of the 16 herds in this study had heifers that were entirely free from infections at calving.

Invasion of the udder by bacteria is by way of the streak canal, but organisms are transferred by the blood in diseases in which septicemia occurs (54). The soft keratin lining of the streak canal plays a role in preventing infections. Murphy (24) subjected 2 teats of each of 10 young cows that were resistant to *Streptococcus agalactiae* infection to various stresses. Removing the keratin from the streak canal with soft plastic cannulae for 3 milkings prior to exposing the teats to *Strep. ag.* organisms completely broke the resistance of the glands to infection. After the infection was removed by antibiotic therapy and sufficient time elapsed for the keratin to regrow, the mammary gland again became resistant to the organisms. It has not yet been possible to identify the chemical components of the keratin material that are responsible for the resistance. The length of the streak canal is not related to the infectability of the glands with *Strep. ag.* (27).

Following invasion of the gland by bacteria, the establishment of an infection depends upon the ability of the organisms to survive and multiply within the udder. Development of clinical mastitis depends upon the ability of the organism to produce substances that are toxic to the glandular tissue (54). Murphy (22) proposed a three-phase concept of udder infection. It includes: invasion, which is the passage of pathogens into the interior of the udder; infection, which is the establishment of the pathogens in the udder; and inflammation, which is the reaction of the tissue to injury by the microorganisms or their products.

As few as 35 *Streptococcus agalactiae* organisms can produce an infection when introduced into the teat cavity. Infections can occur when as few as three *Staphylococcus aureus* organisms and always when 40 or more of these organisms are introduced into the teat cistern. The incidence of infection increases when a large number of streptococci and staphylococci are present on the teats of cows immediately before milking or after the last milking before drying up. In addition, a large proportion of glands in which teat canals had been inoculated with five million *Strep ag.* organisms became infected (16, 26, 37, 39). Prasad and Newbould (55) inoculated teat canals with *S. aureus* organisms and determined the presence of infections thereafter. When the inoculations were made at a depth of 4 mm followed by teat dipping at each subsequent milking, 10 of 16 inoculations resulted in intramammary infections. When the same procedure was followed, but the depth of inoculation was limited to 3 mm, only 3 of 16 inoculations resulted in infection. It would appear that the incidence of infection is in part dependent upon the amount of penetration by the organisms during milking.

The number of leucocytes in the milk is important in whether an infection becomes established in the mammary gland. It is common for an animal to overcome a natural infection unaided by antibiotic therapy (20). Newbould and Neave (41) injected 10 colony-forming units of *S. aureus* into the teat cisterns of cows. They found that there was an inverse relationship between the leucocyte numbers in the milk and the ability to culture staphylococci from the quarter. Schalm et al. (58) introduced streptococci into mammary glands and found that the establishment of an infection was dependent upon the number of organisms introduced and the increase in leucocytes in the milk. A delay of 12-24 hours in the increase in leucocyte numbers in response to the organisms generally permitted survival of the organisms and establishment of an infection. Quarters having existing leucocyte numbers ranging between 200,000 and 500,000 cells per milliliter of fore milk were protected against 100 to 350 streptococcal organisms. It is not possible to readily superimpose an unrelated pathogen upon an existing bacterial infection in lactating mammary glands.

Time of New Infection　Animals are most susceptible to infection during the first month of lactation and during the first few weeks of the dry period. In one study (50), it was found that 11% of the cows became infected for the first time during the first month of lactation and the percentage fell gradually to 1.8% in the 9th month of lactation. In the first month of lactation, 30% of the infected cows showed clinical mastitis, whereas the values for the other months were usually between 10% and 15%. In the average infected herd, approximately 1 to 2 new infections occur per cow per lactation (7, 10).

A large number of new infections occur during the dry period, with most of these occurring in the first 3 weeks of the dry period. Approximately 50% of these infections persist until calving and a like percentage of these produce clinical symptoms within the first 2 weeks after calving. The new infection rate of one herd is shown in Table 15-2 and it will be noted that the infection rate during the early dry period is much higher than that found during lactation (32).

TABLE 15-2
Number of new persisting infections during lactation and the dry period in an 89-cow herd.

	Average period length (weeks)	New persisting infections	Infection rate per week
Lactation period	41	46	1.12
Dry period	14	23	1.64
Early	3	21	7.00
Remaining	11	2	0.18
Period after calving	2	5	2.50

Source: Neave et al. 1950. *J. Dairy Res.* 17:37.

Factors Contributing to Infection A number of conditions have been shown to influence the incidence of udder infection in the early dry period. Among these are high milk yields at drying off, hand stripping during lactation, lower resistance of the cows to infections, and the presence of mastitis organisms on the teats. The incidence of new infections in the early dry period is higher in cows with high daily milk yields at drying-off than in those with lower milk yields. This rise in infection rate is primarily due to an increase in *Streptococcus agalactiae* infections. New dry-period infections are also more numerous in cows that are hand-stripped during lactation than in cows that are machine-stripped. Cows with previous infections have about twice as many new infections during the dry period as cows that have not been infected before (43, 47, 48). The direct effect of the cessation of milking on the new infection rate was shown by Neave et al. (38) in which teats of cows were deliberately contaminated twice daily by dipping them in a suspension of streptococcal and staphylococcal organisms. Half of the quarters were milked and the other half were not milked. Only the unmilked quarters became infected.

Another factor in early dry period infection is the presence of organisms on the teats at that time. *Staphylococcus aureus* organisms can be recovered frequently from the teat skin of animals after the last milking; however, they are seldom recovered after an animal has been dry for 28 days unless an intramammary infection is present (37).

The higher incidence of new infections during early dry period may be related to the high internal udder pressure developed in the udder after drying off. The internal pressure may be sufficient to open the streak canal and allow milk to escape. The milk leaking through the streak canal allows the bacteria easier access to the teat cistern through growth or capillary movement. The pathogens are then less affected by the inhibitory properties of the streak canal epithelium (38, 48).

A number of factors have been shown to be related to the overall infection rate. One of the most common observations is that older cows have a higher incidence of infection and clinical mastitis than younger cows. The increase in infection rate with age is a result of reinfections and persisting infections; however, the rate of first infections does not increase with advancing age. The proportion of infections that give rise to clinical mastitis is about the same for young cows as for old cows. There is a decline in the rate of new infections, reinfections, and total new infections and clinical mastitis in infected quarters with advancing lactation. There are no seasonal trends in the incidence of udder infection or mastitis (50).

It is also a common observation that fast-milking cows have a higher incidence of infection and clinical mastitis than slow-milking cows. This has been shown experimentally by Dodd and Neave (6) who found a high correlation between the rate of milk flow and the incidence of clinical and subclinical mastitis. Of cows with a maximum rate of flow of less than 3 lb/min, only 10% of the cows became infected, whereas 66.7% of the cows with a maximum rate of flow over 6.1 lb/min became infected. A possible explanation for the relationship between fast milking and susceptibility to infection is that bacteria can gain entrance more readily to udders through larger or slacker streak canals. The conformation of the teat, especially the teat end, also influences the incidence of infection. New infections with *Streptococcus agalactiae* are more frequent in teats in which the teat apex is abnormal (35).

Part of the differences in the inheritance of susceptibility to infection and mastitis is due to the differences in milking rate. Several studies have been conducted to measure the heritability of infection rate, resistance to mastitis, and incidence of clinical mastitis (65). Great variations exist in the heritability estimates due to different types of measurements used. From a practical standpoint relatively little progress can be expected in breeding for increased resistance to infection and mastitis. Since fast-milking cows are desired in modern dairy herds, selecting for fast milking will select cows that have a higher susceptibility to mastitis. Other inherited factors that increase the resistance to infection and mastitis have not been defined; therefore, it is impossible to use a single measure to select for resistance.

The number of chaps on the teat skin and other blemishes on the teat influence the infection rate. At any one time 70% of the teat blemishes are infected or contaminated with *Staphylococcus aureus*. This then provides a source of bacteria close to the entrance to the teat (36).

Several milking machine factors and milking techniques have been found to be associated with the level of udder infection. Inadequate vacuum reserve and vacuum fluctuations on the end of the teat appear to increase the incidence of udder infections. Cows milked with bucket machines having a low reserve air capacity and whose teats were exposed to *S. aureus* had a much higher incidence of new infections than the cows milked with a high reserve machine and whose teats were also exposed. The new infection rate of udders exposed to *S. aureus* was also found to be considerably higher when cows were milked with machines with irregular vacuum fluctuations in comparison to quarters milked with a more stable vacuum (45).

Overmilking has often been incriminated as a factor that increases the severity of mastitis. Conflicting evidence for this appears in the literature. In one trial (5), an association was demonstrated between overmilking and the incidence of udder infection and clinical mastitis. In another study, Peterson (51) overmilked quarters of cows for various periods of time and then examined the teats macroscopically and microscopically. Overmilking caused hyperemia, hemorrhage, and edema of the epithelial membrane lining the teat cistern. Inflammatory changes in the epithelium and subepithelial tissue of the streak canal were also observed. However, the infection rate of the quarters of these cows was not measured. Other factors, such as vacuum level, pulsation rate, pulsation ratio, teat cup liners, and management factors may influence the infection rate; but it is impossible to establish a definite relationship between any of the factors and the incidence of infection in controlled experiments (20, 54, 61, 62, 63).

Factors Affecting Clinical Mastitis

An increase in the incidence of clinical mastitis by changes in management, milking or milking machine factors, or physiological changes of the cow can be due either to an increase in the rate of infection or to an increase in the number of infected quarters that become clinical. Any factor that increases the incidence of infections increases the incidence of clinical mastitis, since it has been shown that about one-third of the infections show clinical mastitis during a lactation (14).

High vacuum level is commonly thought to be a major factor that increases the incidence of clinical mastitis. In controlled trials, vacuum levels from 10 to 24 inches Hg have been used and in most cases no relationship has been found between the level of clinical mastitis and the vacuum level (20, 63). The milking machine in these studies was usually removed when the cow was milked out. Considerably more mastitis might result if a high vacuum milking machine was used and accompanied by extensive overmilking.

Increasing the pulsation rate of the milking machine or changing the pulsation ratio has not been shown to affect the incidence of clinical mastitis. A minimum number of pulsations per minute is required to prevent congestion and irritation to the teat end. Cows milked with no pulsations have a much higher infection rate than cows milked with a normal operating machine. Providing air admission holes in the claw has been shown to reduce the incidence of clinical mastitis; however, the research work on this is not very clear-cut (20, 63).

Recent attention has been directed toward the type of milking machine liner. In one trial (9), it was found that cows milked with a moulded liner had a higher incidence of mastitis than cows milked with the extruded liner, however, the new infection rate was similar in both groups of cows. In a further trial by the same authors (28), it was found that there was a slightly higher incidence of infected quarters and clinical mastitis in quarters milked with the extruded liners in comparison to the moulded liners. Other studies have not been able to establish a relationship between the type of liner, the type of mouthpiece on the liner, and the incidence of infection or clinical mastitis. No difference in the incidence of mastitis has been shown between using a floor-type and a suspended-type milking machine or the addition of weights to the teat cup assembly of a floor model milking machine (61, 63).

Factors that have been shown to be related to the incidence of clinical mastitis either through increasing the new infection rate or increasing the incidence of clinical mastitis in infected quarters are incomplete milking, overmilking, and inadequate air reserve capacity. Nyhan (45) found that the cases of clinical mastitis were considerably higher in cows milked with machines having a low air reserve capacity than in cows milked with machines having a high air reserve capacity.

Leaving 2 lb of milk in the udder in addition to the residual milk was shown to increase the severity of clinical manifestations of *Streptococcus agalactiae* infections, but had no effect on quarters shedding staphylococcal organisms (60). Leaving 2 or 4 lb of milk in udders infected with *Streptococcus* organisms other than *agalactiae* and with *Staphylococcus aureus* did not increase the incidence of udder infection or severity of clinical mastitis (62). Eliminating machine stripping has no significant effect on the incidence of infection or incidence of clinical mastitis (13).

Pathology of Mastitis

After the organisms become established in the mammary gland, inflammation may occur. Inflammation is the reaction of the tissue to injury by the organisms or their products. The purpose of the inflammation is to destroy the irritant and prepare the way for repair. Injury of any kind including that caused by the bacteria or their products leads to the death of tissue cells, which results in a release of chemicals from the disintegrating cells. These disintegrating cells attract polymorphonuclear (PMN) leucocytes, which are one of five distinct types of leucocytes. The drawing of the PMN leucocytes from the bloodstream into an area of injury is called "chemotaxis." The leucocyte passes from the blood into the tissue by its amoeboid movement (22, 59).

The PMN leucocytes play a significant role in inflammation in that they engulf bacteria and tissue debris by phagocytosis. Enzymes in the leucocyte digest and destroy the engulfed bacteria. The leucocyte then becomes degranulated, which causes release of chemical substances that increase the permeability of the capillary walls. This in turn allows the escape of fluid and proteins of the blood into the tissues. The PMN leucocytes are responsible for the intense swelling of the gland characteristic of acute mastitis. The leucocytes depress the multiplication of bacteria to sufficiently limit the irritant, and thus prevent complete dysfunction of the gland. During the process a large number of the leucocytes are exudated into the milk. If the injury is extensive, considerable time, such as several weeks to several months, may occur before complete healing results. The leucocyte exudation into the milk may continue for long periods of time after the cause of the inflammation has been removed (59).

Little and Plastridge (17) used the terms interstitial mastitis, exudative mastitis, suppurative mastitis, gangrenous mastitis, and fibrosis to designate tissue changes that occur during and following inflammation. Interstitial mastitis refers to the focal and diffuse cellular infiltration of the interstitial tissue. The cells are primarily reticulo-endothelial cells and lymphocytes. As the severity of the inflation increases, some exudate in the alveoli may be found. The secretory tissue may also show some degenerate changes, such as atrophy of the alveoli (Figure 15-2).

Exudative mastitis is characterized by the accumulation of exudate in the alveoli and ducts, accompanied by degenerative and necrotic changes in the parenchyma. Suppurative mastitis may develop from the exudative type. The affected area appears enlarged and nodular. Within the area, destruction of tissue takes place and encapsulated cavities filled with purulent exudate develop. Necrosis of the tissue and proliferation of the connective tissue take place in order to encapsulate the area. Gangrenous mastitis develops after the entrance of anaerobes, such as *Clostiridium welchii*. The infected gland becomes dark red, bluish, or greenish in color and is cold. The tissue appears dark, soft, and hemorrhagic. Usually the quarter or the entire udder is lost. Fibrosis is a generalized condition that develops during or after the first three types of mastitis. The affected area becomes firm and shows a marked increase in connective tissue.

Within the mammary gland there is a constant battle going on between the infection and the resistant capacities of the gland. When clinical signs of inflammation are apparent, the infecting bacteria are causing injury to the udder and they have overcome the udder's ability to withstand injury. Even if no clinical signs are present, the infections may be causing some damage to the udder (23).

The different types of organisms also show different pathological conditions. For instance, *Streptococcus agalactiae* mastitis is usually found in nonclinical or mild clinical forms but rarely becomes severe clinical, whereas the bacillary mastitis is very often in the severe clinical category. Mastitis due to *Streptococcus dysgalactiae* may be mild or severe and is usually of short duration (23, 54).

Symptoms and Diagnosis

Symptoms   After the mammary gland becomes infected, changes occur in the composition of milk as well as in the gland due to inflammation. These changes are shown in Figure 15-4. The first reaction to an infection is a rise in leucocytes in the infected area and these spill over into the milk. When an abnormality occurs in the mammary gland, the composition of milk tends toward the composition of blood. Blood is higher in chlorine content and has a higher pH, whereas its glucose, casein, and fat contents

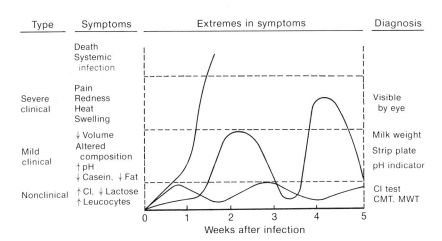

FIGURE 15–4
Symptoms and clinical diagnosis of mastitis. (From Murphy. 1959. Lecture, March 10. Cornell University.)

are considerably lower than those of milk. An increase in the leucocyte count is followed by a rise in the chlorine content and a decrease in the lactose content of milk. These cannot be routinely detected by the dairyman and are classified as nonclinical conditions. The rise in chlorine content is followed by a decrease in the casein and fat contents of milk. Milk from infected glands has a lower concentration of potassium and increased percentages of sodium and noncasein proteins in comparison to normal milk. The pH increases and this is followed by an altered fluid state, such as flakes or clots. If the inflammation is severe enough, a visible drop in milk production occurs. These are referred to as mild clinical symptoms. In severe clinical cases, swelling of the gland is accompanied by increased heat, redness and pain. If the infection causes the entire animal to become affected, systemic or septic mastitis results. The animal has an increased body temperature and usually goes off feed, which may be followed by death in extreme cases. Milk from cows with mastitis has higher histamine and glycogen contents than normal milk. The increased glycogen content is due to the increase in leucocytes (4, 25, 71).

During inflammation, blood vessels in the infected parts become dilated and carry more blood. The blood capillaries become more porous and the rate of blood flow slows down. This allows the blood fluids to pass more easily into the inflamed area. These fluids contain the blood clotting factors and cause coagulation of blood plasma and milk within the alveoli and milk ducts within a few hours after release from capillaries. Casein in the milk is precipitated in some instances, but the coagulation of the blood fluids accounts for most of the flakes and clots in the milk. Rupture of the blood vessels causes release of whole blood into the tissue or milk, which accounts for the presence of blood in the milk (3).

Diagnosis   The diagnosis of mastitis is concerned with the detection of either infection or inflammation, or a combination of the two. The identification of the infectious organisms requires bacteriological cultures of the milk. Fresh, aseptically obtained milk is usually streaked on the surface of a blood agar plate and incubated for a period of time and examined for the presence of various organisms. An infection is usually defined as the presence of the pathogenic bacteria in the milk accompanied by signs of inflammation, such as an increased leucocyte count. Aseptically drawn milk can contain bacteria located in the streak canal, thus the culture does not differentiate between gland and streak canal infections (54).

Barn and laboratory tests are available to measure the degree of inflammation (Figure 15-4). Dairymen commonly use a strip cup or strip plate to detect flakes or clots in the milk. Indicators of pH, such as bromthymol blue, can be used to detect altered pH. Most of the measures of inflammation are related to measuring the leucocyte count of the milk. Milk from normal quarters usually contains less than 500,000 leucocytes per milliliter of milk. Counts higher than 500,000 usually indicate that the quarter is infected. Exceptions are milk from cows that have recently calved and from cows in the terminal phases of lactation. Two common screening tests used to estimate the extent of inflammation are the California Mastitis Test (CMT) and the Whiteside Test. These measure the degree of precipitation or gel formation occurring when the reagents are placed with milk. The degree of precipitation is related to the somatic cell count of the milk. The somatic cell count includes both leucocytes and degenerated tissue cells. Many modifications of these tests have been developed. One of these, the Wisconsin Mastitis Test, quantitatively assesses the degree of gel formation. Physical examination of the udder of milked-out cows can be used to detect the amount of fibrosis within the mammary gland (3, 40, 54, 70).

Laboratory methods of determining leucocyte count include the laborious microscopic examination of stained milk films and the electronic counting of somatic cells in milk. Other laboratory tests are the catalase test and the chlorine test. The catalase test is based on the fact that there is a general relationship between the number of leucocytes and the catalase content of milk (3, 56).

Considerable care must be used in interpreting the indirect tests of inflammation, especially the screening tests. Most of these measure somatic cells, which include leucocytes and somatic cells. Stage of lactation and lactation age influence the somatic cell numbers in milk. As the volume of milk decreases with advancing lactation, cell numbers become concentrated in smaller volumes of fluid. The leucocyte count of milk for a few days before to 2 weeks after calving of uninfected cows is usually high. The leucocyte numbers in milk are lowest just prior to milking, rise sharply in the strippings, remain high during the next 4 hours, and then decrease progressively to a minimum value near the end of the intermilking period (54, 59, 69).

Older cows have a higher leucocyte count than younger cows due to the higher level of mastitis infection in older cows. The average cell count during the first 7 lactations was found to increase progressively from 0.3 to 1.08 million per milliliter of milk and the increase was due mainly to an increase in the number of PMN leucocytes. The increase in the average total cell count with advancing lactation was due to an increase in all cell types (2).

Development of a Control Program

Over the years many types of control programs have been advocated. Attempts have been made to prevent infection by immunization, but it appears that in the near future it is unlikely to be effective even against single pathogens. In the distant future, however, it may be possible to produce useful vaccines to immunize cattle against mastitis (7, 44).

Currently there are no data on which a selective breeding program can be based. Even if there were, the program of breeding resistant cows would have to compete for priority with other selection criteria (7).

Considerable emphasis has been placed on management, especially milking management, in the control of mastitis. Factors such as vacuum fluctuations, inadequate vacuum reserve, and overmilking can influence the rate of infection and clinical mastitis in a dairy herd; however, management *per se* cannot solve the problem. Milking management cannot reduce the incidence of infections or clinical mastitis to such a low level that it can be a basis for an effective control program. It may be a major factor for the differences between herds; however, it has not been possible to define all of the specific factors of milking or milking machines that contribute to infection and mastitis. On the other hand, there are good management reasons why most of the practices in the recommended milking procedures should be carried out and they are probably of some value in controlling mastitis (19). Herds in which excellent milking procedures and machines in good operating condition are used still have mastitis problems. In a field trial (64), it was found that the level of *Streptococcus agalactiae* infection per herd decreased as the production level of the herd increased; however, the infection rate due to other streptococci and to *Staphylococcus aureus* remained about the same.

An effective control system must have the following characteristics: (1) it must be less costly to implement than the costs of disease itself; (2) it must be simple to carry out; (3) there must be good experimental evidence that the control works under a range of conditions; and (4) it must be obvious to the dairyman that clinical mastitis is much reduced (10). A control program based on treatment of clinical mastitis neither reduces the losses of milk yield and secretory tissue due to infection nor prevents the problem of clinical mastitis. An effective control program must *prevent* the problem, i.e., prevent infections. However, a control program is usually initiated in herds where a problem already exists, therefore it must also eliminate the existing infections. No program in existence today will completely prevent all infections, therefore the infections that do become established must also be eliminated.

Sanitation   The most practical way of reducing the new infection rate is to decrease the exposure of cows to pathogenic bacteria. The main reservoir of pathogenic bacteria is infected mammary glands. Mastitis organisms are carried from an infected mammary gland to a noninfected mammary gland primarily by the hands of the milker, udder wash cloths or towels, and teat cup liners. Under strict controlled laboratory conditions the spread of organisms by these routes can be prevented. The common practices usually followed in the dairy barn operation of washing udders with a cloth soaked in disinfectant solution, dipping teat cup liners in a disinfectant between cows, and milking the infected cow last reduce the spread of pathogens to some degree, but they are not adequate to constitute a control program. Large numbers of pathogens can be recovered from the teat skin immediately after washing udders in commonly used disinfectants, from udder cloths after immersion for several minutes in a disinfectant, and from teat cup liners after they have flushed with water or disinfectant (7).

Hygiene procedures can be implemented to reduce the new infection rate in a dairy herd. In one trial (8), two milking regimes were compared for one year. One milking regime consisted of pasteurizing the teat cup liners by flushing hot water (85° C) through them for 5 seconds between cows, washing the udders with individual sterile paper towels dipped in a chlorhexidine solution (100 ppm), and dipping the cow's teats in chlorhexidine (5,000 ppm) after each milking. This regime resulted in a 50% reduction in the new infection rate in comparison to cows milked with no hygiene procedures. The dipping of the teat ends after milking did not prevent the transfer of mastitis pathogens but killed the bacteria present on the teats after milking. In a second field trial (33), a comparison was made between the full hygiene program used in the first trial, a partial hygiene program (full hygiene without teat-cup pasteurization), and a control program with no hygiene procedures. Iosan at 100 ppm was used for udder washing and the teat ends were dipped with 5,000 ppm iodine, which was used for both hygiene regimes. In addition, the dairymen in herds on the full and partial hygiene programs used rubber gloves to provide a smooth surface for disinfection of hands between cows. The full hygiene program reduced the percentage of new infections by 64% and the partial hygiene program reduced the incidence by 53% (Table 15-3).

More effective teat-end dips have recently been found. A 4% chlorine solution is more effective than a 0.5% (5,000 ppm) iodine solution in killing *Staphylococcus aureus* organisms on cow's teats. The chlorine solution has no detrimental effect on the teats if the sodium hydroxide concentration is kept below 0.05%. In fact, it has a small but beneficial effect on teat chaps and sores. Even though the 4% chlorine solution persists from one milking to the next, it can destroy only light bacterial contamination from milk, manure, or mud acquired after milking, thus more effective compounds should be developed. If iodine is used as a

TABLE 15-3
Cases of clinical mastitis and infection rate of cows on three hygiene regimes.

Hygiene	No. of cows	Cases of clinical mastitis with pathogen found	New infection in lactation			
			Total	Staph.	Strep.	Other
Control (No hygiene)	764	410	764	404	332	28
Partial hygiene	732	231	346	187	123	36
Percent reduction from control[a]		41	53	52	61	—
Full hygiene	728	217	265	139	95	31
Percent reduction from control[a]		44	64	64	70	

Source: Neave et al. 1966. *Vet. Record* 78:521.
[a] Ajusted for numbers of cows.

teat-end dip, the phosphoric acid content must be low. Common iodine sanitizers contain about 16% phosphoric acid and high concentrations of iodine with this acid content damage teat ends. If iodine is used, compounds specifically formulated for teat-end dipping should be used. Pine oil has been used, however, it is incapable of killing *S. aureus* organisms. If mastitis organisms do not enter the udder during milking, sterilization of the teat ends after milking should be as effective in reducing the new infection rate as preventing the transfer of bacteria from an infected udder to an uninfected one. Clear-cut evidence that organisms penetrate the mammary gland during milking is lacking (29, 30, 36, 39).

Prevention of new infections during the dry period can also be brought about by teat-end disinfection after the last milking. Immersing teats in a 5% tincture of iodine solution for 20 seconds after drying off and 24 hours later has been found to be effective (49).

Therapy The second portion of a control program is that of eliminating the existing infections. This is a necessary part of a control program since a 50% reduction in the new infection rate reduces the incidence of cows infected by only 14% in 12 months. Antibiotic therapy during lactation can reduce the number of infected quarters as well as the length of time that the infection persists. Lactation therapy has limited value in eliminating infections, since only 30-40% of infections will be detected by the dairyman and would thus be treated. Information on the effectiveness of antibiotics in eliminating infections during lactation is limited since most of the success of a treatment is based upon the disappearance of the clinical signs of the disease. Cloxacillin, a semisynthetic penicillin, has been found to be quite effective. Infected quarters were infused three times at 48-hour intervals with either 0.2 or 0.6 g of sodium cloxacillin. Sixty-nine percent of the infections were eliminated. These preparations eliminated 52% of the *Staphylococcus aureus* infections, 100% of the *Streptococcus agalactiae* infections, 97% of the *Streptococcus dysgalactiae* infections, and 82% of the *Streptococcus uberis* infections. The cloxacillin in the aluminum stearate mineral oil base appeared to be more effective than in the mineral oil base. This compound is not yet sold commercially in the United States (10, 23, 29, 31).

The effectiveness of an antibiotic to eliminate infections is related to the length of time that it stays in the mammary gland. Most antibiotic preparations, however, are formulated to leave the mammary gland within 72–96 hours after the last infusion. Milk must be withheld from the market for this period of time to keep antibiotics out of the milk used for human consumption.

Elimination of existing infections during the dry period has several advantages. The routine treatment of all quarters of cows at drying-off would insure that all infections not detected during the lactation would be treated. Treating cows during the dry period prevents antibiotic contamination of the milk. Treatment during the dry period allows the regeneration of damaged udder tissue before calving and provides that a much higher proportion of cows are likely to be free from infection at the time of the highest milk yield. Therapy at drying-off has the additional advantage of reducing the number of new infections in dry cows, especially during the first 3 weeks after drying-off when the cows are highly susceptible to new infections (10, 57, 68).

Cloxacillin has also been found to be an effective antibiotic for dry-period therapy. Cows receiving 1 g of cloxacillin as the benzathine salt or 0.2 g of cloxacillin as the sodium salt in each quarter at drying-off followed by dipping of teats in 5% available chlorine solution had marked reductions in the number of infections at calving (Table 15-4). The 1-g dose was more effective than the 0.2-g dose in eliminating infections. The 1-g dose eliminated 86% of the infections in quarters at drying-off. The percentage of cows infected at calving in the control group was considerably higher than that of the same group at drying-off. This was due to the high percentage of quarters becoming infected during the dry period. This was greatly reduced with the 0.2-g dose and even more so with the 1-g dose. Five-tenths gram of benzathine cloxacillin in a slow release base followed by teat-end dipping in a 4% available chlorine solution was found to be as effective as the 1-g dose and teat-end dipping (15, 68).

TABLE 15-4
Effect of intramammary antibiotic infusion and teat disinfection on eliminating existing infections and preventing new infections.

			Experimental Treatment			
			0.2 g cloxacillin[a] plus teat dip[c]		1 g cloxacillin[b] plus teat dip	
	Control					
	Cows	Quarters	Cows	Quarters	Cows	Quarters
Number	286	1,144	303	1,212	299	1,196
Percent infected						
At drying-off	53.8	24.2	52.0	27.4	49.9	24.6
At subsequent calving	62.0	30.9	26.0	11.3	15.6	5.4
Percent quarters with new dry-period infection	—	9.5	—	3.3	—	1.7
Percent infections persisting through dry period	—	88.8	—	28.8	—	14.6

Source: Smith et al. 1967. *Vet. Record.* 81:504.
[a] 0.2 g cloxacillin (sodium) in aluminum monostearate base.
[b] 1 g cloxacillin (benzathine) in aluminum monostearate base.
[c] Hypochlorite solution (5% available chlorine).

The persistence of the antibiotic in the dry udder is affected by the solubility of the antibiotic salt, the quantity of antibiotic infused, and the base in which it is formulated. Antibiotics that persist longer in the udder are more effective in reducing infections and preventing new dry period infections. Cloxacillin infused at drying-off and persisting in the udder for one week eliminated 56% of the staphylococcal infections. The same amount of antibiotic infused and remaining in the udder for 3 weeks eliminated 77% of the staphylococcal infections. The infusion of 2 doses of long-acting cloxacillin that persisted in the udder for 6 weeks eliminated 86% of the staphylococcal organisms. All treatments were equally effective in eliminating streptococcal infections. Two-tenths gram of cloxacillin as a sodium salt infused in a 3% aluminum monostearate in mineral oil base after the last milking of lactation persists for less than one week, whereas 0.5 g and 1 g of cloxacillin as the benzathine salt in a similar base persists for 3 weeks (31, 67).

Infected quarters of cows were treated three times at 24-hour intervals at drying-off with randomly selected antibiotics that were commercially available in the United States for mastitis treatment. Results at 14 days after treatment indicated that 88% of the streptococci, 80% of the *Staphylococcus aureus,* and 81% of the nonhemolytic micrococci had been eliminated. However, cultures made 35 or 36 days after treatment indicated that only 51% of the *S. aureus* and 68% of the nonhemolytic micrococci had been eliminated (52).

Combination of Sanitation and Therapy   Elimination of infections has no marked effect on reducing the new infection rate except to reduce the number of pathogens in the environment. A combination of preventing new infections and eliminating existing infections should reduce the incidence of infection on a dairy farm. Trials using a combination of procedures have been carried out at Reading, England and in New York State. One-half of the herds in both trials were on the partial hygiene program as discussed previously (p. 281). The other herds were on a teat-end dip program only. The teat ends of both groups were dipped in a solution of sodium hypochlorite. All cows at drying-off in the British experiment were treated with 0.5 g of benzathine cloxacillin and the teat ends dipped. In the New York experiment, the cows were treated with one million units of penicillin and 1 g of streptomycin and the teats were dipped. Lactation therapy was practiced at the discretion of the dairyman. At the end of 36 months, the British workers found that the quarter infection rate dropped from 27% to 8% (34). Thirty herds and about 2,000 cows were involved in the experiment. The incidence of clinical mastitis dropped by about 40%. During the 36 months of the New York experiment, the infection level dropped from 33% to 10% of the quarters, a 70% reduction in infections. This trial involved 24 herds and approximately 1,800 cows. The results to date are rather dramatic and the program can be carried out with minimal expense to the dairy farmer.

15-2   UDDER EDEMA

Incidence and Symptoms

Udder edema is caused by an excessive accumulation of fluid in the intercellular tissue spaces in the mammary gland. The fluid usually accumulates in the lower parts of the udder and is referred to as caking, udder congestion, or udder swelling. Edema in the dairy cow has been reviewed by Morrow and Schmidt (21). A picture of a cow with severe edema at calving and of the same cow after recovery from edema is shown in Figure 15-5. As fluid accumulates, the udder becomes swollen and hard and the teats become shortened. It causes the cow discomfort, the udder

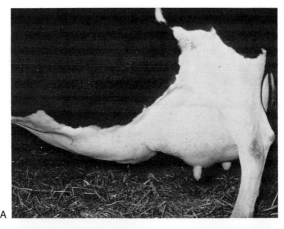

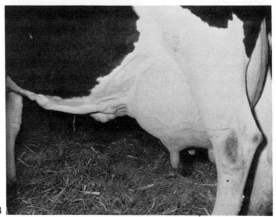

FIGURE 15–5
A. Cow showing severe udder edema at calving.
B. Same cow three weeks later after recovery from
edema. (From Morrow and Schmidt. 1964. CIBA
Veterinary Monograph Series/one. CIBA
Pharmaceutical Company, Summit, New Jersey.)

is more prone to trauma, mastitis, and teat-end injury, and it becomes
difficult to apply the milking machine and to remove normal amounts of
milk.

Edema is of two types, physiological and pathological. Physiological
edema usually develops several days to 2 to 3 weeks prior to parturition
and persists from several days to several weeks after calving. The incidence of physiological edema is much higher in first-calf heifers and in

cows with loosely attached udders. Pathological edema is usually a sequel to physiological edema and may persist for various lengths of time or for an entire lactation. It is more prevalent in cows with pendulous udders.

It is difficult to assess the true incidence of edema, but in one study involving some 12,000 animals the incidence was 18%. Only 100 of these cows required veterinary treatment.

The accumulation of fluid occurs between the secretory tissue and the skin in the bottom parts of the udder. This is shown in Figure 15-6. In more severe cases, the sides of the udder may be involved. The typical case of edema usually involves all four quarters, but in some cases it may involve only half of the udder. It does not appear that the edema penetrates the secretory tissue. In severe cases of physiological edema, the subcutaneous edema may extend from the rear udder up to the vulva and from the fore udder forward to the umbilicus or even to the brisket. The edema usually extends around the base of the teats, which causes the teats to shorten and enlarge and makes them more difficult to milk.

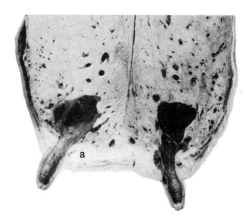

FIGURE 15–6
Accumulation of tissue fluid (a) between skin and secretory tissue causes udder edema. (From Morrow and Schmidt, 1964. CIBA Veterinary Monograph Series/one. CIBA Pharmaceutical Company, Summit, New Jersey.)

Causes

The accumulation of tissue fluid is due to an upset in the balance between the lymph formation in the mammary gland and the movement of the lymph into the circulatory system. Lymph in the mammary gland is similar in composition to blood plasma except lymph has half as much protein as blood plasma. Ruminant mammary gland lymph also has higher concentrations of potassium and chloride and a lower concentration of calcium than blood plasma. Lymph is composed of water and crystaloids that move out of the blood capillaries into the tissue spaces. The movement of the crystaloids from the blood to the tissue is dependent upon the hydrostatic and osmotic pressures of the blood and tissue fluid. Albumin is responsible for approximately 80% of the osmotic pressure in blood and tissue fluid. At the arterial end of the capillary the hydrostatic pressure of the blood is much higher than the hydrostatic pressure of the tissue fluid and the osmotic pressure of the blood vessel. This pressure and the osmotic pressure of the tissue fluid cause water and crystaloids to move out of the capillary. At the venous end of the capillary, the hydrostatic force of the blood is greatly reduced and the osmotic pressure of the plasma is increased. This causes the water and crystaloids to be resorbed. However, in the movement of the blood through the tissue more water and crystaloids are eliminated from the capillaries than are resorbed. The fluid that is not used by the cells for muscular or secretory activity must be returned to the blood by the lymphatic system. If it is not returned, it accumulates and causes edema.

The lymphatic vessels are more permeable than the walls of the capillaries. This allows the larger particles, such as proteins and lipids, to move more easily into the lymph vessels. The movement of the tissue fluid into the lymphatics is primarily dependent upon the pressure differential between the tissue fluid and the lymph vessel.

The movement of fluid in the lymphatics is dependent upon several factors. One is the pressure differential between the small lymph vessels and the thoracic duct. With each inspiration of breathing, the pressure in the thoracic duct is lowered and results in a fluctuating flow of lymph into the blood. Because of their thin walls the lymph vessels are subject to the mechanical action of the visceral organs, muscles and skin, which aids the movement of lymph in the vessels. Lymph vessels also have valves that point towards the thoracic duct and prevent the lymph from moving in the opposite direction.

Factors that cause edema are related to an upset in the balance between the hydrostatic and osmotic pressures in the body, which causes a greater movement of fluid into the tissue spaces. This can be brought about by an increase in capillary pressure resulting from a congestion of the venous blood flow. A lowered osmotic pressure of the blood plasma due to a decrease in protein concentration also causes the movement of tissue fluid out of the capillaries. Similar results occur by damage of the capillary wall. Obstruction of the lymph vessels also prevents the tissue fluid from being returned to the blood. Additional factors that may contribute to edema are low tissue pressure, a high salt intake which helps to retain body fluids in the body, high fluid intake, a warm environment that causes peripheral vasodilation, and a disturbed innervation of the capillaries.

The milk produced by a congested udder is normal in appearance and composition unless sufficient congestion occurs to cause capillary breakdown, which leads to the formation of bloody milk. The edema symptoms usually begin to subside in 2–4 days after parturition and in the reverse order of their onset. The edema near the umbilicus and in the upper parts of the udder regresses first and that in the bottom of the udder is the last to disappear. If the physiological edema persists for a long period of time resulting in pathological edema, the udder becomes larger, firmer, and possibly more pendulous with each successive lactation. It is possible that the lymph accumulation may cause damage to the suspensory apparatus.

Relationship of Feed to Edema

In a number of experiments, it has been found that the type of diet and the amount of feed fed before and after calving have little effect on the severity or incidence of udder edema. These studies have tested various levels of grain feeding before calving and the corn and protein ingredients of the prepartum grain mixtures. However, in one recent experiment (11), it was found that first-calf heifers fed grain for 21 days prepartum had increased severity of edema in comparison to heifers that received no grain. Older cows, however, did not show increased severity of edema when fed grain prior to calving.

Treatment and Prevention

The most effective form of treatment of edema is the use of a diuretic. Most of these cause a decreased resorption of sodium and potassium by the renal tubule of the kidney, resulting in an increased fluid output. The diuretics can be administered orally or parenterally and are effective in reducing the amount of edema and duration of the condition. The addition of a glucocorticoid to a diuretic is more effective than a diuretic alone. Diuretics are not very effective in cows with pendulous udders or in cases of edema complicated with mastitis. No good form of prevention is available. Prepartum milking of cows has not proven to be beneficial in preventing edema.

15-3 SUMMARY

Mastitis

Mastitis is the most costly dairy cattle disease in the United States. Losses up to $1,000,000,000 have been estimated to be caused by losses in milk production, treatment costs, and culling and replacement of cows infected with mastitis. Many cows that do not show clinical mastitis have infections present in the udder and these cause marked decreases in milk production. Clinical mastitis refers to the quarter that produces abnormal milk or shows signs of inflammation. Mammary gland infection refers to the presence of bacteria within the gland.

At least 20 different kinds of organisms cause mastitis, but over 90% of the cases are caused by streptococcal and staphylococcal organisms. In most cases, first-calf heifers are free from mastitis infections when they enter the milking herd. An infection results if the organisms are present near the teat end, if the teat meatus of the cow is susceptible to the entrance of organisms, and if the resistance of the mammary gland cannot overcome the growth of the organisms. The infection can remain as such, develop into clinical mastitis, or be eliminated if the resistance of the udder can destroy the bacteria. In most cases, the clinical quarter receives antibiotic therapy, which causes the clinical mastitis to go back to an infected state. Completely effective antibiotic therapy causes the clinical quarter to revert back to a noninfected state.

Some of the factors related to the establishment of an infection are the number of organisms on the teat, the presence of chaps and blemishes on the teat, the number of leucocytes in the mammary gland, and whether existing infections are present. The highest incidence of new infection rate is in early lactation and in early dry period. High-producing and fast-milking cows are more susceptible to infection. Cows that have been infected previously are more susceptible to reinfection; therefore, older cows have more infections and persisting infections than younger cows.

After the organisms multiply in the mammary gland, inflammation may occur. This is a reaction of the tissue to the irritation caused by the organisms or their products. The inflammation process is accompanied by an increase in the PMN leucocytes, which travel to the inflamed area in an attempt to engulf the bacteria and tissue debris by phagocytosis. This causes a marked increase in leucocyte count of milk during infection, and especially during clinical mastitis.

Symptoms resulting from an infection are an increase in the leucocyte content of milk, an increase in the chlorine content of milk, and a decrease in the lactose content of milk. These cannot be detected by the dairyman and are described as nonclinical conditions. If the infection causes inflammation, definite changes in the milk composition occur. These are a decrease in casein and fat percentages, an increase in pH, and an altered fluid state. A marked drop in milk production also occurs. In severe cases, the quarter develops swelling, and shows heat, redness, and pain. Systemic symptoms and death may occur in extreme cases. Clinical mastitis is usually detected in the barn by a strip cup or plate which shows abnormal clots, flakes, or color in milk.

Barn and laboratory tests, such as the California Mastitis Test (CMT), Modified Whiteside Test, and the Wisconsin Mastitis Test, are used to give an indication of the number of leucocytes in milk. Leucocytes can also be determined directly by microscopic examination of a milk smear. Abnormal milk usually contains over 500,000 leucocytes per milliliter of milk. Bacteriological tests are required to determine the specific bacteria present in the gland.

Considerable attention has been given to the development of control programs. Sanitation procedures and antibotic therapy procedures are proving effective in reducing the incidence of infection and, consequently, the incidence of clinical mastitis. Hygiene procedures have been developed that greatly reduce the spread of the organisms from an infected cow to a noninfected cow. The most important component of the hygiene program appears to be the dipping of teats after milking, which destroys the organisms on the end of the teat. Even though hygiene programs can reduce the new infection rate by 50%, they will reduce the number of infected cows in a herd by only 14% during a 12-month period. The reason for this is that approximately one-half of the cows are infected at the start of a control program and the sanitation procedure does not eliminate existing infections. They are eliminated either by lactation therapy, spontaneous recovery, dry-period therapy, or sale of animals. Dry-period therapy appears to be the most effective of these methods because antibiotic formulations can be infused into mammary glands that will stay there for relatively long periods of time. In addition, the antibiotic infusion in the udder at drying-off prevents a large number of new infections that occur in the early dry period. New antibiotics are being developed that are effective in eliminating a large percentage of the existing infections during the dry period. Lactation therapy is much less effective than dry-period therapy, because smaller amounts of antibiotics must be infused into the udder.

Recent work in England and in New York State indicates that a combination of a sanitation procedure and dry-period therapy reduces the incidence of infections and clinical mastitis on dairy farms.

Edema

Mammary edema is an abnormality that usually occurs shortly before calving and persists for several days to several weeks after calving. It is caused by an excessive accumulation of lymph in the subcutaneous tissue in the ventral portion of the udder. This causes the udder to become hard and swollen and the teats to shorten. In addition to making the cow more uncomfortable and more prone to injury, it also makes the cow more difficult to milk.

The lymph accumulation at calving is a result of an imbalance between the rate of lymph formation and its removal by the blood and lymphatic systems. This can be brought about by increased capillary pressure, decreased blood osmotic pressure, damage to the capillary wall, lymphatic obstruction, or a combination of two or more factors.

In most experiments, it has been found that the level of grain feeding or the composition of the ration fed to the cow prior to parturition has no effect on the incidence or severity of edema. No effective preventive measure has been found. Only a small percentage of cows with edema require treatment, but for those that do, the administration of diuretics has proven beneficial. Most of these cause a decreased resorption of sodium and potassium by the renal tubule of the kidney and, thus, increase the fluid output by the body.

REFERENCES

1. Ashworth, U. S., T. L. Forster, and L. O. Luedecke. 1967. *J. Dairy Sci.* 50:1078.
2. Blackburn, P. S. 1966. *J. Dairy Res.* 33:193.
3. Brown, R. W., H. G. Blobel, W. D. Pounden, O. W. Schalm, L. W. Slanetz, and G. R. Spencer. 1963. *Current Concepts of Bovine Mastitis.* National Mastitis Council, Inc., Hinsdale, Ill.
4. Cecil, H. C., J. Bitman, and J. R. Wood. 1965. *J. Dairy Sci.* 48:1607.
5. Dodd, F. H., A. S. Foot, E. Henriques, and F. K. Neave. 1950. *J. Dairy Res.* 17:107.
6. Dodd, F. H., and F. K. Neave. 1951. *J. Dairy Res.* 18:240.
7. Dodd, F. H., F. K. Neave, and R. G. Kingwill. 1964. *J. Dairy Sci.* 47:1109.
8. Dodd, F. H., F. K. Neave, R. G. Kingwill, C. C. Thiel, and D. R. Westgarth. 1966. *Proc. 17th Internat. Dairy Congr.* A(2):1.
9. Dodd, F. H., J. Oliver, and F. K. Neave. 1957. *J. Dairy Res.* 24:20.

10. Dodd, F. H., D. R. Westgarth, F. K. Neave, and R. G. Kingwill. 1969. *J. Dairy Sci.* 52:689.
11. Emery, R. S., H. D. Hafs, D. Armstrong, and W. W. Snyder. 1969. *J. Dairy Sci.* 52:345.
12. Forster, T. L., U. S. Ashworth, and L. O. Luedecke. 1967. *J. Dairy Sci.* 50:675.
13. Goff, K. R., and G. H. Schmidt. 1967. *J. Dairy Sci.* 50:1787.
14. Kingwill, R. G., F. H. Dodd, and F. K. Neave. 1966. *Esso Farmer* 18:2.
15. Kingwill, R. G., F. K. Neave, F. H. Dodd, and C. D. Wilson. 1967. *Vet. Record* 81:199.
16. Klastrup, N. O. 1956. *Nord. Vet. Med.* 8:193.
17. Little, R. B., and W. N. Plastridge. 1946. *Bovine Mastitis.* New York: McGraw-Hill.
18. McEwen, A. D., and J. M. Samuel. 1946. *Vet. Record* 58:485.
19. Merrill, W. G. 1966. *Ann. Rpt. New York State Assoc. Milk and Food Sanitarians.*
20. Ministry of Agriculture, Fisheries and Food, London. 1959. *Machine Milking.* Bull. 177.
21. Morrow, D. A., and G. H. Schmidt. 1964. *Udder Edema.* CIBA Veterinary Monograph Series/one.
22. Murphy, J. M. 1947. *Amer. J. Vet. Res.* 8:29.
23. Murphy, J. M. 1956. *J. Dairy Sci.* 39:1768.
24. Murphy, J. M. 1959. *Cornell Vet.* 49:411.
25. Murphy, J. M. 1959. Lecture, Cornell University, March 10.
26. Murphy, J. M., and O. M. Stuart. 1953. *Cornell Vet.* 43: 290.
27. Murphy, J. M., and O. M. Stuart. 1955. *Cornell Vet.* 45:112.
28. National Institute for Research in Dairying, Shinfield, England. *Ann. Rpt.* 1957.
29. National Institute for Research in Dairying, Shinfield, England. *Ann. Rpt.* 1965.
30. National Institute for Research in Dairying, Shinfield, England. *Ann. Rpt.* 1966.
31. National Institute for Research in Dairying, Shinfield, England. *Ann. Rpt.* 1967.
32. Neave, F. K., F. H. Dodd, and E. Henriques. 1950. *J. Dairy Res.* 17:37.
33. Neave, F. K., F. H. Dodd, and R. G. Kingwill. 1966. *Vet. Record* 78:521.
34. Neave, F. K., F. H. Dodd, R. G. Kingwill, D. R. Westgarth, and T. K. Griffin. 1970. *Proc. XVIII Internatl. Dairy Congr.,* Sydney, Australia. 1E:581.
35. Neave, F. K., T. M. Higgs, D. Simpkin, J. Oliver, and F. H. Dodd. 1954. *J. Dairy Res.* 21:10.
36. Neave, F. K., F. H. Dodd, R. G. Kingwill, and D. R. Westgarth. 1969. *J. Dairy Sci.* 52:696.
37. Neave, F. K., and J. Oliver. 1962. *J. Dairy Res.* 29:79.
38. Neave, F. K., J. Oliver, F. H. Dodd, and T. M. Higgs. 1968. *J. Dairy Res.* 35:127.
39. Newbould, F. H. S. 1965. *Canadian Vet. J.* 6:29.
40. Newbould, F. H. S., and D. A. Barum. 1964. *Ontario Department of Agriculture Publ.* 525.
41. Newbould, F. H. S., and F. K. Neave. 1965. *J. Dairy Res.* 32:157.

42. Newbould, F. H. S., and F. K. Neave. 1965. *J. Dairy Res.* 32:163.
43. Newbould, F. H. S., and F. K. Neave. 1965. *J. Dairy Res.* 32:171.
44. Norcross, N. L., and D. M. Stark. 1969. *J. Dairy Sci.* 52:714.
45. Nyhan, J. F. 1969. *Proceedings of the Symposium on Machine Milking.* National Institute for Research in Dairying, Reading, England. p. 71.
46. O'Donovan, J., F. H. Dodd, and F. K. Neave. 1960. *J. Dairy Res.* 27:115.
47. Oliver, J., F. H. Dodd, and F. K. Neave. 1956. *J. Dairy Res.* 23:197.
48. Oliver, J., F. H. Dodd, and F. K. Neave. 1956. *J. Dairy Res.* 23:204.
49. Oliver, J., F. H. Dodd, and F. K. Neave. 1956. *J. Dairy Res.* 23:212.
50. Oliver, J., F. H. Dodd, F. K. Neave, and G. L. Bailey. 1956. *J. Dairy Res.* 23:181.
51. Peterson, K. J. 1964. *Amer. J. Vet. Res.* 25:107.
52. Philpot, W. N. 1966. *J. Dairy Sci.* 49:730.
53. Philpot, W. N. 1967. *J. Dairy Sci.* 50:978.
54. Plastridge, W. N. 1958. *J. Dairy Sci.* 41:1141.
55. Prasad, L. B. M., and F. H. S. Newbould. 1968. *Canadian Vet. J.* 9:107.
56. Read, R. B. Jr., A. L. Reyes, J. G. Bradshaw, and J. T. Peeler. 1967. *J. Dairy Sci.* 50:669.
57. Roberts, S. J., A. M. Meek, R. P. Natzke, R. S. Guthrie, L. E. Field, W. G. Merrill, G. H. Schmidt, and R. W. Everett. 1969. *J. Amer. Vet. Med. Assoc.* 155:157.
58. Schalm, O. W., J. Lasmanis, and E. J. Carroll. 1966. *Amer. J. Vet. Res.* 27:1537.
59. Schalm, O. W., and J. Lasmanis. 1968. *J. Amer. Vet. Med. Assoc.* 153:1688.
60. Schalm, O. W., and S. W. Mead. 1943. *J. Dairy Sci.* 26:823.
61. Schmidt, G. H., R. S. Guthrie, and R. W. Guest. 1963. *J. Dairy Sci.* 46:1064.
62. Schmidt, G. H., R. S. Guthrie, and R. W. Guest. 1964. *J. Dairy Sci.* 47:152.
63. Schmidt, G. H., R. S. Guthrie, R. W. Guest, E. B. Hundtoft, A. Kumar and C. R. Henderson. 1963. *Cornell Agr. Expt. Sta. Bull.* 983.
64. Schmidt, G. H., W. G. Merrill, and R. S. Guthrie. 1964. *Cornell Agr. Expt. Sta. Bull.* 996.
65. Schmidt, G. H., and L. D. Van Vleck. 1965. *J. Dairy Sci.* 48:51.
66. Smith, A., F. H. Dodd, and F. K. Neave. 1968. *J. Dairy Res.* 35:287.
67. Smith, A., F. K. Neave, F. H. Dodd, A. Jones, and D. N. Gore. 1967. *J. Dairy Res.* 34:47.
68. Smith, A., D. R. Westgarth, M. R. Jones, F. K. Neave, F. H. Dodd, and G. C. Brander. 1967. *Vet. Record* 81:504.
69. Smith, J. W., and W. D. Schultze. 1967. *J. Dairy Sci.* 50:1083.
70. Thompson, D. I., and D. S. Postle. 1964. *J. Milk Food Tech.* 27:271.
71. Wheelock, J. V., J. A. F. Rook, F. K. Neave, and F. H. Dodd. 1966. *J. Dairy Res.* 33:199.

UNDESIRABLE FLAVORS AND CONTAMINANTS IN MILK

16-1 UNDESIRABLE FLAVORS

Good quality raw milk is a rather bland food having a faint characteristic flavor, which is due to low molecular weight compounds, such as acetone, acetaldehyde, methyl sulfide, traces of C_4-C_{10} fatty acids, methyl ketones, and lactones. These compounds give milk a slightly sweetish taste, with a suggestion of saltiness. Good quality milk is neither bitter nor sour, has very little or no odor, and evokes a smooth, rich feel in the mouth (15, 26).

Milk is unstable and very susceptible to many flavor defects. Because milk is bland in nature, low amounts of undesirable constituents readily result in detectable off flavors. The off flavors can arise from two sources. The internal off flavors are present in the milk when it comes from the cow and these flavors do not intensify in storage. The external off flavors develop in the milk during storage due to either microbiological, enzymatic, or chemical deterioration (26).

Feed, Weed, Cowy, Barny, and Unclean Flavors

Internal off flavors arise through one of three routes of transmission. They are the respiratory route, the digestive route, or from eructated gases. Odors from the feed and the environment pass from the air into the cow's lungs. The odors are then picked up by the blood and transported to the mammary gland epithelial cells, where they diffuse into the milk. The flavors arising by the digestive route are absorbed from the digestive tract by the blood draining it and are then transmitted to the milk. Other off flavors are produced by the partial digestion of feeds in the rumen resulting in volatile substances, which are eructated or belched from the rumen, inhaled into the lungs, and transferred to the milk by the blood (26).

The time of appearance of an undesirable flavor in the milk after cows are exposed to it is dependent upon the pathways by which the flavor enters the bloodstream. Dougherty et al. (4) found that some chemicals produced flavors in the milk within 15 minutes after they were introduced via the respiratory route. When these same chemicals were added to the digestive tract, it took up to 60 minutes before they were present in the milk. If the eructated gases from the rumen were allowed to enter the lungs, the flavor showed up in the milk within 30 minutes after feeding.

The undesirable flavors of milk can be eliminated by a reversal of the three pathways. The concentration of the off flavor in milk is dependent upon the concentration of flavor components in the blood, which is in turn dependent upon the amount being supplied to the cow's lungs or rumen. As the amount going into the blood is reduced, the concentration in the blood becomes lower than that of the milk and the flavors diffuse from the milk to the blood. Eventually all of the off flavors due to feed and undesirable environment are excreted or exhaled (26, 29).

The most common off flavor of milk is caused by feed. In one study (16), it was found that the feed flavor was present in 88.4% of all milk samples taken from a university dairy herd over a 4-year period. Some of the feed flavors, however, are present in milk of acceptable quality to most consumers. Dunkley (5) states that there are at least 46 weeds and 10 feeds that cause off flavors in milk if they are fed during a 5-hour period prior to milking. Among these are: ragweed, buttercup, onions, garlic, turnip, kale, and silage. Most of the flavor compounds in silage are transmitted to the milk. The common management recommendation to eliminate these flavors from milk is to withhold the feeds producing off flavors in milk for 4 to 5 hours before milking. Weeds that cause off flavors should be removed from the cow's rations, because most of these flavors persist for longer than 12 hours (26, 29).

Barny and unclean flavors appear in the milk when cows are housed in barns with inadequate ventilation systems. These off flavors are most prevalent in the winter months and can be avoided by proper ventilation of the barn. The cowy flavor is usually the result of ketosis, which causes the blood and milk to have a high concentration of ketone bodies (acetone, acetoacetic acid, and β-hydroxybutyric acid) (26). If this flavor presents a problem in a dairy herd, the milk from ketotic cows should be eliminated from the bulk milk supply.

Oxidized Flavor

The most important flavor defect to the consumer of nonhomogenized milk is oxidized flavor. This is also described as a metallic, cardboardy, cappy, papery, oily, or tallowy flavor. The oxidized flavor is brought about by the accumulation of carbonyl compounds, which are produced by an auto-oxidation of unsaturated fatty acids in the milk phospholipids. The milk phospholipids are concentrated in the fat globule membrane. The oxidation of the unsaturated fatty acids is catalyzed by copper in the presence of a pro-oxidant, ascorbic acid (vitamin C) (26).

There is great variation among cows in the susceptibility of milk to oxidized flavor. Milk has been classified according to its oxidative stability into three categories: (1) spontaneous—milk that oxidizes within 48 hours after milking without any treatment; (2) susceptible—milk that oxidizes in the presence of 0.5–5.0 ppm of copper or iron within 48 hours after milking; and (3) resistant—milk that does not oxidize on storage even in the presence of copper or iron (26).

A number of factors affect the oxidative stability of milk. In general, milk with a low bacteria count is usually more susceptible to an oxidative deterioration than high count milk. The bacteria apparently protect the milk against oxidation either by directly competing for available oxygen or by producing reducing substances during metabolic activity (30). The storage of milk at low temperatures results in lower bacterial activity, thus it is more susceptible to oxidation. Milk produced on alfalfa hay is more susceptible to oxidation than milk produced from grass hay. In general, pasture and green succulent feeds give milks that are less susceptible to oxidation than do dry feeds. The influence of feeds on the oxidative stability is probably the result of their effects on the constituents of milk involved in oxidation, such as copper, ascorbic acid, tocopherol, carotene, and on the degree of unsaturation of the lipids (26).

The metallic and oxidized flavors of milk occur more frequently in early stages of lactation (16, 30). This susceptibility may be due to changes in the copper content of milk, since King and Dunkley (14) found that the natural copper content of milk was much higher in early lactation than in late lactation. The variation in the susceptibility to oxidation is partially dependent upon the composition of milk. Smith, Dunkley, and Ronning

(31) found that an increase in the linoleic acid content of the phospholipids of milk was associated with an increased susceptibility to copper-induced oxidation.

The role of ascorbic acid seems to be twofold. The oxidation of milk is catalyzed by copper in the presence of ascorbic acid; however, high levels of ascorbic acid can also act as an antioxidant. Levels of 50–100 mg of ascorbic acid per liter act as an effective antioxidant, whereas low levels (10–20 mg/liter) function as a pro-oxidant. On the other hand, tocopherol and, to a certain extent, carotene act as natural antioxidants to help increase the resistance to oxidation (26). Even though there are great differences in the susceptibility of milk to oxidation as it leaves the cow, Shipe (30) concluded that the development of oxidized flavor is probably more dependent upon what happens after the milk leaves the cow than on what the cow does.

Copper and iron are strong catalysts of lipid oxidation and copper is the stronger of the two. If milk is exposed to any of these metals during handling, oxidation occurs. This has resulted in the widespread use of stainless steel equipment for handling milk. However, copper can still be absorbed on the stainless steel surfaces from the water supply or from white metal fittings during circulation cleaning. Control measures that are effective in reducing the susceptibility of milk to oxidized flavor are homogenization and high-heat treatment of milk. Chemical antioxidants are effective in preventing oxidation; however, the addition of antioxidants is not permitted in most states (26).

Another type of oxidized flavor can be induced by exposure of milk to light. The light-activated flavor is detectable in as few as 10 minutes of sunshine exposure. The oxidized flavor due to light can be controlled by providing a minimum of exposure of milk to light during distribution. This can be done by placing homogenized milk in amber- or ruby-colored bottles and/or the placing of milk in light-proof boxes on the consumers' doorsteps (26).

Cooked flavor of milk is unique to high-heated milk. The heat treatment activates the sulfhydryl (SH) group with the liberation of volatile sulfides, especially hydrogen sulfide. The sulfides result from the heat denaturation of the serum proteins, especially β-lactoglobulin and the fat globule membrane. The critical temperature for a serum protein denaturation is slightly above conventional pasteurization. The presence of the cooked flavor disappears on storage due to the oxidation of the SH groups. The cooked flavor in heated milk also provides protection against oxidized flavor development, because it results in a lowering of the oxidation-reduction potential of the milk due to the presence of the SH groups (26).

Rancid Flavors

One of the highly objectionable off flavors in raw milk is rancid flavor, which is due to the hydrolysis of milk fat triglycerides by the lipases that are normally present in milk. The rancid flavor can also be caused by microbial lipases. The hydrolysis of the triglycerides is termed lipolysis, which liberates free fatty acids. The short-chain fatty acids, especially butyric acid, are the compounds responsible for the rancid flavor in milk. Other terms used to describe the rancid flavor in milk and milk products are goaty, dirty, or soapy.

The short-chain fatty acids in milk give rise to a bitter taste. These odors and tastes become more apparent when the sample is warm or hot since the fatty acids are volatile. Only a very limited degree of lipolysis is required for the flavor to develop. Two milk lipases have been described, one being a membrane lipase that is absorbed to the fat globule membrane. The other is a plasma lipase, which remains in the plasma and is associated with a casein fraction of milk. Milk lipases are always present in freshly drawn milk, but are inactive in the udder at the time of milking, because the triglycerides are protected by the fat globule membranes surrounding them. Lipolysis proceeds at a slow rate unless thermal or mechanical activation treatment is applied. Pasteurized milk usually does not exhibit lipolysis, because the lipase system is inactivated by conventional pasteurization (26).

Cow's milk varies in its susceptibility to lipolysis. Spontaneous rancidity does occur in some cows in which the milk becomes rancid simply by cooling the fresh milk and aging it without any further treatment. The incidence of spontaneous rancidity in milk is higher in cows in late lactation and in cows to which no dry feed is fed (32). Spontaneous rancidity in this milk can be prevented by mixing it with three parts of normal milk within one hour after milking (26).

The activation of lipolysis is, to a large extent, dependent upon alteration of the fat globule membrane, which provides protection to the fat droplet. Homogenization of warm milk containing fat induces rancidity by destroying the fat globule membrane, which allows the lipase to come in contact with the triglycerides. Rancid flavor is also induced when small amounts of raw milk are mixed with homogenized pasteurized milk. Agitation of milk also induces rancidity, especially if foam formation accompanies agitation. Thus, it is important for milk to receive minimum agitation prior to homogenization. This is especially true when milk is transferred in pipeline milkers. This has led to the common recommendation that risers should be avoided in pipeline milking installations (26).

Temperature manipulation can also induce rancidity. It was found that lipolysis was induced by warming cooled milk to 30° C followed by cooling it to 10° C (17).

Other Off Flavors

Large numbers of other off flavors have been described in milk. Some of these are due to chemical or foreign materials, primarily as a result of contamination after the milk leaves the cow. Certain salves and disinfectants containing phenol that are used for treatment of teat sores and udder abrasions cause milk to have a slight phenolic flavor. The phenolic flavor is intensified in the presence of chlorine, which produces a characteristic chlorophenol flavor. Chlorine contamination of milk resulting from its use as a sanitizer may also produce off flavors. Detectable amounts can be picked up by the taste if 6–8 ppm available chlorine are present in the skim milk. Iodophores may also produce off flavors in milk. If skim milk contains 2–5 ppm of available iodine, a medicinal or chemical flavor occurs in the milk (26).

Salty flavor has an internal origin. The slight sweetness of normal milk is due to an equilibrium between the sweet taste of lactose and the salty taste of chlorine concentration. If a marked increase in the chlorine content occurs, as in advanced lactation or mastitis, a slightly salty taste occurs (5).

Some of the common off flavors are caused by microbial fermentation. Usually large numbers of microorganisms are present in the milk before detectable off flavors can be recognized. Some of the common off flavors due to microbial fermentation are sour or high-acid flavor, which is a result of the fermentation of lactose by various genera of bacteria that convert lactose into lactic acid. The malty flavor of milk is produced when the amino acid leucine is fermented to produce the aldehyde 3-methylbutanal by the organism *Streptococcus lactis,* variety maltigenes. The organism is not heat-resistant, therefore pasteurized milk is not susceptible to this defect. A bitter flavor is a result of a hydrolysis of milk proteins by microorganisms, resulting in an accumulation of polypeptides (26).

16-2 PESTICIDES

In the past twenty years, a large number of pesticides have been developed to control pests of both cattle and plants. The control of pests is important for the production of crops and livestock. The dairy cow is an important source of human food, and can thus be a major source of pesticides in the human diet.

Chlorinated Hydrocarbons

One of the early and most important pesticides is DDT. Relatively high levels of DDT are found in the milk (2.5 ppm of milk fat) if the cows or barns are treated with DDT or if cows consume DDT-contaminated feeds. The pesticide appears in the milk within a few hours after the feeding of a high level of DDT. The use of DDT around the milking barns has been prohibited for a number of years. The dairy industry is faced with the problem that a general low ($\pm$ 0.02 ppm) DDT background contamination of the environment now exists. This is due to the heavy, worldwide use of DDT, its high stability in the environment, its transmission from the contaminated soil and water to plants, its assimilation and retention in the body fat of animals, and its transfer from body fat to the blood and in turn the milk of the cow. The Food and Drug Administration of the United States government has set a maximum tolerable amount of DDT in the milk at 0.05 ppm in milk (1.25 ppm on a milk-fat basis). The levels of DDT found in human food have not yet presented a health problem to the humans. The human body fat levels of DDT have either declined or shown no increase over the past 10 to 15 years (18).

The use of DDT in the environment has, however, had an adverse effect on fish and wildlife populations. DDT has been banned for use against most pests.

DDT is a chlorinated hydrocarbon with a chemical formula of 2,2-bis (p-chlorophenyl)-1,1,1-trichloroethane. Cows treated with DDT, either by spraying or dipping, or fed DDT-contaminated feed, absorb the pesticide and store it in adipose tissue. The DDT absorption occurs through the alimentary and respiratory tracts and through the epidermis. Cows then secrete a portion of it or its metabolites in the milk. The two common metabolites are DDE [2,2-bis (p-chlorphenyl) 1,1-dichloroethylene)] and DDD [2,2-bis (p-chlorophenyl) 1,1-dichloroethane)]. DDD is produced from DDT by microorganisms in the rumen and by breakdown in the liver. Extensive transformation of DDT to DDE occurs by metabolic action that is separate from the rumen, and the liver is probably the site of transformation (18, 35, 37).

Because DDT is absorbed by the adipose tissue, the amount of DDT in the milk closely follows the body fat levels. The rate of depletion of body fat stores of DDT in lactating dairy animals is about 8–10% per week in early weeks of the feed-off period (the time after the DDT is withdrawn from the diet). Nonlactating animals have even slower rates of depletion. Thus the elimination of the DDT from the body due to a single accidental feeding of a high dose or brought about by a low level feeding over a long period is a very slow process. The rate of depletion of DDT appears to be independent of the rate of body fat mobilization. Generally, the use of feeding regimes of low-energy rations or thyroprotein have not been successful in increasing the rate of removal of DDT from the body fat (18).

Dieldrin is another chlorinated hydrocarbon that is used for pest control. Cows continue to excrete dieldrin in the milk for long periods of time after use of the pesticide is discontinued, because it is also stored in the body fat. Decreasing the energy level did not increase the rate of dieldrin decontamination; however, thyroprotein feeding increased the rate of this pesticide disappearance slightly (3).

Tests have been made to determine the presence in milk of many other chlorinated hydrocarbon pesticides, if they are a contaminant of the feed. It appears that all of them act similarly to DDT and dieldrin in that they become part of the body fat and then are excreted into the milk for long periods of time after the contaminated feed is withdrawn from the cow. The use of electron capture detectors in the analysis of pesticide residues by gas chromotography has made it possible to detect small amounts of residue in the feed and milk. In one study (8), cows received roughage containing 5 and 20 parts per billion (ppb) of either heptachlor epoxide or Telodrin. Small but detectable amounts (0.4–7.7 ppb) of both pesticides appeared in the milk within 5 days after their feeding and they were detectable in milk for 10 weeks after the termination of feeding.

Organic Phosphate Compounds

Organophosphate pesticides used to protect plants against pests apparently do not enter the milk of cows when they are fed as a contaminant of feed. Among those tested are Imidan, Bidrin, Dursban, and Supracide. None of these appeared in the milk at levels that could be detected by procedures that are now available (9, 10, 11, 27).

16-3 RADIONUCLIDES

The advent of nuclear fission and the resultant bombs and nuclear testing have led to concern about radioactive fallout. Milk and milk products serve as major routes for radionuclide contamination of man. Among the isotopes that are considered to be the most potentially dangerous to man are ^{131}iodine, ^{90}strontium, and ^{137}cesium. Even though some of these radioactive isotopes enter the milk, they have not yet created a human health problem.

The Federal Radiation Council (33) has prepared Radiation Protection Guides (RPG), which are the radiation doses that should not be exceeded. The RPG on a continuous daily intake in picrocuries (pCi) for the radionuclides are as follows: ^{90}Sr, 200; ^{131}I, 100; and ^{137}Cs, 3,600. From December 1967 to November 1968, the monthly averages of the three radionuclides range from 0–26 pCi ^{90}Sr, 0–15 pCi ^{131}I, and 0–117 pCi ^{137}Cs per liter of milk. In all but one of the 63 reporting stations, the ^{131}I values were below the practical reporting level. Since milk is a major source of the dietary intake of radionuclides, it can be seen that the consumption of 1 liter of milk per day usually provides less than 10% of the daily RPG.

Radionuclide contamination could become a very serious problem in case of a nuclear war or in a local area where a nuclear fission accident occurred. Considerable progress is being made to remove the isotopes from the milk in the dairy plant operation by ion-exchange systems (24).

^{90}Strontium is potentially the most dangerous nuclide that is formed in the fission reaction. It has a half-life of 28 years and is produced in relatively high yields in the fission reaction. It follows calcium metabolism and is deposited in the bones. Because of its long half-life, there is the danger that the accumulation of large amounts of ^{90}Sr in the bone may lead to bone disease, especially cancer. Plant sources are biologically more important sources of ^{90}Sr than is milk. The dairy cow ingesting feed containing ^{90}Sr discriminates against ^{90}Sr in favor of calcium. This discrimination takes place in the gut, kidney, placenta, and mammary gland. As the amount of calcium available to the organ increases in relation to the ^{90}Sr, the organ absorbs more calcium per unit of ^{90}Sr. For this reason, milk has a much lower amount of ^{90}Sr per unit of calcium than does the nonmilk portion of the diet. Increasing the calcium consumption of the cow thus lowers the amount of ^{90}Sr per gram of calcium. Comparable discrimination occurs in the human so that the amount of ^{90}Sr per gram of calcium deposited in the bone is about one-fourth of that in the diet. Increasing the calcium consumption by humans decreases the ^{90}Sr per gram of calcium deposition in the bones even further. People in primarily milk-consuming areas are acquiring lower levels of ^{90}Sr in their bones than people in primarily plant-consuming areas (19, 20, 21).

^{137}Cesium is another important product produced by nuclear fission. It has a long half-life of 27 years. It is related chemically to potassium and is distributed in the body somewhat like potassium, being found in the muscles, blood, and other soft tissue. It is produced in slightly greater abundance than ^{90}Sr in nuclear fission and is metabolically more likely to be found in plants and animals than ^{90}Sr. The contamination of cow's milk is associated with the contemporary fallout rate since the soil uptake is negligible. The fallout rate is in turn dependent upon the amount of rainfall and latitudinal location. Even though ^{137}Cs has a long half-life, its potential danger to the body is minimized because it has a biological half-life in the body of 200 days (12, 21, 34).

Radioactive iodine, ^{131}I, accumulates in the thyroid of the animal or human. It is not a great potential hazard because it has a very short half-life of 8 days. If animals consume pastures contaminated with ^{131}I, the amount of ^{131}I in the milk can be rapidly decreased by changing them to stored feed. Feeds that have been contaminated can be stored for 45 or more days and nearly all of the ^{131}I disappears. Milk is the most important avenue of disappearance of ^{131}I from the lactating animal. The goat has a much greater ability to concentrate ^{131}I in the milk than the cow. Even though the mammary gland of the goat has a more efficient iodine trap than the cow, the mechanisms of concentration of iodine in the milk appear similar in both animals (2, 22).

Another radionuclide that has resulted from radioactive fallout is ^{54}manganese. It is a neutron activation product with a half-life of 310 days. The transfer of ^{54}Mn to milk is extremely low, however, because manganese is poorly absorbed from the intestinal tract (36).

16-4   ANTIBIOTICS AND DRUGS

Antibiotics have been used extensively in dairy cattle management, especially in the treatment of mastitis. This has led to problems with the antibiotic contamination of milk. This was reviewed by Albright et al. (1) in 1961. The antibiotic contamination of milk is largely the result of improper use of the antibiotic for the treatment of mastitis or the failure to withhold the milk from sale for the specified periods of time.

Public health officials are concerned about antibiotic contamination of milk for three major reasons. First, some people have a very high sensitivity to antibiotics, particularly penicillin. Allergic dermatitis reactions have been reported in humans consuming small amounts of penicillin in contaminated milk. Secondly, the continued consumption of antibiotics in the milk may cause certain bacteria to develop resistance to the antibiotics and thus become refractive to treatment. A third concern is the possibility that dairy products made from milk containing antibiotics may at times contain antibiotic-resistant strains of infectious bacteria. Even though it is of no immediate concern to public health officials, the presence of antibiotics in milk is of concern to dairy plants that manufacture fermented dairy products. Fermented dairy products cannot be produced from antibiotic-contaminated milk because the antibiotics inhibit the growth of bacteria in the culture.

Proper use of antibiotics largely eliminates the contamination problem. The reduction in the incidence of antibiotic-contaminated milk has been brought about by the education of the dairy farmer in the use of the antibiotics and to their potential danger, by testing for antibiotics and the enforcement of shipping antibiotic-free milk by milk plants, and by lowering the concentration of penicillin in mastitis preparations. Since 1957, the maximum permissible quantity per dose of antibiotic used for lactation therapy is 100,000 units of penicillin. An example of the progress that can be made is shown in a New York study. At the beginning of a 4-month period in 1959 and 1960, 6.5% and 5.1% of the milk from can and bulk tank producers tested showed the presence of antibiotics. During the period, 10,000 samples from 4,000 farms were tested and the farmers were made aware of the findings. At the end of the period, less than 0.5% of the samples showed the presence of antibiotics.

A dilemma exists in the use of antibiotics for the treatment of clinical mastitis and infections. In order to eliminate the infectious pathogens from the gland, it is desirable to have relatively large amounts of antibiotics in the gland for a long period of time. From a production standpoint, it is desirable to have the antibiotic leave the gland as rapidly as possible so that it does not contaminate the milk to be sold.

The portion of the antibiotic that is not absorbed by the udder tissue is voided in the milk. The amount voided varies from cow to cow, but the length of time that the cow eliminates antibiotics in the milk is dependent upon concentration of antibiotics injected, the amount of milk produced by the cow, and the carrier of the antibiotics. High injection doses and low levels of milk production cause the penicillin to remain in the udder for longer periods of time. In most cases, antibiotic contamination of milk is avoided if the dairyman withholds the milk from the market for the period specified on the label of each antibiotic tube. Most products have a withholding period of 72 hours after infusion into the udder, but some are as short as 36 hours and some require 96 hours.

Intramammary infusion of an antibiotic into one quarter may lead to the presence of the antibiotic in the milk of the other three quarters. With penicillin the transfer is slight and of short duration, and, consequently, it usually presents no problem. Intramuscular or subcutaneous injections of antibiotics also produce a contaminated product. The antibiotics appear in the milk for up to 72 hours after injection. The length of time that the intramuscular injection is present in the milk is dependent upon the same factors that apply to the intramammary infusion. The oral administration of antibiotics can create a milk contamination problem if high levels are fed. Levels of penicillin used for the prevention of bloat do not produce detectable levels of penicillin in the milk.

Rasmussen (28) reviewed the comprehensive literature on the mammary excretion of drugs and pesticides in animals and humans. Among the drugs that have been shown to appear in the milk following oral, cutaneous, or parenteral administration are: alkaloids—atropine, chinine, colchicine, ergot, ergotamine, heroine, hydrastinine, morphine, nicotine, physostigmine, pilocarpine, strychnine, theobromine; anthelmintics—hexachloraethane, phentiazine, Promintic®, tetrachloraethylene, tetrachlormethane, thiabendazole; anthraquinone derivatives—aloe, cortex rhamni purshianae, dianthone, rheum; antihistamines—antazoline, diphenhydramine, mepyramine; barbiturates—diemale, ibomale, mebumale, Medomin®, phenamale; chemotherapeutics—diphenylsulfone, isoniazide, nitrofurans, pyrimethamine, and most of the sulfa drugs; diuretics—bendroflumethiazide, and furosemide; and numerous miscellaneous drugs.

The drugs in milk occur in either the aqueous phase, in the milk fat, or are bound to the proteins of milk. For instance, the sulphonamides are dissolved in the aqueous phase, whereas some barbiturates occur in part dissolved in the milk fat. The barbiturate, barbitone, which has a low lipid-solubility is found in the aqueous phase and pentobarbitone, which is highly lipid-soluble, is bound primary to the milk fat. The nonprotein bound and un-ionized fractions of drugs are in equal concentrations in the blood plasma and the concentration in the milk is independent of the volume of milk produced. The fractions of drugs apparently enter the milk by diffusion across the epithelial cells. The movement of drugs from the mammary gland to the blood take place by diffusion of the un-ionized fraction at a rate dependent upon the lipid-solubility of the fraction.

The concentration of the partially ionized drugs in milk is dependent upon the pH of the milk and the nature of the drug. Drugs of an acid character have a higher concentration in the blood than in the milk at a normal milk pH (6.5 to 6.8) but move toward an equal concentration in blood and milk when the pH of milk moves toward that of blood (7.4). Drugs of an alkaline nature have a higher concentration in milk than in blood, but the concentration is reduced to a concentration equal to that of blood as the pH of milk increases.

16-5 TOXIC METALS

The two metals that cause the most problems as toxic agents to animals are lead and arsenic. Consumption of either of these in large quantities cause illness and death of animals. Both lead (Pb) and arsenic (As) concentrations in milk increase when large amounts are consumed.

The average lead content of market milk tested in 59 North American cities ranged from .023 to 0.79 ppm. The weighted average was .049 ppm (25). In one trial (23), cows fed up to 12.95 mg Pb/100 lb body weight for 126 days produced milk that contained less than 0.05 mg Pb/l. In contrast to this, milk from two cows surviving in a dairy herd that consumed two feedings of concentrate contaminated with lead oxide contained 2.26 and 0.15 ppm/kg 12 days later. At 122 days after the lead feeding, the milk contained .028 and 0.030 ppm (13). It appears that the level of lead in the milk is more dependent upon the body burden of the element than on the daily intake of it.

Bovine milk contains between 0.032 and 0.060 mg As/l; colostrum has a higher concentration (23). Grimmett (7) reported that milk samples of cows contained from 0.8 to 1.5 mg As/l in areas where the soil and water are contaminated with arsenic, and illness and death of the cattle was attributed to its toxicity. The feeding of arsenic up to 468 mg/100 lb body weight daily for 126 days did not increase the arsenic content above 0.05 mg/1 (23). In one trial, one lactating heifer was drenched with 0.3428 g of $As_2 O_3$ as sodium arsenite for 3 days and the level of arsenic in the milk was not increased over the predrenching level of 0.23–0.27 mg/l. Eleven days later, the same animal was drenched with 1.367 g of As_3O_3 daily for 3 days and the milk contained from 0.34 to 0.47 mg/l prior to her death (6). The amount of arsenic in the milk is thus dependent upon the amount consumed and may also be dependent upon the body burden of the element.

16-6 SUMMARY

Undesirable Flavors

Off flavors in milk can occur from a variety of sources. Since milk is a bland food, it is very susceptible to off flavors because small amounts of a contaminant can impart a flavor to the milk. The most common flavors in milk are those due to feeds and the unclean environment of the cow. These arise in the milk by being inhaled by the lungs, being absorbed from the rumen, or from volatile substances that are eructated from the rumen and absorbed by the lungs. These flavors are carried to the udder via the blood and there diffuse into the milk. Since most of these are volatile substances, the concentration in the milk is dependent upon their concentration in the blood. As the blood concentration is reduced after the inhalation or ingestion of the flavor-producing substance, the milk concentration is likewise reduced. These flavors can be prevented by not feeding flavor-producing feeds for 5 hours before milking and providing proper ventilation in the barns.

Oxidized flavors are the result of the oxidation of fatty acids in the milk phospholipids. Much variation exists in the susceptibility of cow's milk to oxidized flavor. Oxidized flavors are more prevalent in early lactation and in cows receiving alfalfa hay. Milk that is exposed to copper- and iron-containing equipment or exposed to sunlight becomes very susceptible to oxidation. This had led to the almost exclusive use of stainless steel milk-handling equipment. Oxidation can be prevented by homogenization and high-heat treatment of milk. After bottling, the milk should not be exposed to sunlight.

The rancid flavor of milk is caused by the hydrolysis of milk fat triglycerides by lipase that is present in the milk. Fresh milk ordinarily does not develop a rancid flavor because the fat globule membrane surrounding the triglycerides prevents the lipase from coming in contact with them. Destruction of the fat globule membrane by agitation of milk in places such as risers in a pipeline or through the homogenization process brings about the rancidity. In normal processing, the homogenization does not produce rancidity because the milk is also pasteurized, a process that destroys the lipase enzyme.

Contaminants

Chlorinated hydrocarbon pesticides used for the treatment of pests on the cow, her environment, or on the forage she consumes, appear in the milk. They continue to be excreted by the cow long after the pesticides are withdrawn from her feed because the pesticides become absorbed by the body adipose tissue and are depleted at a very slow rate. Organic phosphate pesticides apparently are not excreted into the milk.

Radionuclides that might present a problem as milk contaminants in case of a nuclear war or a nuclear fission accident are ^{90}strontium, ^{137}cesium, and ^{131}iodine. ^{90}Strontium follows calcium metabolism but is discriminated against in the gut, kidney, placenta, and mammary gland in favor of calcium. Increasing the calcium intake of the cow lowers the amount of ^{90}Sr per gram of calcium absorbed at each site of discrimination, so that the amount of ^{90}Sr per gram of calcium deposited in the bone is about one-fourth of that in the diet.

^{137}Cesium follows potassium metabolism and is found in the muscles, blood, and soft tissue. The potential danger of ^{137}Cs to the body is minimized because of its relatively short body biological half-life. ^{131}Iodine accumulates in the thyroid of the animal and human. Because of its very short half-life, it does not stay in the feed supply of cows very long and ceases to be a problem.

Antibiotic contamination of milk is largely due to the improper use of antibiotics in the treatment of disease, especially mastitis, and the failure to withhold antibiotic-contaminated milk from the milk sold for human consumption. Antibiotic-contaminated milk creates problems in some humans who are extremely sensitive to antibiotics, especially penicillin. Antibiotic contamination of milk can be eliminated, for the most part, by the judicious use of antibiotics for dairy cow therapy and by withholding the milk from antibiotic-treated cows from the bulk milk supply for the period of time specified on the label of the antibiotic tube.

Many of the drugs used to treat animals appear in the milk either in the aqueous phase, in the milk fat, or bound to the proteins of milk. Drugs that are lipid-soluble are bound to the milk fat. Nonprotein and un-ionized drugs apparently cross the epithelial cells by diffusion and are found in equal concentrations in the blood plasma and in milk. Ionized drugs move into the milk according to their own pH and the pH of milk. Acid drugs are in higher concentration in the blood than in the milk; whereas alkaline drugs are in higher concentration in the milk than in the blood. Both types of drugs move toward equal concentrations in blood and milk as the pH of milk increases to that of blood.

High levels of either arsenic or lead consumption increase the amount of these metals found in the milk. The level in the milk appears to be a function of the body burden of the element instead of its daily intake.

REFERENCES

1. Albright, J. L., S. L. Tuckey, and T. G. Woods. 1961. *J. Dairy Sci.* 44:779.
2. Allen, R. S. 1966. *J. Dairy Sci.* 49:889.
3. Braund, D. G., L. D. Brown, J. T. Huber, N. C. Leeling, and M. J. Zabik. 1969. *J. Dairy Sci.* 52:172.
4. Dougherty, R. W., W. F. Shipe, G. V. Gudnason, R. A. Ledford, R. D. Peterson, and R. Scarpellino. 1962. *J. Dairy Sci.* 45:472.
5. Dunkley, W. L. 1964. Factors Affecting Milk Quality. In *Dairying in California.* California Agr. Expt. Sta. Manual.
6. Fitch, L. W. N., R. E. R. Grimmett, and E. M. Wall. 1939. *New Zealand J. Sci. Technol.* 21:146a.
7. Grimmett, R. E. R. 1939. *New Zealand J. Agr.* 58:383.

8. Hardee, D. D., W. H. Gutenmann, G. I. Keenan, G. G. Gyrisco, D. J. Lisk, F. H. Fox, G. W. Trimberger, and R. F. Holland. 1964. *J. Econ. Entomology* 57:404.

9. Johnson, J. C., Jr., and M. C. Bowman. 1968. *J. Dairy Sci.* 51:1225.

10. Johnson, J. C., Jr., M. C. Bowman, and D. B. Leuck. 1969. *J. Dairy Sci.* 52:1253.

11. Johnson, J. C., Jr., R. S. Lowrey, M. C. Bowman, D. B. Leuck, E. W. Beck, and J. C. Derbyshire. 1968. *J. Dairy Sci.* 51:1219.

12. Johnson, J. E., D. W. Wilson, and W. L. Lindsay. 1966. *Soil Sci. Soc. Amer. Proc.* 30:416.

13. Kehoe, R. A., J. Cholak, and R. V. Story. 1940. *J. Nutr.* 19:579.

14. King, R. L., and W. L. Dunkley. 1959. *J. Dairy Sci.* 42:420.

15. Kinsella, J. E., S. Patton, and P. S. Dimick. 1967. *J. Amer. Oil Chem. Soc.* 44:449.

16. Kratzer, D. D., C. F. Foreman, A. E. Freeman, E. W. Bird, W. S. Rosenberger, and F. E. Nelson. 1967. *J. Dairy Sci.* 50:1384.

17. Krukovsky, V. N., and B. L. Herrington. 1939. *J. Dairy Sci.* 22:137.

18. Laben, R. C. 1968. *J. Animal Sci.* 27:1643.

19. Larson, B. L. 1960. *J. Dairy Sci.* 43:1.

20. Larson, B. L. 1963. *J. Dairy Sci.* 46:759.

21. Larson, B. L., and K. E. Ebner. 1958. *J. Dairy Sci.* 41:1647.

22. Lengemann, F. W. 1970. *J. Dairy Sci.* 53:165.

23. Marshall, S. P., F. W. Hayward, and W. R. Meagher. 1963. *J. Dairy Sci.* 46:580.

24. Marshall, R. O., E. M. Sparling, B. Heinemann, and R. E. Bales. 1968. *J. Dairy Sci.* 51:673.

25. Murthy, G. K., U. Rhea, and J. T. Peeler. 1967. *J. Dairy Sci.* 50:651.

26. O'Sullivan, A. C. 1965. *Irish Agr. Creamery Rev.* 16:4 (Aug. 1965) and 16:6 (Sept. 1965).

27. Polan, C. E., J. T. Huber, C. N. Miller, and R. A. Sandy. 1969. *J. Dairy Sci.* 52:1384.

28. Rasmussen, F. 1966. *Studies on the Mammary Excretion and Absorption of Drugs.* Commissioned by Carl Fr. Mortensen, Copenhagen.

29. Shipe, W. F. 1964. *Proc. Cornell Nutr. Conf.*, p. 108.

30. Shipe, W. F. 1964. *J. Dairy Sci.* 47:221.

31. Smith, L. M., W. L. Dunkley, and M. Ronning. 1963. *J. Dairy Sci.* 46:7.

32. Tarassuk, N. P., and E. N. Frankel. 1957. *J. Dairy Sci.* 40:418.

33. U. S. Dept. of Health, Education, and Welfare. 1969. *Radiological Health Data and Reports* 10:103.

34. Ward, G. M., H. F. Stewart, and J. E. Johnson. 1965. *J. Dairy Sci.* 48:38.

35. Whiting, F. M., S. B. Hagyard, W. H. Brown, and J. W. Stull. 1968. *J. Dairy Sci.* 51:1612.

36. Wilson, D. W., and G. M. Ward. 1967. *J. Dairy Sci.* 50:592.

37. Witt, J. M., F. M. Whiting, W. H. Brown, and J. W. Stull. 1966. *J. Dairy Sci.* 49:370.

INDEX